Lecture Notes in Computational Vision and Biomechanics

Volume 8

For further volumes:
http://www.springer.com/series/8910

This book is the eighth volume to be published in the Book Series "Lecture Notes in Computational Vision and Biomechanics (LNCV&B)".

The research related to the analysis of living structures (Biomechanics) has been a source of recent research in several distinct areas of science, for example, Mathematics, Mechanical Engineering, Physics, Informatics, Medicine and Sport. However, for its successful achievement, numerous research topics should be considered, such as image processing and analysis, geometric and numerical modelling, biomechanics, experimental analysis, mechanobiology and enhanced visualization, and their application to real cases must be developed and more investigation is needed. Additionally, enhanced hardware solutions and less invasive devices are demanded.

On the other hand, Image Analysis (Computational Vision) is used for the extraction of high level information from static images or dynamic image sequences. Examples of applications involving image analysis can be the study of motion of structures from image sequences, shape reconstruction from images and medical diagnosis. As a multidisciplinary area, Computational Vision considers techniques and methods from other disciplines, such as Artificial Intelligence, Signal Processing, Mathematics, Physics and Informatics. Despite the many research projects in this area, more robust and efficient methods of Computational Imaging are still demanded in many application domains in Medicine, and their validation in real scenarios is matter of urgency.

These two important and predominant branches of Science are increasingly considered to be strongly connected and related. Hence, the main goal of the LNCV&B book series consists of the provision of a comprehensive forum for discussion on the current state-of-the-art in these fields by emphasizing their connection. The book series covers (but is not limited to):

- Applications of Computational Vision and Biomechanics
- Biometrics and Biomedical Pattern Analysis
- Cellular Imaging and Cellular Mechanics
- Clinical Biomechanics
- Computational Bioimaging and Visualization
- Computational Biology in Biomedical Imaging
- Development of Biomechanical Devices
- Device and Technique Development for Biomedical Imaging
- Experimental Biomechanics
- Gait & Posture Mechanics
- Grid and High Performance Computing for Computational Vision and Biomechanics
- Image Processing and Analysis
- Image Processing and Visualization in Biofluids
- Image Understanding
- Material Models
- Mechanobiology
- Medical Image Analysis
- Molecular Mechanics
- Multi-Modal Image Systems
- Multiscale Biosensors in Biomedical Imaging
- Multiscale Devices and Biomems for Biomedical Imaging
- Musculoskeletal Biomechanics
- Multiscale Analysis in Biomechanics
- Neuromuscular Biomechanics
- Numerical Methods for Living Tissues
- Numerical Simulation
- Software Development on Computational Vision and Biomechanics
- Sport Biomechanics
- Virtual Reality in Biomechanics
- Vision Systems

In order to match the scope of the LNCV&B book series, each book must include contents relating to or combining both Image Analysis and Biomechanics. Proposals for new books are welcome and should be submitted to the editors of the book series.

The Editors would like to take this opportunity to thank once again to all members of the Advisory Board for their support in the establishment and scientific managing of this book series, and also to Nathalie Jacobs and Anneke Pot for their assistance.

João Manuel R. S. Tavares
R. M. Natal Jorge
(LNCV&B book series editors)

João Manuel R. S. Tavares
Renato M. Natal Jorge
Editors

Topics in Medical Image Processing and Computational Vision

Springer

Editors
João Manuel R. S. Tavares
Renato M. Natal Jorge
Departamento de Engenharia Mecânica
Faculdade de Engenharia
Universidade do Porto
Porto
Portugal

ISSN 2212-9391 ISSN 2212-9413 (electronic)
ISBN 978-94-017-8180-0 ISBN 978-94-007-0726-9 (eBook)
DOI 10.1007/978-94-007-0726-9
Springer Dordrecht Heidelberg New York London

Printed on acid-free paper

Springer is part of Springer Science+Business Media (www.springer.com)

Preface

This book presents novel and advanced Topics in Medical Image Processing and Computational Vision in order to solidify knowledge in the related fields and define their key stakeholders.

The sixteen chapters included in this book were written by invited experts of international recognition and address important issues in Medical Image Processing and Computational Vision, including: Object Recognition, Object Detection, Object Tracking, Pose Estimation, Facial Expression Recognition, Image Retrieval, Data Mining, Automatic Video Understanding and Management, Edges Detection, Image Segmentation, Modelling and Simulation, Medical Thermography, Database Systems, Synthetic Aperture Radar and Satellite Imagery.

Different applications are addressed and described throughout the book, comprising: Object Recognition and Tracking, Facial Expression Recognition, Image Database, Plant Disease Classification, Video Understanding and Management, Image Processing, Image Segmentation, Bio-structure Modelling and Simulation, Medical Imaging, Image Classification, Medical Diagnosis, Urban Areas Classification and Land Map Generation.

Therefore, this book is of crucial effectiveness for Researchers, Students, End Users and Manufacturers from several multidisciplinary fields, as the ones related with Artificial Intelligence, Bioengineering, Biomechanics, Computational Mechanics, Computational Vision, Computer Sciences, Human Motion, Mathematics, Medical Image, Medicine, Pattern Recognition and Physics.

The Editors would like to take this opportunity to thank all invited authors for sharing their works, experiences and knowledge, making possible their dissemination through this book.

João Manuel R. S. Tavares
Renato M. Natal Jorge

Contents

Learning a Family of Detectors via Multiplicative Kernels

Quan Yuan, Ashwin Thangali, Vitaly Ablavsky and Stan Sclaroff

Abstract Object detection is challenging when the object class exhibits large within-class variations. In this work, we show that foreground-background classification (detection) and within-class classification of the foreground class (pose estimation) can be jointly learned in a multiplicative form of two kernel functions. Model training is accomplished via standard SVM learning. When the foreground object masks are provided in training, the detectors can also produce object segmentations. A tracking-by-detection framework to recover foreground state in video sequences is also proposed with our model. The advantages of our method are demonstrated on tasks of object detection, view angle estimation and tracking. Our approach compares favorably to existing methods on hand and vehicle detection tasks. Quantitative tracking results are given on sequences of moving vehicles and human faces.

Keywords Object recognition · Object detection · Object tracking · Pose estimation · Kernel methods

Q. Yuan (✉)
Ventana Medical Systems, 919 Hermosa CT, Sunnyvale, CA 94085, USA
e-mail: yq.bu.edu@gmail.com

A. Thangali · S. Sclaroff
Department of Computer Science, Boston University, 111 Cummington Street, Boston, MA 02215, USA
e-mail: tvashwin@cs.bu.edu

S. Sclaroff
e-mail: sclaroff@cs.bu.edu

V. Ablavsky
EPFL IC-CVLab, BC 309 Station 14 CH-1015 Lausanne, Switzerland
e-mail: vitaly.ablavsky@epfl.ch

J. M. R. S. Tavares and R. M. Natal Jorge (eds.), *Topics in Medical Image Processing and Computational Vision*, Lecture Notes in Computational Vision and Biomechanics 8,
DOI: 10.1007/978-94-007-0726-9_1,

1 Introduction

A computer vision system for object recognition typically has two modules: a detection module [10, 55] and a foreground state estimation module [1, 3, 46]. The detection module is often implemented as a scanning window process where each window location in an image is evaluated by a binary classifier, i.e., foreground class versus background class. The invocation of the foreground state estimation module is conditioned on the detection of an instance of the foreground class; in other words, the second module is tuned to the variations within the foreground class. This second module can be implemented in numerous ways. For discrete state spaces—for example, face ID, hand shape class, or vehicle type—estimation can be framed as a multi-class classification problem [42]: given an input feature vector, produce an estimate of the class label. For continuous state spaces—for example, face age, hand joint angles, vehicle orientation—estimation can be formulated in terms of regression [1]: map a given input feature vector to its most likely location in the foreground state space. Another common approach for foreground state estimation is to use nearest neighbor methods [3, 46].

In any case, when object classes exhibit large within-class variations, detection and foreground state estimation can be chicken-egg problems. Assuming the objects are detected and segmented from the background, foreground state estimation is relatively straightforward. Assuming specific variations of the foreground class, detection can be achieved as in [41]. However, if neither the foreground state nor detection is given, then challenges arise. For example, it is difficult for a single detector to cope with all variations of the foreground class, while at the same time providing reliable discrimination between the foreground and background—especially in applications where there are widely varying, or even unconstrained backgrounds.

A common strategy in this setting is divide-and-conquer [27, 36, 54, 57]: divide the foreground class into subclasses by partitioning the space of within-class variations, and then train a separate detector for each partition. Thus, a set of detectors is trained, where each detector discriminates between the background class and its subset of the foreground class. This strategy has been employed in hand detection [36], multi-pose vehicle detection [57] and multi-pose face detection [27, 54]. An additional advantage of such a strategy is that coarse estimation of the object pose can also be obtained during the detection process. For example, in multi-pose face detection, the detector of the correct face pose tends to have a high response. However, in a divide-and-conquer strategy, the partitioning of a foreground class is oftentimes arbitrary. Moreover, to keep ample training examples in each subclass, the partitioning of the foreground class is usually coarse, which limits the ability of pose estimation.

We propose a different strategy that avoids explicit partitioning of the foreground class in this paper: learning a family of detectors, where the detectors themselves are parameterized over the space of within-class variations. Our formulation utilizes a product of two kernel functions: a within-class kernel k_θ to handle foreground state variations and feature sharing, and a between-class kernel k_x to handle foreground-background classification. This kernel formulation is used in a Support Vector Machine (SVM) [8] training algorithm that outputs support vectors and their weights, which can be used to construct a family of detectors that are tuned to foreground variations. After SVM training, a sample set of detectors can be generated, where each detector is associated with a particular foreground state parameter value. All the samples from the detector family share the same support vectors, but the weights of these support vectors vary depending on the within-class state value. A useful side effect of this support vector sharing is that features are implicitly shared across the whole detector family.

The formulation is useful in solving detection, state estimation, and tracking problems. For detection using a scanning window process, an image window can be classified as foreground if at least one of the detectors in the family produces a score that is above a predefined threshold. For a given image window, the foreground state can be estimated simply by examining the state values associated with detectors that produce the highest responses for that input. For particle filter-based tracking methods, like Condensation [21], importance sampling from the detector family can be driven by a dynamical model at each frame, where the objects are allowed to undergo a range of state variations over time.

With proper nonparametric kernel functions, our formulation can be extended to nonparametric cases, when explicit parameter annotation of the foreground class examples is too expensive to obtain. A mode finding method is proposed that selects a representative subset of samples from the detector family in the nonparametric case. This generally reduces the number of detectors to be invoked, and thereby makes detection more efficient. If state estimation or tracking is desired, then the user can label the state for each sample in the representative subset. This alleviates the burden of assigning ground truth states for the complete training set, and instead focuses only on labelling the smaller representative subset.

The proposed framework is evaluated in three application areas. The first involves hand detection, segmentation, and shape estimation for images taken from videos of Flemish and American Sign Language. There is a wide variation of hand shapes and orientations in these videos. The framework is also tested in estimating index finger angles. The second application involves detection, orientation estimation and tracking of vehicles driving on highways, and the more challenging case of race cars careening on dirt roads. The third application focuses on the problem of detecting and tracking multiple human faces, while simultaneously estimating the left-right rotation angles under illumination variations.

2 Related Work

A large amount of work in computer vision has been proposed to handle the issue of detecting an object class that exhibits large appearance variations. For instance, generative models were proposed in [31, 39] to learn a set of low-dimensional representations (eigenspaces) that cover a broad range of appearance variations. Given a novel input image, the position of its projection on these eigenspaces determines its state.

Recent work in multi-view face detection builds detectors for different head pose ranges. In [26, 54], subclasses according to the face orientation are created and corresponding detectors are learned for each subclass. In [18, 27], coarse to fine hierarchies (trees) of face orientation are created. Each non-leaf node in the hierarchy is a face subclass and is further partitioned into subclasses. At each node a detector is learned for this subclass. During detection, an input is examined by the detectors of a sequence of nodes, starting from the root. If the input is classified by the detector of the current node as from the corresponding face subclass, it is passed to its children (one or multiple) to be examined; otherwise it is rejected as from the background class. The annotation of the leaf node at the end of the sequence determines the face orientation of the input, if it passes all detectors along the sequence.

Similar approaches that partition the foreground class according to foreground state annotation [51] or via unsupervised clustering [15, 25, 36, 45, 57] are employed in pedestrian and human hand detection. However, the trained subclass detectors have limited power when there are too few training samples in each subclass. A large foreground training set is required to handle a large number of foreground subclasses.

To make the best use of limited training data, feature sharing is important for multi-class detection. Explicit feature sharing approaches proposed in [52, 59] improve detection accuracy, but they also tend to make training more expensive due to the combinatorial complexity in choosing classes or training examples to share features. In both works, greedy strategies to select sharing classes or training examples of each feature are employed as a tradeoff for training speed.

Given the above mentioned issues, hybrid methods that unify detection and foreground state estimation are of great interest. Some approaches combine bottom-up part-based detectors with top-down geometric constraints [14, 19, 38, 49]. These methods are applied to handle large appearance variations of articulated objects like the human body. However, the number of possible configurations exhibits combinatorial complexity in terms of the number of detected parts. The search for satisfactory part configurations can be expensive in practice. A recent work [13] applies the idea of part-based model in a latent-SVM formulation. The detection accuracy is improved with this discriminatively trained model on various object detection tasks. However, in this model each part may not necessarily correspond to a meaningful object part. Body pose or foreground state information is not directly available from the detection result.

Some other approaches employ a recognition-verification strategy (e.g., [43]), where a one-to-many mapping is used to produce estimates of body pose (bottom-up), and then recognition models are used to verify pose estimates (top-down). Nevertheless, bottom-up recognition from images with background clutter remains difficult, and the verification step cannot correct an error when the recognition is already wrong.

Other approaches use probabilistic methods to learn a generative model to predict a human pose and then verify it [5, 12, 50] using a recognition model. In [5], a generative model of the background class is also obtained. However, for recognition, generative models may not be as robust as discriminative models. One of the major reasons is that generative models often make conditional independence assumptions that are not well justified (not supported by the data).

Some other works [11, 30, 53] propose kernel combinations or kernel parameter optimization to improve the performance of kernel methods. In these works, kernel combinations are used for a single classification or regression task, but not both; whereas in our approach, both the foreground-background classification and foreground state estimation problems are jointly solved.

A recent approach [20] jointly solves human body localization and pose estimation by a structural SVM using a product kernel. In this work, both localization and pose estimation are defined as continuous parameter estimation problems that can be solved via nonlinear optimization. However, the optimization process still needs help from a traditional localization method and a greedy scheme, due to the non-convexity of the model.

3 Problem Definition and Our Approach

Given a feature vector $\mathbf{x} \in \mathbb{R}^{\ltimes}$ computed for an image patch[1], our goal is to decide whether or not the image patch depicts an instance of the object with parameter $\theta \in \mathbb{R}^{>}$, which parameterizes certain variations of the foreground object class, e.g., object pose, view angle, or latent factors that can be obtained via unsupervised learning. Basically, we want to have following outputs given an input $\mathbf{x}$: (1) *if* $\mathbf{x}$ *is a foreground object, the output is an estimate of the foreground parameter*, and (2) *if* $\mathbf{x}$ *is a background patch, the output is simply a label "background."*

In a traditional multi-pose object detection approach, e.g., multi-pose face detection [27], the foreground class is first partitioned in to subclasses. Each subclass is associated with a rotation angle, e.g., $\theta \in \{0°, 20°, 40°, \ldots, 180°\}$. Then a set of detectors $C_0(x), C_{20}(x), C_{40}(x), \ldots, C_{180}(x)$ is trained with corresponding training examples. The detection process is organized into a hierarchy for efficiency. Because the detector of the correct rotation angle tends to have the highest response, a rotation angle estimate can be obtained by comparing detection scores from all detectors.

In our work, we aim to learn a unified function $C(\mathbf{x}, \theta)$ that tells whether $\mathbf{x}$ is an instance of the object with parameters θ,

$$C(\mathbf{x}, \theta) \begin{cases} > 0, \mathbf{x} & \text{is an instance of the object with } \theta, \\ \leq 0, & \text{otherwise.} \end{cases} \tag{1}$$

[1] In this paper, all vector variables are column vectors.

The function $C(\mathbf{x}, \theta)$ can be viewed as a global function to "generate" individual detectors $C_0(x), C_{20}(x), C_{40}(x), \ldots, C_{180}(x)$ by plugging in a θ value into $C(\mathbf{x}, \theta)$. These individual detectors can be regarded as points in a space of detectors. The main idea of our approach is to learn the detector space as a function of θ, rather than learning individual detectors separately. During detection, we use a discretization of the continuous model to generate discrete samples in θ space and apply corresponding detectors on an input. Rather than considering a sample set of detectors, it is possible to optimize $C(\mathbf{x}, \theta)$ for a given $\mathbf{x}$; however, in practice, this optimization-based approach tends to be slower than running a sampled set of detectors that are just linear classifiers. We experimentally compare the performance of the detector optimization versus sample set approaches in Sect. 7.2.

3.1 Multiplicative Kernel Construction

Assume $C(\mathbf{x}, \theta)$ can be factorized into the product of two Hilbert space representations $\phi_x(\mathbf{x})$ and $\phi_\theta(\theta)$ with a matrix $\mathbf{V}$,

$$C(\mathbf{x}, \theta) = \phi_x(\mathbf{x})^T \mathbf{V} \phi_\theta(\theta). \tag{2}$$

If we use the kernel trick, the dual of the primal formulation in Eq. 2 is

$$C(\mathbf{x}, \theta) = \sum_{i \in SV} \alpha_i k_\theta(\theta_i, \theta) k_x(\mathbf{x}_i, \mathbf{x}), \tag{3}$$

where $k_\theta(\theta, \theta') = \phi_\theta(\theta)^T \phi_\theta(\theta')$ and $k_x(\mathbf{x}, \mathbf{x}') = \phi_x(\mathbf{x})^T \phi_x(\mathbf{x}')$. α_i is the weight of the ith support vector. To apply a standard SVM classifier training algorithm on Eq. 3, we can virtually concatenate θ with $\mathbf{x}$ into a single variable:

$$C([\mathbf{x}, \theta]) = \sum_{i \in SV} \alpha_i k_c([\mathbf{x}_i, \theta_i], [\mathbf{x}, \theta]), \tag{4}$$

where $k_c([\mathbf{x}_i, \theta_i], [\mathbf{x}, \theta]) = k_\theta(\theta_i, \theta) k_x(\mathbf{x}_i, \mathbf{x})$. The product of two positive semi-definite functions is still a positive semi-definite function. Each training example is a tuple $(\mathbf{x}, \theta)$ in our method, with a label $y \in \{+1, -1\}$. We give details of SVM training process in Sect. 4.

There is also an interesting interpretation of feature sharing if we combine α_i with $k_\theta(\theta_i, \theta)$,

$$C(\mathbf{x}, \theta) = \sum_{i \in SV} \alpha'_i(\theta) k_x(\mathbf{x}_i, \mathbf{x}), \tag{5}$$

where $\alpha'_i(\theta) = \alpha_i k_\theta(\theta_i, \theta)$. Feature sharing is implicitly achieved by sharing support vectors. When $k_\theta(\cdot, \cdot)$ is strictly non-negative, e.g., a radial basis function (RBF) kernel, Eq. 5 can be interpreted as re-weighting the support vectors so that only those having parameters similar to θ are assigned high weights. Fewer support vectors have to be taken into account in a local subregion in θ space.

3.2 Construction of Individual Detectors when k_x is Linear Kernel

We are particularly interested in the case when k_x is linear kernel, because linear classifiers are fast in practice. Furthermore, when the foreground variation is fixed to a particular θ (e.g., faces of a fixed rotation angle 45°), a linear classifier is usually good enough as a detector.

When k_x is a general linear kernel, a linear classifier $\mathbf{w}(\theta)$ can be constructed as a weighted sum of support vectors following Eq. 5:

$$\begin{aligned} C(\mathbf{x},\theta) &= \sum_{i \in SV} \alpha_i'(\theta) k_x(\mathbf{x}_i, \mathbf{x}) \\ &= \sum_{i \in SV} \alpha_i'(\theta)(\hat{\mathbf{x}}_i^T \hat{\mathbf{x}}) = \mathbf{w}(\theta)^T \hat{\mathbf{x}}, \end{aligned} \tag{6}$$

where $\mathbf{w}(\theta) = \sum_{i \in SV} \alpha_i'(\theta)\hat{\mathbf{x}}_i^T$ and $\hat{\mathbf{x}} = [1, \mathbf{x}^T]^T$. Thus, a set $\{\mathbf{w}(\theta_1), \mathbf{w}(\theta_2), \ldots, \mathbf{w}(\theta_s)\}$ can be precalculated at the off-line stage, and used in the detection stage as subclass detectors in a partition based method. The set of $\{\theta_k\}$ can be sampled denser in our approach than in a partition based method, because we do not need to partition the foreground class and maintain ample training examples for each subclass. The details of the sampling process for generating a set of detectors are given in Sect. 5. Note that once this set of detectors is constructed, the within-class kernel k_θ does not have to be evaluated during detection. Only the dot products between $\mathbf{w}(\theta_k)$ and input $\mathbf{x}$ are evaluated during detection as in Eq. 6.

3.3 An Example on a Synthetic Data Set

Figure 1 illustrates the basic idea of our approach using a synthetic data set, where the foreground class of brown points is parameterized by an angle θ. In the multiplicative formulation, k_θ is a Gaussian RBF kernel and k_x is a linear kernel. The local linear boundary (Eq. 6) can be reconstructed as a weighted sum of support vectors in x_1, x_2 space. The figure shows two constructed linear classifiers $\mathbf{w}(\mathbf{23}^\circ)$ and $\mathbf{w}(-\mathbf{30}^\circ)$. Ideal local linear classifiers in this case are tangent lines to the circular boundary, and our result follows the tangent lines very well.

To illustrate the effect of reweighting support vector weights (Eq. 5), we plot support vectors with $\alpha'(\theta) > 0.5$ as circles for each of the two linear boundaries. For each of the two example linear classifiers, the highest weighted support vectors are always those close to the boundary and have similar angles to the chosen angles 23 and $-30°$.

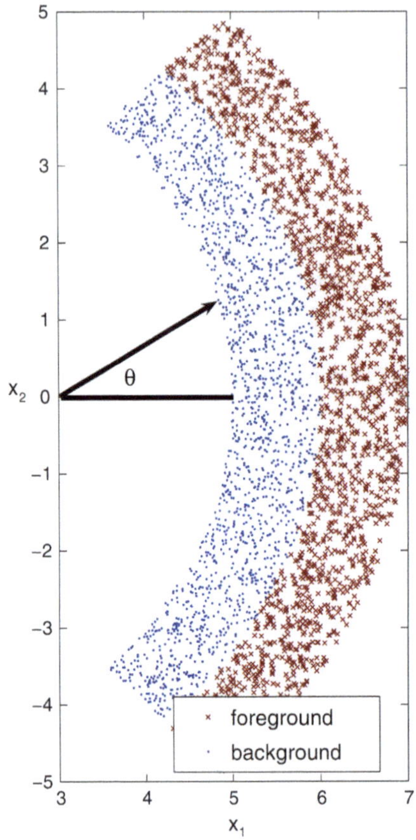

(a) The original data

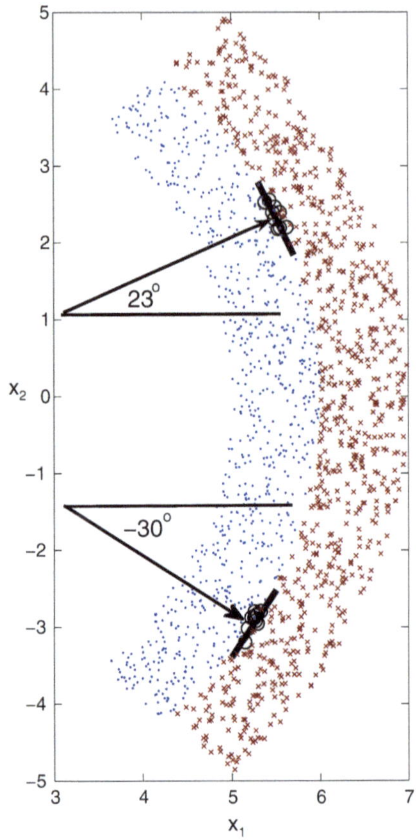

(b) Two example detectors

Fig. 1 An experiment on synthetic data. A family of multiplicative kernel classifiers is learned, where k_θ is a RBF kernel defined on θ, and k_x is a linear kernel defined on $\mathbf{x} = (\mathbf{x_1}, \mathbf{x_2})^\mathbf{T}$. The linear boundaries for example detectors $\mathbf{w}(\mathbf{23}^\circ)$ and $\mathbf{w}(-\mathbf{30}^\circ)$ are shown on the *right*. The *circle points* along each linear boundary are the reweighted support vectors (Eq. 5) of weights > 0.5. These synthetic "foreground" and "background" classes were chosen to illustrate the idea that local discriminants can be learned jointly via multiplicative kernels, and then constructed at a given θ

3.4 Nonparametric k_θ

In some problems, parametric forms of foreground within-class variations may not be readily available. For example, there are numerous degrees of freedom in the human hand and the human body. Manual annotation of a large real image data set of hand shapes or body poses can be very expensive, tedious, and prone to errors. For such cases, we propose a nonparametric formulation for the within-class kernel k_θ.

To understand the usage of the nonparametric k_θ we need to examine the role of the parametric k_θ in feature sharing as outlined in Sect. 3.1. When k_θ is defined over continuous θ, two training samples with close θ values should obtain a high k_θ score, and thus are more likely to share features. Conversely, training samples that are far from each other in θ space are less likely to share features, and should obtain a small k_θ score. The nonparametric formulation attains the same behavior. Another way to understand the usage of the nonparametric k_θ is by considering k_θ as it varies the weights of support vectors. Intuitively, different foreground examples may have different "confusing" background examples. Thus, a support vector from the background class may not be globally useful for all foreground examples. The k_θ only gives higher weights to the most the useful support vectors for a particular foreground state.

We define a kernel $k_\theta(i,j)$ on a finite set I, which is the set of indices of foreground training examples. According to the Moore-Aronszajn theorem, there is a unique Hilbert space of functions $\phi_\theta(i)$ on I for which $k_\theta(i,j)$ is a reproducing kernel, as long as $k_\theta(i,j)$ is a symmetric positive definite kernel on I. Thus, as long as we can define a symmetric positive definite kernel $k_\theta(i,j)$ on I, we can carry on the SVM training process just like the parametric case in Sect. 3.1.

A straightforward design of a symmetric positive definite kernel k_θ employs a nonparametric similarity/distance measure, e.g., bidirectional chamfer edge distance [3, 15] or shape context distance [4]. These distance metrics have been used successfully to measure within-class similarities for object classes like hand shape and body pose. Based on a distance measure D, a kernel function can be defined [34],

$$k_\theta(i,j) = exp\big(-\eta D(\mathbf{z_i}, \mathbf{z_j})\big), \tag{7}$$

where $\mathbf{z_i}$ and $\mathbf{z_j}$ are representations (e.g., edge images) of the foreground training samples indexed by i and j to calculate distance D. The representation $\mathbf{z}$ is selected to be suited for describing within-class variations. By adjusting η, we can make k_θ symmetric positive definite on all pairs $i,j \in I$. Note when this $k_\theta(i,j)$ is not defined on a finite set I, it may not always be a valid Mercer Kernel. Because the $k_\theta(i,j)$ defined in Eq. 7 is not guaranteed to be positive semi-definite on any $\mathbf{z_i}$ and $\mathbf{z_j}$. Thus, this nonparametric kernel representation cannot be used in a conventional SVM classifier. But when it is defined on a finite set as a within-class kernel in our approach, it can be made a valid Mercer kernel by selecting proper η.

When k_x is a general linear kernel, we can obtain a linear classifier $\mathbf{w(i)}$ for a particular training sample indexed by i:

$$\begin{aligned} C(\mathbf{x}, \mathbf{i}) &= \sum_{j \in SV} \alpha_j k_\theta(i,j) k_x(\mathbf{x_j}, \mathbf{x}) \\ &= \sum_{j \in SV} \alpha'_j(i)(\hat{\mathbf{x}}_j^T \hat{\mathbf{x}}) = \mathbf{w}(i)^T \hat{\mathbf{x}}. \end{aligned} \tag{8}$$

After SVM training we are able to construct linear classifiers $\mathbf{w}(i)$, for any foreground example i. This can be regarded as an extreme case of a partition-based method where each subclass is a singleton of just one foreground example. However, there may exist redundancy among $\mathbf{w(i)}$, since some of $\mathbf{w(i)}$'s may be very similar to each other. One representative will be enough for a group of similar $\mathbf{w(i)}$'s. We discuss mode finding methods in Sect. 5 to handle this issue.

4 Detector Training

In this section, we give details on how to train the model defined in the previous section. A constraint generation process for SVM learning is described first. Then, we describe how to incorporate image masks in training, if they are available. This can help reduce the influence of background clutter and can also enable foreground object segmentation during detection.

4.1 Constraint Generation Process

The training samples are in the form of tuples. In the following paragraphs, we present formulations in the parametric case when θ is available in training. Thus, the tuples are in the form $(\mathbf{x}, \theta)$. The nonparametric case has a similar formulation by replacing θ with foreground example index i. The constraints in the SVM formulation are as following:

$$\begin{aligned} & min \ \frac{1}{2}||\mathbf{V}||_2^2 + C\sum_k \xi_k \\ & s.t. \ \xi_k \geq 0, \forall k \\ & \qquad y_k[\phi_x(\mathbf{x_k})^{\mathbf{T}}\mathbf{V}\phi_\theta(\theta_\mathbf{k})] \geq \mathbf{1} - \xi_\mathbf{k}, \forall \mathbf{k}, \end{aligned} \tag{9}$$

where $||\mathbf{V}||_2$ is the Frobenius norm and $y_k \in \{+1, -1\}$ is the annotation of a training tuple $(\mathbf{x_k}, \theta_\mathbf{k})$, assigned by the definition in Eq. 1. Because we use a linear kernel for k_x, the constraint in Eq. 9 can be simplified:

$$\begin{aligned} y_k\hat{\mathbf{x}}_k^T\mathbf{w}(\theta_\mathbf{k}) \geq 1 - \xi_k, \forall k, \\ \mathbf{w}(\theta_k) = \mathbf{V}\phi_\theta(\theta_k). \end{aligned} \tag{10}$$

Each foreground training sample $\mathbf{x}$ is associated with its corresponding ground-truth θ to make a positive tuple. By definition, a background training sample $\mathbf{x}$ can be associated with any θ to make a negative tuple. The number of such combinations (constraints) is huge. We therefore employ a constraint generation process to add violated constraints as new constraints iteratively until convergence. Note we only use θ values that appear with foreground training examples. Thus, the total number of constraints is still finite. A similar constraint generation process has been employed in [6] for structured output regression.

The training process starts with assigning each background feature vector $\mathbf{x}$ a randomly selected θ from foreground training examples to form initial constraints. Then in each iteration all constraints are evaluated to find most violated ones, which are added as new constraints in the next iteration of SVM training. Note we are able to evaluate all of the constraints with the current model via the product in Eq. 10, although we cannot include all constraints at the same time in SVM quadratic programming. The pseudo code for the this process is given in Fig. 2. In the pseudo code, the degree of a constraint violation is given by $e_k = 1 - y_k \hat{\mathbf{x}}_k^T \mathbf{w}(\theta_\mathbf{k})$. Violated constraints are ranked by their e_k values and the top N_s of them are added in each iteration. The number N_s may depend on the size of training set. A rule of thumb used in our experiment is that N_s equals one tenth of the total number of background training examples.

When the constraint generation process stops with all constraints satisfied ($\xi_k = 0$ for those constraints not included in the final round of SVM optimization), we can show that the obtained model $\mathbf{V}_c$ is equivalent to the model $\mathbf{V}_a$ that is optimized using all constraints in one batch. Let D_c, D_a denote the sets of constraints that are taken into account in training of $\mathbf{V_c}$ and $\mathbf{V_a}$, respectively. Let g_c and g_a denote the final goal values after the model is optimized with D_c and D_a, respectively. By definition $D_c \subseteq D_a$. Because g_a is the minimized goal value with more constraints, we have $g_c \leq g_a$. On the other hand, although both $\mathbf{V_c}$ and $\mathbf{V_a}$ satisfy all the constraints D_a, $\mathbf{V_a}$ is the one that is explicitly optimized with D_a to achieve the minimal goal value g_a. Thus, $g_a \leq g_c$. So we have $g_a = g_c$. Since SVM training is a convex optimization (quadratic programming), the optimal solution is unique and both $\mathbf{V_c}$ and $\mathbf{V_g}$ achieve it. So the two models are equivalent.

Given
Foreground training samples $X_f = \{\mathbf{x}_{f_1}, \ldots, \mathbf{x}_{f_n}\}$,
Background training samples $X_b = \{\mathbf{x}_{b_1}, \ldots, \mathbf{x}_{b_n}\}$,
Parameters of foreground training samples $\Theta = \{\theta_{f_1}, \ldots, \theta_{f_n}\}$.

Initialize
Assign each foreground training sample $\mathbf{x}_{f_i}$ its actual parameter θ_{f_i}, and each background training sample $\mathbf{x}_{b_i}$ a random value from Θ to form tuples $(\mathbf{x}, \theta)$. If object masks are available for foreground examples, the mask of θ is applied on $\mathbf{x}$.
While

1. Compute Gram matrix K_c of current tuples, where $k_c([\mathbf{x}_i, \theta_i], [\mathbf{x}_j, \theta_j]) = k_\theta(\theta_i, \theta_j) k_x(\mathbf{x}_i, \mathbf{x}_j)$.
2. Carry out SVM training using K_c.
3. Examine all possible tuples to find violated constraints (tuples).
4. If it converges or the max number of iterations reached, break.
5. Add a fixed number N_s of mostly violated constraints (tuples) as new tuples.

End

Fig. 2 Pseudo code for bootstrap training with parametric within-class kernel k_θ. For the case of nonparametric k_θ, the set is replaced by the set of indices of foreground training samples

4.2 Including Object Masks in Training

There are situations in practice when object masks can be obtained during training data acquisition, for instance, when the background is known. In such cases, masks can be exploited to reduce the influence of background regions inside the detection window during both training and testing. Ideally, whether a training object is captured with a highly textured background or with a smooth background should have minimum impact on the final classifier. However, when the bounding box is not tight, features from textures of background regions may be included in a foreground training example. For instance, in gesture recognition, many training hand images may be captured in front of a fixed camera. The same background region behind the hand may be included in hand images for many frames. There is a risk that the texture from the same background regions will be reinforced as features from "hand" during training of a hand classifier.

When each training sample has a foreground mask, features from outside the mask can be ignored. For instance, to calculate the color histogram of a foreground object, only those pixel colors from inside the mask region may be considered. When the features have local support and are ordered according to their spatial arrangement, e.g., HOG features [10] or Haar wavelet features [55], applying object masks in feature extraction means that the feature components that have support from outside the object masks have zero values.

To be consistent, masks should also be applied to the background training samples during feature extraction. As mentioned earlier, each background training sample is associated with a foreground parameter θ or an index i of a foreground training sample. Therefore, the mask of the foreground training sample with θ or i is applied to this background training sample during training.

Since a mask is associated with a θ or i, each detector $\mathbf{w}(\theta)$ or $\mathbf{w}(\mathbf{i})$ can be associated with a corresponding mask. In our approach, the image mask of a detector is calculated as a weighted sum of image masks from foreground support vectors using the support vector weights α_i'. This mask of continuous values can be binarized by a threshold, when a binary image mask is required. For instance, segmentation can be produced by superimposing the detector's binary image mask onto a detected object.

Because applying a linear SVM classifier is equivalent to summing up dot products between support vectors and $\mathbf{x}$, the masks of support vectors are implicitly applied on $\mathbf{x}$ during this linear classification $\mathbf{w}^{\mathrm{T}}\mathbf{x}$. More precisely, masks do not have to be explicitly applied on a test input when both of the following two conditions are met:

1. The features have local support like HOG [10] or Haar wavelet features [55].
2. $k_x(\mathbf{x}_1, \mathbf{x}_2)$ is based on the dot product $\mathbf{x}_1^{\mathrm{T}}\mathbf{x}_2$, e.g., the linear or polynomial kernels.

Object masks or shape priors were also used in previous work [7, 23, 56, 58, 60]; however, in our method no decomposition of the image mask into local edgelets or parts is needed. If available, context cues may help the detection process, e.g., following [10, 17].

5 Detection and Foreground State Estimation

After training as described in Sect. 4, we are able to construct a linear classifier as a detector for any parameter θ or any foreground sample index i. However, in a real world application like multi-view face detection, neither object locations (there could be multiple faces or none in an image) nor object foreground states are known. Thus, during detection, a scanning window process is employed using detectors associated with a predefined representative set of θ or i, which covers typical foreground state variations. The foreground state annotation θ associated with the detector of the highest detection score is assigned to a detected object as a foreground state estimate. As will be described in the rest of this section, there are a number of ways to determine the representative set of θ or i that is used in generating the set of detectors. We will focus on two methods: uniform sampling over the training set, and finding representative samples via mode finding (clustering).

5.1 Generating a Sample Set of Detectors

Assume that the training set provided a fair and representative sampling of the foreground class. If the foreground states are annotated as parameters θ, e.g., view angles or rotation angles, a representative set of θ can be obtained by uniformly sampling from the parameters of foreground training examples. In special cases when prior information about the parameter distribution is provided, e.g., in object tracking where temporal information is propagated from frame to frame, importance sampling can be employed instead to draw parameter samples to comprise a representative set of θ. In our experiments, we obtain satisfactory results via uniform sampling for detection and parameter estimation applications, and via importance sampling for tracking.

In the nonparametric case, uniform sampling over the foreground training samples can also be used to generate the detector family, assuming that the training set provides a fair and representative sample of the foreground class. However, we have found that a mode finding technique is more effective in practice.

5.2 Mode Finding for Nonparametric Detectors

In the nonparametric case, we can use mode finding to reduce the redundancy in the detector set. Clustering is a straightforward option for mode finding. We define a similarity measure S_α on the support vector weights $\alpha'(i)$ of foreground examples,

$$S_\alpha(i,j) = \frac{\alpha'(i)^T \alpha'(j)}{||\alpha'(i)|| \cdot ||\alpha'(j)||}, \tag{11}$$

where $\alpha'(i) = \left[\alpha'_1(i), \alpha'_2(i), \ldots, \alpha'_n(i)\right]^T$ are the support vector weights for i, as defined in Eq. 8. Each cluster is regarded as a mode that represents a variation of the foreground class. The proper number of modes is decided via cross validation to obtain acceptable detection accuracy. The cluster centers comprise the representative set used in the online stage.

Note our clustering process is different from that in a partition based method. In a partition based method, the training examples are clustered before subclass detectors are trained. In our approach, the detectors are first trained and then clustered are identified.

Interestingly, annotation of training examples can be made efficient with mode finding, because we can start with an unannotated foreground class to train detectors first, and then after mode finding only the representative set needs to be annotated with foreground states. The complete training process with a nonparametric kernel is as follows:

1. Train the model with a nonparametric kernel. At this step, no foreground state annotations are needed. Only labels of foreground (+1) vs background (−1) and a distance D are required. After training, each detector $\mathbf{w}(\mathbf{i})$ is associated with a unique foreground example, as in Eq. 8.
2. Use mode finding to find clusters in the foreground class. Only those $\mathbf{w}(\mathbf{i})$ of cluster centers will be employed in detection.
3. Annotate the cluster centers (foreground examples) with foreground states. The foreground states can be continuous variables like rotation angles and pose parameters, or nominal values like "standing", "walking" and "running."

An obvious advantage of this strategy is that only a small portion of the foreground training data must be annotated. This can save a significant amount of effort that might be needed to label all training samples for the same purpose.

6 Tracking with Multiplicative Kernel Detectors

Tracking objects that undergo large appearance changes is challenging, e.g., tracking articulated objects like human hands or multi-view objects like faces and vehicles. Commonly used cylinder models [48] or edge templates [51] usually require strong temporal models and manual initialization to achieve robust tracking, particularly in cluttered scenes.

One way to cope with a cluttered background is to use detectors that are trained against representative background examples. Such a strategy was employed in the in "tracking-by-detection" approaches of [2, 28, 35], where the tracking performance is enhanced by using the detectors that handle cluttered background and variations of the foreground class.

Our detectors trained with multiplicative kernels can be also employed in a tracking-by-detection framework. A brute force way to implement tracking with parametric detectors that are trained with multiplicative kernels is via frame by frame detection. Although the object locations and foreground states can be recovered in this way, it can be expensive to run a dense scan on each frame with all detectors. We instead propose a tracking approach that incorporates temporal information to make the tracking process more efficient.

We formulate the tracking process in a standard prediction-update framework as in particle filtering and Condensation [21]. For an existing object, given its observations $\mathbf{Z_t} = (\mathbf{z_1}, \ldots, \mathbf{z_t})$ up to time t, we estimate the current state $\mathbf{s_t}$ by the following steps:

1. Prediction: $p(\mathbf{s_t}|\mathbf{Z_{t-1}}) = \int \mathbf{p}(\mathbf{s_t}|\mathbf{s_{t-1}})\mathbf{p}(\mathbf{s_{t-1}}|\mathbf{Z_{t-1}})\mathbf{ds_{t-1}}$,
2. Update: $p(\mathbf{s_t}|\mathbf{Z_t}) \propto \mathbf{p}(\mathbf{z_t}|\mathbf{s_t})\mathbf{p}(\mathbf{s_t}|\mathbf{Z_{t-1}})$.

We define $\mathbf{s_t} = (\mathbf{l_t}, \theta_\mathbf{t})$, where $\mathbf{l_t}$ is the location (including scale) and θ_t is the pose parameter. We assume independence between $\mathbf{l_t}$ and θ_t. Thus,

$$p(\mathbf{s_t}|\mathbf{s_{t-1}}) = \mathbf{p}(\mathbf{l_t}|\mathbf{l_{t-1}})\mathbf{p}(\theta_\mathbf{t}|\theta_\mathbf{t-1}). \tag{12}$$

During importance sampling, $\mathbf{s_t}$ is factorized into $\mathbf{l_t}$ and θ_t to reduce the number of dimensions of samples. In practice such factorization is reasonable, since position and θ tend to be independent. We also assume zero mean Gaussian distributions for both $p(\mathbf{l_t}|\mathbf{l_{t-1}})$ and $p(\theta_t|\theta_{t-1})$, i.e., $\mathbf{l_t} - \mathbf{l_{t-1}} \sim \mathbf{N}(\mathbf{0}, \Sigma_\mathbf{l})$ and $\theta_t - \theta_{t-1} \sim N(0, \Sigma_\theta)$. The covariance matrices Σ_l and Σ_θ are chosen according to the typical state changing speed of foreground objects. The Gaussian distribution assumption follows a common choice for the proposal distribution in the particle filtering framework [21].

In the update step, $p(\mathbf{z_t}|\mathbf{s_t})$ is evaluated using our detectors, i.e., given a sample $\hat{\mathbf{s_t}} = (\hat{\mathbf{l_t}}, \hat{\theta}_t)$, the detector associated with $\hat{\theta}_t$ is evaluated at location $\hat{\mathbf{l_t}}$ to give a score $C(\hat{\mathbf{z_t}}, \hat{\theta}_t)$ that determines whether the observation $\hat{\mathbf{z_t}}$ at location $\hat{\mathbf{l_t}}$ should be accepted or rejected as an instance of the object with parameter $\hat{\theta}_t$. The sample $\hat{\mathbf{s_t}}$ is discarded if the detector classifies it as from the background class. We define $p(\mathbf{z_t}|\mathbf{s_t}) = \frac{1}{\mathbf{1+exp(C(z_t,\theta_t)+r)}}$ as a sigmoid function, which has been shown in [40] to fit well as a probability model of SVM classification scores. r is determined by classification scores on the training examples.

Our posterior distribution is represented as a mixture over detector modes. Thus, the number of particles drawn for a mode is proportional to the weight of the mixture, which is set to be equal to the weight of the mode. The sum of sample weights is normalized to one in each iteration. Non-maximum suppression is applied on locations of accepted samples to produce a set of putative locations for tracked objects in the current frame.

In our tracker implementation, to deal with the entrance of new objects, exhaustive detection is triggered at every k frames. The parameter k is selected according to the expected entrance rate for new objects. Once a foreground object is detected during exhaustive detection, a tracking process starts to track it until it exits the scene. Exitance of objects is also automatically handled; once an object exits the scene, samples that are not located on foreground objects in the next frame will be rejected by the detectors.

7 Experiments

In this section we describe the evaluation of the proposed method in three applications: hand detection and shape estimation, multi-view vehicle detection and tracking, and multi-view face detection and tracking. For the purpose of these experiments, HOG [10] features are employed for $\mathbf{x}$ on all data sets; while other features could be possible, we chose the HOG feature representation since it is widely used. The detectors of our method are trained using a modified version of SVMlight [22] with multiplicative kernels. The between-class kernel k_x is always a linear kernel, and the within-class kernel k_θ is a Gaussian RBF kernel or a nonparametric kernel (Eq. 7) depending on the data set. Our results are compared with results obtained via methods proposed in [36, 52, 57, 59]. All approaches are implemented in Matlab, and run on a 2.6 GHz AMD Opteron 852 processor.

The parameters of HOG features are the same as [10]. The only difference is the detection window size for different objects. We use a 48 by 48 window on hand data sets, 90 by 90 window on the vehicle data set and 60 by 60 window on the multi-pose face data set.

In our experiments, we use two clustering techniques in our approach for mode finding: agglomerative clustering and spectral clustering [47]. Agglomerative clustering is a greedy algorithm that runs faster but may create clusters of unbalanced sizes. Spectral clustering creates balanced clusters but runs slow for large numbers of examples. We use agglomerative clustering on the hand data set and spectral clustering on the vehicle data set, mainly because of the sizes of the foreground training set.

7.1 Hand Detection and Segmentation with Nonparametric k_θ

We first conduct an experiment in hand detection for sign language data. The hand data set is collected from two sources of sign language video sequences: Flemish

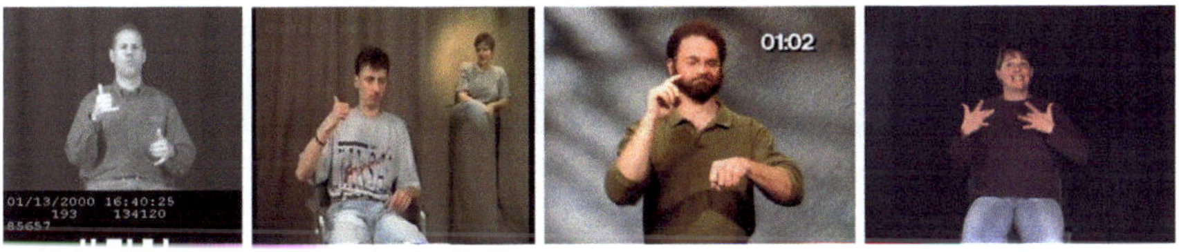

Fig. 3 Example sign language sequences from which the training and test hand images are obtained

Sign Language data [9] and American Sign Language data [32].In total there are 17 signers. The data set comprises a training set of 3,005 hand images and a test set of 2,270 hand images. The test set and training set are disjoint. The hand images are not annotated with hand shape parameters. For the training images, corresponding hand silhouettes are also provided. About 70 % of the hand silhouettes are automatically segmented by skin color models or simple background models. The rest are obtained manually. Example frames are shown in Fig. 3. This data set is available for download.[2]

The background image set contains images of outdoor and indoor scenes. This set is separated into disjoint training and test sets, which contain 300 images each. 5,000 image patches are collected as samples from each image set to be used as training or testing background samples.

Training of detectors is done as described in Sect. 4. k_x is a linear kernel. For the within-class kernel k_θ, the nonparametric form of Eq. 7 is used, since parameter annotations are unavailable for the training images. The distance measure D is the bidirectional chamfer edge distance [15] between hand images. With $\eta = 1$, the Gram matrix of k_θ is positive definite on the training set. In total about 14,300 tuples $(\mathbf{x}, \mathbf{i})$ are selected as support vectors during training. This is still a small portion of all possible training tuples, which can be as many as $3005 + 3005 \times 5000$. Because each background example $\mathbf{x}$ can be combined with different i (foreground example index) to make a training tuple $(\mathbf{x}, \mathbf{i})$. Agglomerative clustering is used in the mode finding process to generate the detector sample set of 1,242 hand modes. The number of modes is determined by the stopping criterion in agglomerative clustering, when the similarity measure of Eq. 11 between any two clusters is below a threshold value 0.7. The total training time is about 30 mins on a single 2.6 GHz AMD Opteron 852 processor.

Three out of the 1,242 hand clusters are illustrated in Fig. 4. The figure shows three images for each cluster: the image of the cluster medoid, the positive weights of the detector associated with the cluster medoid, and the mask for the medoid. The positive weights of a detector demonstrate how local edge orientations are weighted. The image mask of a cluster is computed as a weighted sum of image masks of support vectors for the top 50 weights, and then thresholded to obtain a binary image. While there could be different ways to construct an image mask, in

[2] available at http://cs-people.bu.edu/yq/projects/mk.html.

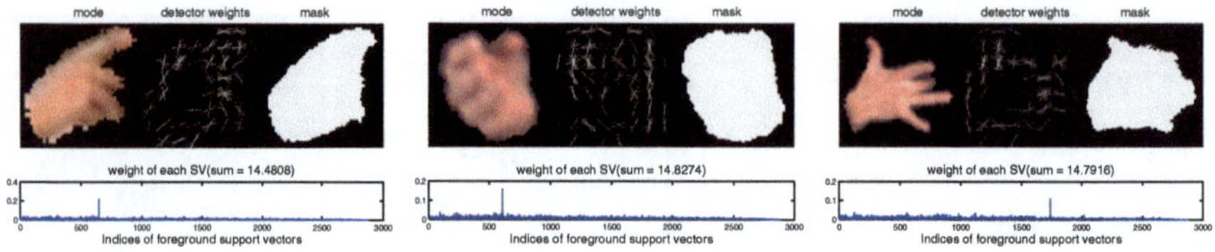

Fig. 4 Three hand clusters are displayed with their cluster medoids, positive detector weights and hand masks. For each cluster the weights of foreground support vectors are displayed at bottom

our experiment, the resulting masks have appropriate sizes and shapes for this setting.

For each cluster medoid shown in Fig. 4, a graph shows the distribution of support vector weights α'. Interestingly, although the weights have peaks on a few foreground support vectors, the sum of weights from low weight support vectors is substantial. This indicates that the contributions to the detector of a particular foreground variation come from a broad range of training samples, although each contribution may be small. One explanation is that very different hand shapes may still share segments of finger or palm boundaries.

Examples of the combined detection and segmentation results obtained with our method are shown in Fig. 5b. The segmentation result is obtained by applying the mask associated with the detector of the highest score on a detected hand. The segmentation obtained in this way is only approximate; nonetheless, the shapes are matched well and the segmentation is obtained at nominal extra cost. The segmentation result from our method can be used to mask the image for a hand shape estimation module in sign language analysis or used as initialization to a method that requires segmented input.

When the detectors are applied on the frames of the Flemish and American sign language sequences [9, 32], they can detect most of the hand shapes in the test set correctly. The detectors may fail to detect a hand when there is strong motion blur or it is partially occluded. False positives happen occasionally in regions of strong textures.

For experimental comparison, a partitioning-based method [36] is trained as follows: first clustering of hand subclasses is obtained via k-means with Euclidean distance of HOG features, then the detector for each subclass is trained using SVM with a RBF kernel. The η of the RBF kernel is 0.1, which is chosen empirically to maximize the accuracy. Each subclass is also associated with a mask, which is the union of all training masks belonging to this subclass. The features from outside a subclass mask are ignored during detection. The accuracy of the partition based method improves until the number of partitions increases to about 50 partitions. Further increases of the number of partitions do not yield significant improvement. We also implemented another version of our approach using RBF kernel in HOG features space as within-class kernel k_θ. It gives results that are comparable with our method when the chamfer edge kernel is used.

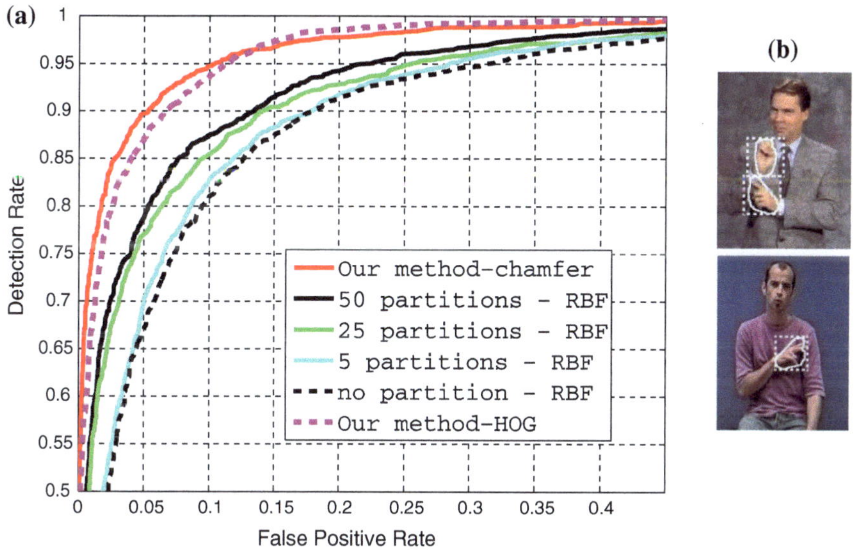

Fig. 5 Hand detection results: **a** ROC curves of different detectors for hand detection. "Our method-chamfer" uses the k_θ defined by chamfer edge distance. "Our method-HOG" uses the k_θ defined using RBF kernel in HOG feature space. **b** Example detection and segmentation results on the sign language test images

The detection accuracy of the different methods is summarized in the ROC curves of Fig. 5a. As can be seen in the graph, our method outperforms the partition-based methods by a clear margin on this data set. Compared to the best partition-based method (50 partitions), our method using the chamfer edge kernel improves detection rate from 80 to 90 % at a false positive rate of 5 %. At the detection rate of 80 % our method reduces the false positive rate from 5.3 to 1.7 %. We report the rate of false positives per window instead of false positives per image mainly because of the varying sizes of test images. The smallest image size is 98 by 58 and the largest is 640 by 480.

To better understand the accuracy tradeoff in using the representative subset of detectors determined via mode finding, we compared performance against using all detectors. The detectors are trained using the chamfer edge kernel. At a fixed false positive rate of 5 %, when all detectors are used (3,005 in total), the detection rate is 90.1 %. With our mode finding approach, the detection accuracy is 90.0, 88.4 and 83.5 % with 1,242 modes, 938 modes and 300 modes, respectively. The online detectors used in our approach (1,242 detectors) achieve the same accuracy, while reducing the number of detector evaluations by about two thirds. In contrast, when we use uniform sampling to obtain 1,242 online detectors, the average detection accuracy over ten trials is 88.1 % with a standard deviation of 0.49 % at the false positive rate of 5 %.

7.2 Hand Detection and Shape Estimation with Parametric k_θ

In the second experiment, we detect instances of a hand shape class that is parameterized by two angles from a cluttered background and estimate the two angles simultaneously. In the hand shape data set of [59], each hand image is given two angles within the range [0,90]: one for the angle of the index finger, the other one for the in-plane rotation. There are 1,605 hand images for training and 925 for testing. There are also 5,500 background training samples and 50,000 background test samples, cropped from real background images or hand images of other hand shapes not included in the target hand shape class.

In our method, HOG features are computed in the same way as [59]. The two angle parameters θ_1 and θ_2 are both normalized to $[0, 1]$. The within-class kernel k_θ is a Gaussian RBF kernel in the two-dimensional parameter space, with $\frac{1}{\sigma^2} = 10$. The change of margin during constraint generation process is plotted in Fig. 6a. After SVM training, 200 parameter values θ with corresponding detectors are uniformly sampled from the 1,605 parameter values associated with foreground training examples. This number of online detectors is determined to be adequate via cross-validation using training examples. These 200 detectors are used at the online stage.

We compare the performance of our formulation with a boosting-based approach [59]. The ROC curves of the detection result (hand vs. background) are shown in Fig. 6b. As can be seen from the ROC curves, our method consistently outperforms [59]. At a false positive rate of 2×10^{-4}, our approach improves the true positive rate from 94 to 99 %. The partition-based method of [36] is compared in [59] on the same data set. With 25 subclasses, it achieves a true positive

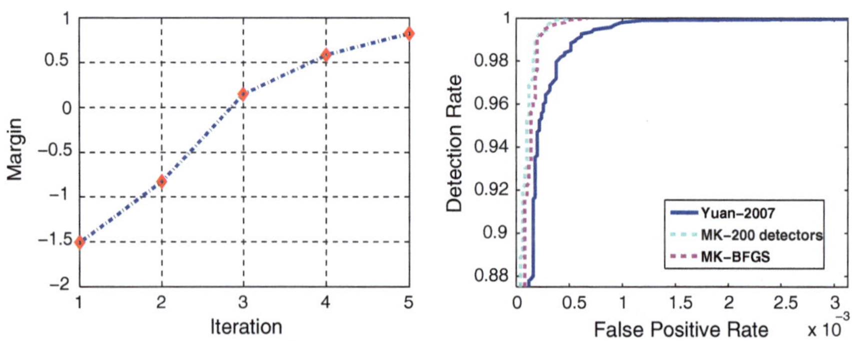

(a) Margin change **(b)** ROC comparision

Fig. 6 Training and test performance of the proposed approach on the hand shape data set [59]: **a** The change of margin during the iterative training process. The margin is defined as the minimum classification score of positive training tuples minus the maximum score of all negative training tuples at an iteration. **b** Comparison of ROC curves on the hand shape data set with two-dimensional parameters [59]. The detection rate is in the range between 88 and 100 %

rate of 91 % at the false positive rate 2×10^{-4}. Thus, our work is indirectly compared with [36]. In terms of training time, the multiplicative kernel based method is about 10 times faster than the boosting based method [59].

As noted earlier, it is possible to use nonlinear optimization of $C(\mathbf{x}, \boldsymbol{\theta})$ to determine the best $\boldsymbol{\theta}$ for a given input $\mathbf{x}$. We conducted a comparison of the sample-based versus optimization approach on this data set. Nonlinear optimization was accomplished in Matlab using a BFGS [33] quasi-Newton method with cubic polynomial search for the optimal step size. Because the multiplicative kernel may have multiple local minima, the (θ_1, θ_2) are initialized at 36 evenly distributed grid points in the box defined by the bottom left corner $(0, 0)$ and the top right corner $(90, 90)$. The ROC curve for this approach is included in Fig. 6b. The detection accuracy of BFGS is similar to using a sample set of 200 detectors, but BFGS runs much slower. On average it takes about 8.2 gradient descent iterations to converge at each of the 36 initial points.

Our approach also estimates two parameters on each hand image. The mean absolute errors (MAE) of θ_1 and θ_2 are 6.7 and 4.6° respectively by using a sample set of 200 online detectors, in contrast to 9.0 and 5.3° in [59]. The BFGS optimization achieves better MAEs of 6.5 and 3.7°. The partition-based approach [36] with 25 subclasses does not produce a parameter estimate, but a subclass label that is within a range of 18°.

7.3 Multi-View Vehicle Detection

In the next experiment we look at a multi-view vehicle detection problem. We evaluate the performance of the proposed method in two vehicle detection tasks, with comparison to previous approaches [52, 57]. In the first task, we detect vehicles appearing in city scenes. In the second task, we detect vehicles on highways.

For the first task, we use a multi-view vehicle data set [24], which is a subset of LabelMe [44] database. This subset contains 1,297 vehicles images. Each vehicle image also has a binary segmentation mask converted from the LabelMe annotation polygon. In [24], the data is split up into seven subcategories for car viewpoints approximately 30° apart. Because of vehicle symmetry, the labelled angles cover a half circle from approximately −30 to 180°. Example images from this data set are shown in Fig. 7. These 1,297 vehicle images are separated into a training set of 866 images and a test set of 431 images.

We collected background training and test image sets, which contain 432 and 344 outdoor street scene images, respectively. Most of the background images are from street scene images used in [10]. The rest are downloaded from web. The background image data sets are available for download.[3]

[3] available at http://cs-people.bu.edu/yq/projects/mk.html.

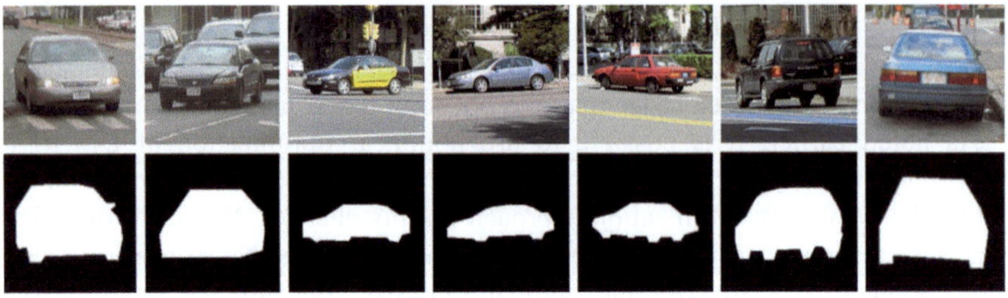

Fig. 7 Example images and their binary segmentation masks from the multi-view vehicle data set used in [24]

The rotation angles only have 8 distinct values at 30° apart, which is too coarse for a continuous model. Therefore, in our approach, a nonparametric kernel is adopted. The nonparametric within-class kernel k_θ is an RBF kernel defined with an Euclidean distance between HOG features. The kernel parameter $\eta = 0.2$. We implemented two versions of our approach. One is trained with binary image masks and the other one is without image masks. For both versions, the training process takes 10 iterations. For both versions, 280 modes are obtained by spectral clustering (normalized cuts [47]) after training. The number of modes is again determined by cross-validation of detection accuracy.

Performance is compared with Torralba's feature sharing method [52], Wu-Nevatia's tree based detector [57] and a RBF kernel SVM classifier with $\eta = 0.2$. In each method, the parameter settings were determined to optimize detection accuracy. For [52], the view angle subcategory labels of training images are provided in training since it is a multi-class detection method. In training it adds 4,000 weak classifiers in total and outputs seven subclass detectors. Each subclass detector is for a view angle subclass. In [57] the tree structure is mainly controlled by a splitting threshold θ_z. The best θ_z is found at 0.95 by cross validation, which produces a tree of eight leaf nodes. The final numbers of weak classifiers in these eight subclass detectors are between 2,032 and 2,213. We tested our implementation of [57] on the pedestrian data set [10] and obtained comparable results to those reported in [57]. At a false positive rate 10^{-4}, our implementation of [57] has a detection rate 93.4 %.

In training, a bootstrap method is employed to collect non-trivial background examples for all methods, in the same way as in [10]. First a linear SVM classifier is trained with an initial set of 10,000 training background patches. Then we exhaustively search all the background training images with this linear SVM classifier to collect false positive image patches ("hard examples"). In the scanning process, a total of 2,211 false positive patches are collected. They are added to the initial 10,000 background training samples as the background training set for all methods. In total there are about 8,300 tuples selected as support vectors in our method that utilizes image masks.

The detection performance of all methods in the first task is shown in the ROC curves of Fig. 8a. Compared with [57], our method with image masks improves the detection rate from 96.7 to 99.0 % at the false positive rate of 5×10^{-3}. At the detection rate of 99.5 %, our method reduces the false positive rate from 5 to 0.8 %. On average, it takes 1.85×10^{-4} s for our method to evaluate a test example, and 4.40×10^{-4} and 2.46×10^{-4} s for [52] and [57], respectively. However, the speed difference between all methods is not significant and we do not claim classification speed as an advantage of our approach.

In Fig. 8b, c, we show some false negative examples and false positive examples of our approach on the first task. The false negatives are collected at a fixed false positive rate of 10^{-3}. The false positives are collected at a fixed detection rate 95 %. Because the HOG features are based on gradient orientations and vehicles have symmetric shapes when viewed from certain angles, the false positive examples also show symmetric patterns and strong edges.

In the second part of this experiment, we test our method on detecting vehicles on a highway. Different from the first task where the vehicles are mostly captured in urban scenes, test sequence 5 of PETS 2001 vehicle data set is captured by two moving cameras on a highway, one facing the front and the other one facing the back of the vehicle. Example frames from the two cameras are shown in Fig. 9. In total there are 2,867 frames for each camera. The frame size is 768×576.

In these two test sequences, the vehicles that are moving in the same direction with the cameras (i.e., vehicles bound in same direction) tend to be close to the cameras, and they are imaged at good pixel resolution. It is more challenging to detect the vehicles that are moving in the opposite direction, on the other side of the highway. These vehicles appear at smaller pixel resolutions and are partially occluded by the highway guard rail. For evaluation purposes, we manually annotated vehicles of sizes no smaller than 45 by 45 and occluded by less than one third, in every 10th frame of each camera sequence.

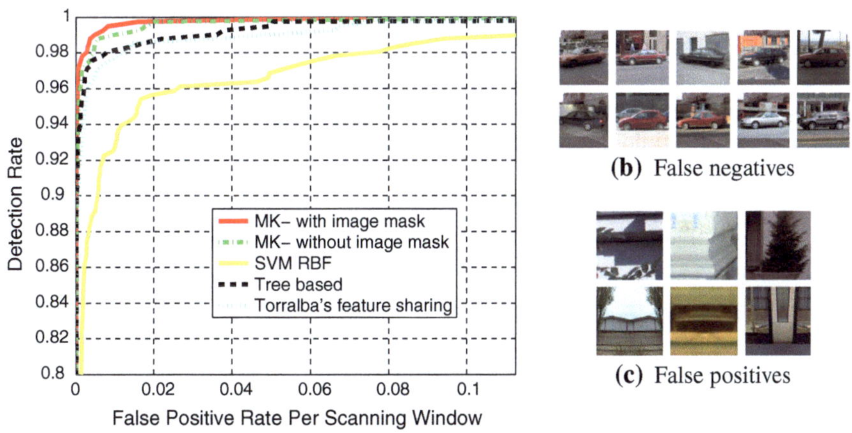

(a) ROC curves

(b) False negatives

(c) False positives

Fig. 8 Vehicle detection result on data set [24]: **a** ROC curves. **b** False negative examples of our method. **c** False positive examples of our method

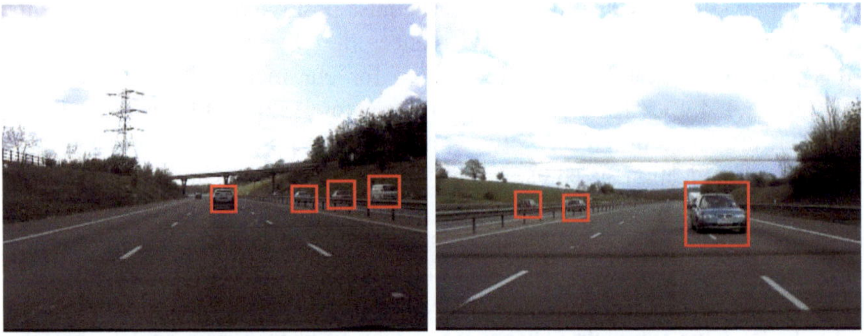

(a) Camera 1 **(b)** Camera 2

Fig. 9 Example frames and ground truth annotations of two cameras in test sequence 5 of the PETS 2001 data set. Although vehicles running close to the cameras have good resolutions, the actual challenges come from the vehicles running at the opposite direction across the fence. They usually have small resolutions and are partially occluded. Detection accuracy of these vehicles is a decisive factor in the ROC curves

As before, comparison is conducted between our approach and [52, 57]. For the purpose of fair comparison, we compared these methods with our detector without tracking. All methods detect vehicles frame by frame without temporal information. All 1,297 vehicle images from [24] with their horizontally flipped images are used as training samples. The settings of our method are the same as in the first task. For the tree based method [57], the best splitting threshold is found again at 0.95, which produces a tree that has 19 leaf nodes. For the feature sharing method [52], view categories are provided and 4,000 weak classifiers are collected in training.

For evaluation, we consider a detection window as correct if it overlaps with the ground-truth annotation by more than 50 % using the intersection-over-union criterion [29]. The detection performance of the three methods is summarized in Fig. 10. Compared with Torralba's method [52], our approach improves the detection rate from 40 to 60 % for Camera 1 and 63 to 82 % for Camera 2, both at the false positive rate of one per frame. The tree-based method [57] yielded consistently inferior performance to both [52] and our approach.

With our approach, most of the mis-detections are due to small object scales and occlusions. False positives happen in textured regions, e.g., along the highway guard rail.

7.4 Vehicle Tracking and View Angle Estimation

In this experiment, we measure the vehicle orientation estimation accuracy in tracking. For evaluation, eight test vehicle sequences were downloaded from Google video, and provided in the supplemental materials. The test sequences are

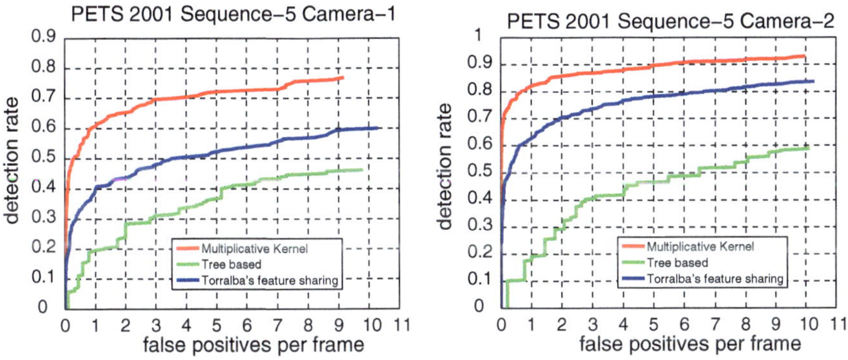

Fig. 10 Vehicle detection rate versus false positive rate on sequence 5 of PETS 2001 data set. The proposed approach (Multiplicative Kernel) is compared with Wu-Nevatia's tree based detector [57] and Torralba's feature sharing method [52]

of low frame rate—about 5 to 10 frames per second, with a pixel resolution of 320 by 240. These sequences exhibit strong motion blur artifacts and fast changes in object scale. There are eight distinct vehicles in the sequences, and each vehicle has at least 90° view angle change. Most of the vehicles run on dirt roads and three of them are race cars. The vehicles in the test sequences are annotated with view angles at 5° apart, by having a user compare vehicles in the video sequences with images of a synthetic car model rotated at different angles.

In this experiment, our multiplicative kernel detector is the same detector trained for the first vehicle detection task in the previous section. However, the original view angle partition is too coarse for view angle tracking. Thus, we use the mode finding approaches in Sect. 5 and annotate the 280 detector modes (cluster centers) with angles that are quantized to 5-degree steps. Note in total there are 866 vehicle training examples, but with our approach only fewer than one third must be annotated for the purpose of angle estimation.

We apply the tracking process explained in Sect. 6 on this data set. In this test, we assume that there is at most one vehicle in a sequence. Thus, extensive search with detectors is triggered at the first frame, and then triggered again when the tracker loses the target. The view angle estimate in a no-detection frame is linearly interpolated from previous and later view angle estimates. The number of particles is 3,000 in this experiment.

Example tracking results in four test sequences are shown in Fig. 11. The resulting angle estimation accuracy during tracking is summerized in Table 1. The median of absolute error is in the range from 5 to 15° for the eight test sequences. The mean of absolute errors is in the range from 7.62 to 26.29°. Two main causes of errors are motion blur and view angles that are not covered in the training examples. Although the tracker may lose the target due to these two reasons, the detectors can recover the target location and view angle automatically in later frames when observations are better presented. The online tracking speed is about 2 seconds per frame, including the HOG feature extraction and detector evaluation,

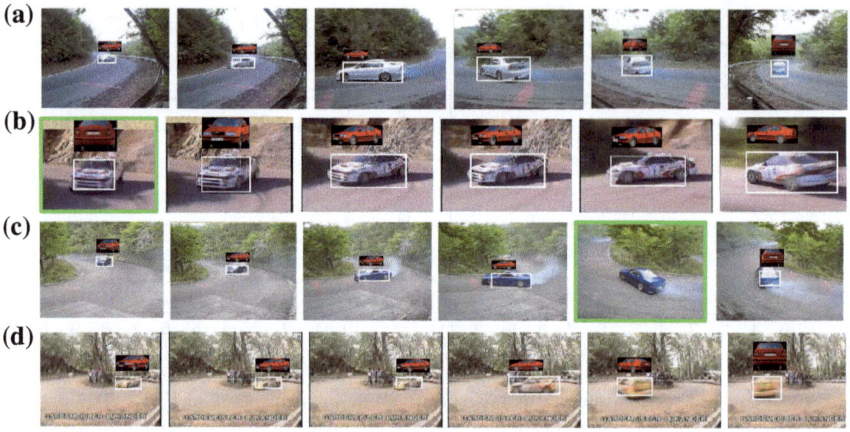

Fig. 11 Four example sequences of car tracking. Sequences (**a–d**) correspond to sequence IDs 3,8,1 and 7 respectively in Table 1. Synthesized views of tracked cars are displayed on the top of a car. *Green boxes* highlight the errors in these sequences. In sequence (**b**), the initial detection in the first frame assigns the detected car a rear view, due to the ambiguity between *front view* and *rear view*. The error is corrected at subsequent frames when more frames are evaluated during temporal propagation. In sequence (**c**), the car is missed at frame 25 because the view point elevation is much higher than those in training images

Table 1 View angle estimation accuracy in tracking vehicles in eight different test sequences

Sequence ID	1	2	3	4	5	6	7	8
# frames	32	31	39	64	40	16	59	43
Mean-AE	24.38	26.29	15.71	17.10	7.62	11.25	18.73	19.42
Median-AE	10	10	15	15	5	10	10	15

which were both implemented in Matlab without special optimization. The HOG feature extraction takes about 70 % of the CPU time.

7.5 Multi-View Face Angle Estimation and Tracking

Multi-view face detection is challenging due to the variation of face appearances at different view angles, in addition to other variations due to changes in illumination and facial expressions. A commonly used approach to detecting multi-view faces is to divide the view space into partitions and train a different detector for each partition. In previous work [18], multi-view face detection is achieved via partitioning the face class into subclasses according to face view angles. In [37] a face manifold is learned by encoding the face view angles to detect multi-view faces. Both approaches, however, require a huge amount of training images (30,000 in [37] and 75,000 in [18]). Manual annotation of such a large amount of data is expensive and both face training sets in [18, 37] are not publicly available. In contrast, our multi-view face detectors can be trained with much fewer training examples because of implicit feature sharing.

In this experiment, we train and test our approach with a subset of the recently released CMU Multi-PIE data set [16]. The complete Multi-PIE data set contains face images from 337 subjects, imaged under 15 view points and 19 illumination conditions in up to four recording sessions. We use a subset of 13 views and 10 illuminations of the first 32 subjects. In total there are 8,320 face images in the subset. The 13 view points are 30° apart. Face regions are manually annotated by us. Background training samples are collected from 1,000 background images, containing indoor and outdoor images.

Our multiplicative kernel detector is trained with a nonparametric RBF kernel k_θ. The RBF is defined over the Euclidean distance of HOG feature vectors, with $\eta = 0.1$. For comparison, subclass detectors for 13 view angle subclasses are trained by Torralba's feature sharing method [52], with 2000 boosting iterations.

We evaluate the performance of face view angle estimation by 4-fold cross validation on 32 subjects. That is, every time we train on 24 subjects and test on the remaining 8 subjects. Mean absolute error (MAE) is used as an evaluation metric for angle estimation accuracy. The comparison result is shown in Fig. 12. The overall MAE of our approach is 2.1°, in contrast to 3.0° of Torralba's feature sharing method. With our approach, 0.2 % of the test samples have errors greater than or equal to 15°. In contrast, 0.6 % of the test samples have errors greater than or equal to 15° with Torralba's feature sharing method.

To demonstrate our tracking approach in this setting, we collected two video sequences with multiple faces in a lab environment. There are 117 frames in the first sequence and 179 frames in the second sequence. The frame size is 480 by 360 pixels for the first sequence and 648 by 488 pixels for the second sequence. In each sequence there are up to three faces in a frame. The faces make left-right out-of-plane rotations and slight in-plane rotations. For evaluation purposes, we manually annotated all face locations and their left-right rotation angles in every other frame of the test sequences. During annotation, the faces in the test sequences are compared with face images from Multi-PIE training set to find matching face rotation angles.

We apply the tracking algorithm of Sect. 6 with multiplicative detectors on the two sequences. The training set for detectors that are used in tracking are the 4160 face images of first 32 subjects and first 5 illumination variations in Multi-PIE data set. During tracking, the frames are rotated up to 15° at 5-degree increments to compensate for in-plane rotations. The number of particles is 6,000 in our approach. The tracking process is fully automatic. Exhaustive search with all detectors is triggered at every 5 frames in the first sequence and every 10 frames in the second sequence to reset the tracker. The reset rate was determined to match roughly the entrance rate of faces. The number of faces is determined by exhaustive search. Example frames of the tracking result are shown in Fig. 13. Most faces are detected correctly when their pitch angle is within the range [−90, 90] degrees. Most of the missed detections are due to large in-plane orientations or yaw angles.

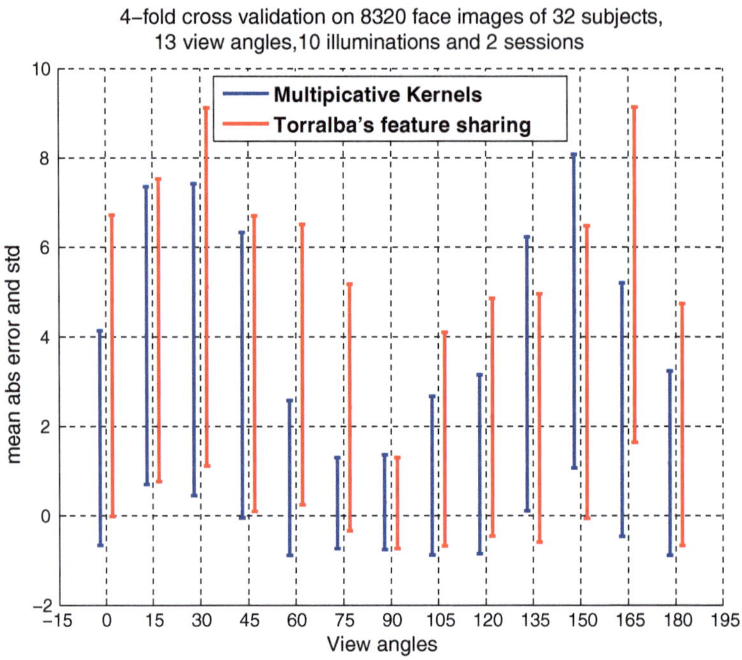

Fig. 12 Face view angle estimation result on Multi-PIE data set. For each view angle subclass, we plot the mean and standard deviation of the errors on test samples. The overall mean absolute errors are 2.1 and 3.0° for our method and Torralba's feature sharing method [52], respectively

At a false positive rate of 0.1 false positives per frame, our method achieves a detection rate of 77 % on the first sequence and 90 % on the second sequence. This difference might be attributed to the fact that faces are rotated outside the range [−90,90] in pitch angle more frequently in the first sequence. The MAEs of view angle estimation on detected faces are 3.08° on the first sequence and 3.68° on the second sequence.

The online tracking speed is about 10 seconds per frame on the first sequence and 17 seconds per frame on the sequence sequence. Extensive search takes about 5 minutes per frame on the first sequence and 14 minutes per frame on the second sequence, using un-optimized Matlab code. About 74 % of the total time is spent in HOG feature extraction.

8 Discussion and Future Work

An observation in our experiments is that the knowledge of variations within the foreground class helps the detection task. Both partition based approaches [36, 52, 57] and our method are doing better than a single foreground-background classifier. Compared with partition based approaches, our method can model more

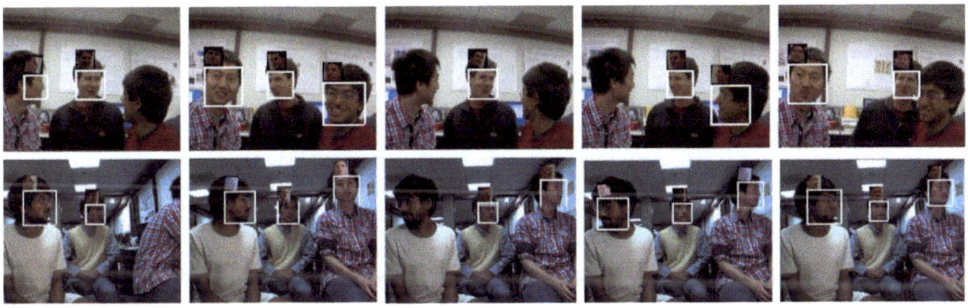

Fig. 13 Example tracking result in two test sequences. *First row* is from sequence 1. *Second row* is from sequence 2. On *top* of each tracked face, a training example with the same face orientation is displayed. The tracker stops tracking when *left-right* rotation of a face is larger than 90° from a frontal face. A face is missed in the fifth example frame of the first sequence and the third example frame of the second sequence

detailed variations like continuous rotation angles and distances/similarities between individual training examples. At the same time, feature sharing is strong during joint optimization of multiplicative kernels. These two factors may explain why our model does better than previous approaches in detection tasks.

The proposed approach is reasonably efficient given the fact that it uses a whole bank of detectors. Furthermore, our formulation does not preclude the use of a multi-level cascade structure. One possible extension is to add early detection stages to reject trivial background patches quickly. The detection speed may be further improved by a quick online process to determine a small subset of detectors to apply for a given input.

Acknowledgments This paper reports work that was supported in part by the U.S. National Science Foundation under grants IIS-0705749 and IIS-0713168.

References

1. Agarwal A, Triggs B (2004) 3D human pose from silhouettes by relevance vector regression. In: Proceedings of the IEEE conference on computer vision and pattern recognition
2. Andriluka M, Roth S, Schiele B (2008) People-tracking-by-detection and people-detection-by-tracking. In: Proceedings of the IEEE conference on computer vision and pattern recognition
3. Athitsos V, Sclaroff S (2003) Estimating 3D hand pose from a cluttered image. In: Proceedings of the IEEE conference on computer vision and pattern recognition
4. Belongie S, Malik J, Puzicha J (2002) Shape matching and object recognition using shape contexts. IEEE Trans Pattern Anal Mach Intell 24(24):509–522
5. Bissacco A, Yang M, Soatto S (2006) Deteing humans via their pose. In: Proceedings of advances in neural information processing systems
6. Blaschko MB, Lampert CH (2008) Learning to localize objects with structured output regression. In: Proceedings of the European conference on computer vision
7. Borenstein E, Ullman S (2002) Class-specific, top-down segmentation. In: Proceedings of the European conference on computer vision

8. Cortes C, Vapnik V (1995) Support vector networks. Mach Learn 20:273–297
9. Crasborn O, van der Kooij E, Nonhebel A, Emmerik W (2004) ECHO data set for sign language of the Netherlands. Technical report Department of Linguistics, University Nijmegen
10. Dalal N, Triggs B (2005) Histograms of oriented gradients for human detection. In: Proceedings of the IEEE conference on computer vision and pattern recognition
11. Damoulas T, Girolami MA (2008) Pattern recognition with a Bayesian kernel combination machine. Pattern Recogn Lett 30(1):46–54
12. Enzweiler M, Gavrila DM (2008) A mixed generative-discriminative framework for pedestrian classification. In: Proceedings of the IEEE conference on computer vision and pattern recognition
13. Felzenszwalb PF, Girshick RB, McAllester D, Ramanan D (2009) Object detection with discriminatively trained part based models. IEEE Trans Pattern Anal Mach Intell (to appear)
14. Felzenszwalb PF, Huttenlocher DP (2005) Pictorial structures for object recognition. Int J Comput Vision 61:55–79
15. Gavrila DM (2000) Pedestrian detection from a moving vehicle. In: Proceedings of the European conference on computer vision
16. Gross R, Matthews I, Cohn J, Kanade T, Baker S (2008) Multi-PIE. In: Proceedings of the IEEE international conference on face and gesture recognition
17. Hoiem D, Efros AA, Hebert M (2008) Putting objects in perspective. Int J Comput Vision 80(1):3–15
18. Huang C, Ai H, Li Y, Lao S (2007) High-performance rotation invariant multiview face detection. IEEE Trans Pattern Anal Mach Intell 29(4):671–686
19. Ioffe C, Forsyth D (2001) Probabilistic methods for finding people. Int J Comput Vision 43(1):45–68
20. Ionescu C, Bo L, Sminchisescu C (2009) Structural SVM for visual localization and continuous state estimation. In: Proceedings of the IEEE conference on computer vision and pattern recognition
21. Isard M, Blake A (1998) CONDENSATION: Conditional density propagation for visual tracking. Int J Comput Vision 29(1):5–28
22. Joachims T (1999) Making large-scale SVM learning practical. In: Scholkopf B, Burges C, Smola A (eds) Advances in Kernel methods—support vector learning. MIT Press, Cambridge
23. Kumar MP, Torr PHS, Zisserman A (2005) Obj Cut. In: Proceedings of the IEEE conference on computer vision and pattern recognition
24. Leibe B, Cornelis N, Cornelis K, Gool LV (2007) Dynamic 3D scene analysis from a moving vehicle. In: Proceedings of the IEEE conference on computer vision and pattern recognition
25. Leibe B, Leonardis A, Schiele B (2007) Robust object detection with interleaved categorization and segmentation. Int J Comput Vision 77(1):259–289
26. Li S, Fu Q, Gu L, Scholkopf B, Cheng Y, Zhang H (2001) Kernel machine based learning for multi-view face detection and pose estimation. In: Proceedings of the IEEE international conference on computer vision
27. Li S, Zhang Z (2004) Floatboost learning and statistical face detection. IEEE Trans Pattern Anal Mach Intell 26(9):1112–1123
28. Li Y, Ai H, Yamashita T, Lao S, Kawade M (2008) Tracking in low frame rate video: a cascade particle filter with discriminative observers of different life spans. IEEE Trans Pattern Anal Mach Intell 30(10):1728–1740
29. Everingham M et al (2006) The 2005 PASCAL visual object class challenge. In: Machine learning challenges—evaluating predictive uncertainty, visual object classification, and recognising textual entailment, Springer
30. Marszalek M, Schmid C, Harzallah H, van de Weijer J (2007) Learning object representations for visual object class recognition. In: Visual recognition challange workshop, in conjunction with ICCV
31. Murase H, Nayar SK (1995) Visual learning and recognition of 3D objects from appearance. Int J Comput Vision 14(1):5–24

32. Neidle C (2003) ASLLRP signstream databases. Boston University, Boston. http://ling.bu.edu/asllrpdata/queryPages
33. Nocedal J, Wright SJ (2006) Numerical optimization. Springer, New York
34. Oikonomopoulos A, Patras I, Pantic M (2006) Kernel-based recognition of human actions using spatiotemporal salient points. In: Workshop on vision for human computer interaction
35. Okuma K, Taleghani A, Freitas ND, Little J, Lowe D (2004) A boosted particle filter: multitarget detection and tracking. In: Proceeedings of the European conference on computer vision
36. Ong E, Bowden R (2004) A boosted classifier tree for hand shape detection. In: Proceedings of the IEEE international conference on face and gesture recognition
37. Osadchy R, Miller M, LeCun Y (2004) Synergistic face detection and pose estimation with energy-based model. In: Proceedings of advances in neural information processing systems
38. Papageorgiou C, Poggio T (2000) A trainable system for object detection. Int J Comput Vision 38(1):15–33
39. Pentland A, Moghaddam B, Starner T (1994) View-based and modular eigenspaces for face recognition. In: Proceedings of the IEEE conference on computer vision and pattern recognition
40. Platt J (1999) Probabilistic outputs for support vector machines and comparisons to regularized likelihood methods. In: Smola A, Bartlett P, Scholkopf B, Schuurmans D (eds) Advances in large margin classifiers. MIT Press, Cambridge
41. Ramanan D, Forsyth DA, Zisserman A (2005) Strike a pose: tracking people by finding stylized poses. In: Proceedings of the IEEE conference on computer vision and pattern recognition
42. Rifkin R, Klautau A (2004) In defense of one-vs-all classification. J Mach Learn Res 5:101–141
43. Rosales R, Sclaroff S (2002) Learning body pose via specialized maps. In: Proceedings of advances in neural information processing systems
44. Russell BC, Torralba A, Murphy KP, Freeman WT (2005) LabelMe: a database and web-based tool for image annotation. Technical report, MIT Press, Cambridge
45. Seemann E, leibe B, Schiele B (2006) Multi-aspect detection of articulated objects. In: Proceedings of the IEEE conference on computer vision and pattern recognition
46. Shakhnarovich G, Viola P, Darrell T (2003) Fast pose estimation with parameter-sensitive hashing. In: Proceedings of the IEEE international conference on computer vision
47. Shi J, Malik J (1997) Normalized cuts and image segmentation. In: Proceedings of the IEEE conference on computer vision and pattern recognition
48. Sidenbladh H, Black MJ, Fleet DJ (2000) Stochastic tracking of 3D human figures using 2D image motion. In: Proceedings of the European conference on computer vision, pp 702–718
49. Sigal L, Bhatia S, Roth S, Black M, Isard M (2004) Tracking loose-limbed people. In: Proceedings of the IEEE conference on computer vision and pattern recognition
50. Sminchisescu C, Kanaujia A, Metaxas D (2006) Learning joint top-down and bottom-up processes for 3D visual inference. In: Proceedings of the IEEE conference on computer vision and pattern recognition
51. Stenger B, Thayananthan A, Torr P, Cipolla R (2003) Filtering using a tree-based estimator. In: Proceedings of the IEEE international conference on computer vision
52. Torralba A, Murphy K, Freeman W (2004) Sharing features: Efficient boosting procedures for multiclass object detection. In: Proceedings of the IEEE conference on computer vision and pattern recognition
53. Varma M, Ray D (2007) Learning the discriminative power-invariance trade-off. In: Proceedings of the IEEE international conference on computer vision. Rio de Janeiro, Brazil
54. Viola P, Jones M (2003) Fast multi-view face detection. In: Proceedings of the IEEE conference on computer vision and pattern recognition
55. Viola P, Jones M (2004) Robust real time object detection. Int J Comput Vision 57(2):137–154

56. Wang L, Shi J, Song G, Shen I (2007) Object detection combining recognition and segmentation. In: Proceedings of Asian conference on computer vision
57. Wu B, Nevatia R (2007) Cluster boosted tree classifier for multi-view multi-pose object detection. In: Proceedings of the IEEE international conference on computer vision
58. Wu B, Nevatia R (2007) Simultaneous object detection and segmentation by boosting local shape feature based classifier. In: Proceedings of the IEEE conference on computer vision and pattern recognition
59. Yuan Q, Thangali A, Ablavsky V, Sclaroff S (2007) Parameter sensitive detectors. In: Proceedings of the IEEE conference on computer vision and pattern recognition
60. Zhu L, Chen Y, Lin C, Yuille AL (2007) Rapid inference on a novel and/or graph: detection, segmentation and parsing of articulated deformable objects in cluttered backgrounds. In: Proceedings of advances in neural information processing systems

Facial Expression Recognition Using FAPs-Based 3DMMM

Hamimah Ujir and Michael Spann

Abstract A 3D modular morphable model (3DMMM) is introduced to deal with facial expression recognition. The 3D Morphable Model (3DMM) contains 3D shape and 2D texture information of faces extracted using conventional Principal Component Analysis (PCA). In this work, modular PCA approach is used. A face is divided into six modules according to different facial features which are categorized based on Facial Animation Parameters (FAP). Each region will be treated separately in the PCA analysis. Our work is about recognizing the six basic facial expressions, provided that the properties of a facial expression are satisfied. Given a 2D image of a subject with facial expression, a matched 3D model for the image is found by fitting them to our 3D MMM. The fitting is done according to the modules; it will be in order of the importance modules in facial expression recognition (FER). Each module is assigned a weighting factor based on their position in priority list. The modules are combined and we can recognize the facial expression by measuring the similarity (mean square error) between input image and the reconstructed 3D face model.

Keywords Modular PCA · 3D Morphable model · 3D Facial expression recognition

H. Ujir (✉)
Universiti Malaysia Sarawak, Kota Samarahan, Sarawak, Malaysia
e-mail: uhamimah@fit.unimas.my

M. Spann
University of Birmingham, Birmingham, UK
e-mail: m.spann@bham.ac.uk

J. M. R. S. Tavares and R. M. Natal Jorge (eds.), *Topics in Medical Image Processing and Computational Vision*, Lecture Notes in Computational Vision and Biomechanics 8,
DOI: 10.1007/978-94-007-0726-9_2,

1 Introduction

Facial expression recognition (FER) deals with the application of facial motion and facial feature deformation into abstract classes that are purely based on visual information [1]. Facial expression studies are beneficial to various applications. Among the applications are physiological studies, face image compression, synthetic face animation, robotics as well as virtual reality.

In this chapter, we propose a novel approach for FER called 3D Modular Morphable Model (3DMMM) that combines three advances in the face processing field: 3D Morphable Model (3DMM), Modular Principle Component Analysis (MPCA) and Facial Animation Parameters (FAP).

There have been numerous works in this area. However, our work has the following differences with others: (1) the fitting of 3D shape is done according to the modules and therefore each module has their own eigenvalues and eigenvectors; and (2) each module are given priority in the fitting process which depends on its importance in recognizing facial expression.

The outline of the chapter is as follows: In the second section, the three separate advances are discussed. The framework of this work is explained by the flowchart can be found in the third section. In the fourth section is about the database description. The experiment as well as its analysis is presented in fifth section. Finally, we give the conclusion as well as the limitations and future works.

2 Related Works

2.1 Modular PCA

Using PCA, a face is represented by a linear combination of physical face geometries, S_{mode} and texture images, T_{mode} and both models are within a few standard deviations from their means. PCA is indeed a promising approach in for face analysis. It is fast, reliable and able to produce good results. However, according to Mao et al. [2], PCA does not cope well with variations of expression, facial hair, and occlusion. Thus, we chose a slightly different PCA version which is MPCA to cover all variations of six basic facial expressions.

A similar concept used in this chapter can be found in Tena et al. [3] where they also used a collection of PCA sub-models that are independently trained but share boundaries. The segmentation of the face is a data-driven where the correlation and connection of the vertices are rated based on the range of motion, emotional speech and FAC sequences. The highly correlated and connected vertices form compact regions and compressed by PCA. Their findings strengthen the hypothesis that region-based model is better than holistic approach. However, no FER results recorded as this work is developed for animation purpose.

Zhao et al. [4] state that face recognition using eigenmodules (i.e. mouth, nose and eyes) showed improvement in facial recognition compared to using only eigenfaces. Other work using MPCA showed a significant result especially when there are large variations in facial expression and illumination is by Gottumukkal and Asari [14].

Most work in face processing is based on linear combination approach. Employing PCA on one whole face is like learning a face as one big module. In other word, the local features and its holistic information are not being taken full advantage of.

One major prominent feature of MPCA is it yields new modules to recognize different facial expressions which could be the new addition to the existing facial expression in the training set. The new modules here are the combination of different modules. Besides that, with MPCA, a smaller error is generated compared to conventional PCA as it pays more attention to the local structure [5].

However, according to Gottumukkal and Asari [14], MPCA is known as not giving a significant advancement in pose and orientation problem. It also requires the location of each facial feature to be identified initially. In their work, they also stated that if the face images are divided into very small regions the global information of the face may be lost and the accuracy of this approach is no longer acceptable. Thus, choosing the number of modules to represent a face is also important. MPCA in their work has been employed in face recognition area.

King and Xu [5] divided a face into 4 modules; centre-of-the-left-eye, centre-of-the-right-eye, tip-of-the-nose and centre-of-the mouth feature points. According to them, MPCA generates a smaller error as it pays more attention to the local structure. Chiang et al. [6] used 5 modules which include the left eye, the right eye, the nose, the mouth, and the bare face with each facial module identified by a landmark at the module centre. In this work, a face is divided into several modules according to different facial features which are categorized based on the Facial Animation Parameters (FAPs).

2.2 Facial Animation Parameters

A facial expression is about the deformation of facial features and muscles. Different combination of facial features and muscles produces different type of facial expressions. For instance, how to differentiate between the true smile and polite smile since both types of smile share the same action unit (AU) deformation which is the lip corner puller. In this case, the cheek raiser AU needs to be checked; if it's in action, the true smile is performed and vice versa.

Different works state different AUs are involved in six basic facial expressions which can be found in Appendix 2. Ekman and Friesen [7] introduced the basic AUs involved and in time, other researchers add/deduct certain AUs to represent the facial expressions. We believed this has to do with the intensity of the facial expressions itself, for instance different works might focused on true smile while others focused on polite smile. However, no report about this matter is found to date. Zhang et al. [8] divided the AUs into two, the primary and auxiliary type. The primary AUs are the AUs that strongly pertinent to one of the facial expressions without ambiguity while the supplementary cues are the auxiliary type.

FAPs are a set of parameters, used in animating MPEG-4 models that define the reproduction emotions, expressions and speech pronunciation. It gives the measurement of muscular action relevant to the AU and it provides temporal information that is needed in order to have a life-like facial expression effect [8]. Figure 1 shows FAPs and feature points on a neutral face and both define Facial Animation Parameters Unit (FAPU).

FAPs represent a complete set of basic facial actions, such as stretch nose, open or close eyelids, and therefore allow the representation of most natural facial expressions. In order to relate the FAPs and AUs, a mapping between both can be found in Appendix 1. The red coloured numbers in Appendix 1 denote that the AUs which are present for that expression in all previous works. Since different works defined different AUs for the basic facial expressions, hence it is affecting the decision on which FAPs to be monitored. In this work, we followed Ekman and Friesen's [7] work where only 13 AUs were considered.

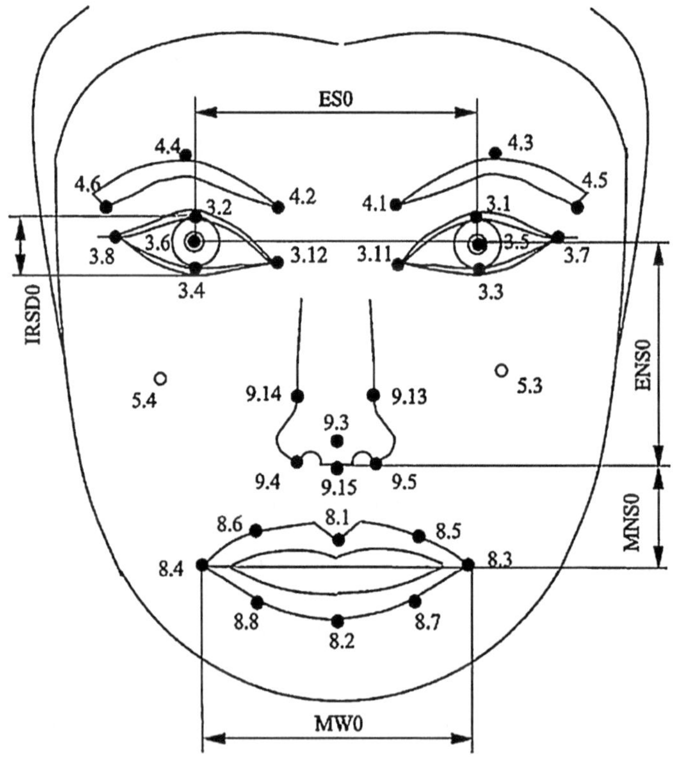

Fig. 1 A neutral face with FAPs and feature points to define FAPU [15]

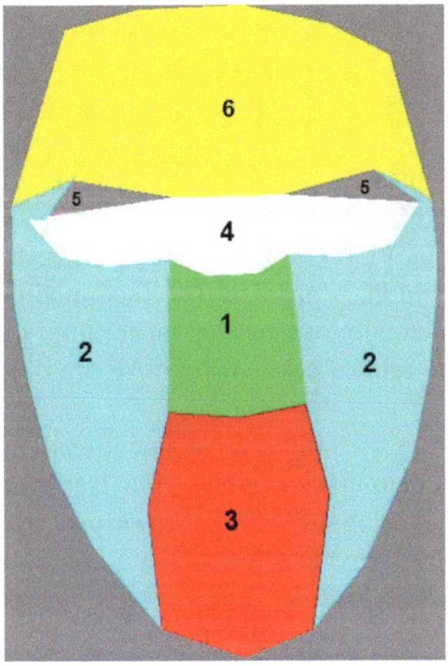

Fig. 2 Facial modules of a face

Table 1 Face modules based on FAPs group

Module	Facial Animation Parameters (FAP)
1	stretch_l_nose, stretch_r_nose
2	lift_l_cheek, lift_r_cheek
3	open_jaw, raise_b_midlip, stretch_r_cornerlip, raise_l_cornerlip, raise_r_cornerlip, push_b_lip, stretch _l_cornerlip, depress_chin, raise_b_midlip_o, stretch_r_cornerlip_o, raise_l_cornerlip_o, raise_r_cornerlip_o, stretch _l_cornerlip_o
4	close_t_r_eyelid, close_t_l_eyelid, close_b_r_eyelid, close_b_l_eyelid
5	raise_r_i_eyebrow, raise_r_i_eyebrow, squeeze_r_eyebrow, raise_l_i_eyebrow, raise_l_o_eyebrow, squeeze_l_ eyebrow

Figure 2 shows different colours for every module and each colour defined the modules priority. In this work, six FAP-based modules are used to represent a whole face, see Table 1. Each module contains the facial features that correspond to the FAP in that module. Forehead module is not mentioned in Table 1 as no FAPs involved in six facial basic emotions come from this region. However we also include this module in this work because the end outcome needs to have a complete face as well as to see how it influences each of the expression. In group one, the two FAPs only exists in disgust and anger expression and when there is a change for these two parameters, it means the subject is showing the disgust or anger expression.

2.3 FAPs-Based 3D MMM

3D MM is based on a series of 3D scans example represented in an object centred system and registered to a single reference [9]. It will be used for MPCA-based representation of faces; this combination of algorithms will then be named as the 3D Modular Morphable Model (3D MMM).

In this work, a Modular PCA (MPCA) is implemented where each face module is treated separately in the PCA process. The face modules are decided based on the facial features which are categorized according to the Facial Animation Parameters (FAP). Basic related concepts of FAP are described in Lavagetto and Pockaj [10].

The training of MPCA is similar to conventional PCA with the algorithm applied to each of the six groups in Table 1. For convenience, six disjoint sets of facial features are denotes as $P \in \{forehead, eyebrows, eyes, mouth, cheeks, nose\}$. The training examples are stored in terms of *x, y z*-coordinates of all vertices in the same modules of a 3D mesh. The following is the example of the nose module:

$$S_{\text{nose}} = \{x_1, y_1, z_1, x_2, y_2, z_2, \ldots\ldots\ldots, x_n, y_n, z_n\} \tag{1}$$

$$S_{\text{nose}} = \bar{S}_{\text{nose}} + \sum_{i=1}^{n} a_i s_i \tag{2}$$

The linear space of face geometries is denoted in Eq. 2 and it assumes a uniform distribution of the shapes. a_{nose} is the coefficients that determine the variation between 3D nose modules for all faces in the training set.

In this work, our aim is to experiment the decomposition of 3D face shape. Therefore, for appearance part, one modular approach is implemented. Accordingly, the texture vectors are formed from the red, green and blue of all vertices and b (in Eq. 4) is the appearance coefficient that determine the appearance variation for all faces in the training set.

$$T = \{r_1, g_1, b_1, r_2, g_2, b_2, \ldots\ldots\ldots, r_n, g_n, b_n\} \tag{3}$$

$$T = \bar{T} + \sum_{i=1}^{n} b_i t_i \tag{4}$$

3 Our Framework

PCA algorithms produce a set of values of uncorrelated variables called principal module (PC). All PCs are then ordered so that the first few retain most of the variation in all of original variables while the rest of the modules contain the remaining original variables after all correlation with the preceding PCs has been subtracted out. The number of PCs is normally chosen to explain at least 90 % of the variation in the training set.

The fitting process of a new image to the model involved projecting the 2D image onto the subspace (which is called the "face space") and then finding the minimum of the distance all of the faces stored in the database and the closest matching one is recognised. With the number of subjects involved, as well as large variation of expressions, poses and illumination in the training set, the number of PCs to be considered is rather high as it needs to cover all variation of faces in the dataset. Rationally, the linear computational cost is linear with the number of PCs. With MPCA, the number of PCs to be considered for each module is lower when compared to calculating PCs for a whole face.

Figure 3 describes our 3D Modular Morphable Model Framework. For 3D shape data in training set, they were all decomposed into six modules then each module will go through PCA calculation. However, the appearance data will go straight to PCA process without decomposition process.

Given a 2D image of a subject with facial expression, a matched 3D model for the image is found by fitting them to our 3D MMM. Again, the 3D shape of a probe image is decomposed into six modules, then the matching shape for each modules are found by projecting each modules into their respected face modules space.

As mentioned before, the 3D shape fitting is done according to the modules; it will be in order of the importance modules in FER. Each module is assigned a weighting factor based on their position in priority list. For instance, three modules are involved to decide the new 3D facial landmarks for eyes module which are the eyebrows, cheeks and nose. Nose will be given a higher weighting factor because of its position in priority list and then followed by cheeks and eyebrows. While for appearance, the fitting is done for a whole face, similar to a conventional PCA fitting. Finally, a 3D shape and a texture are combined and a new 3D face model is generated.

4 Database Description

A multi-attribute database developed by Savran et al. [18] from Bogazici University, Turkey called The Bosphorus Database is used. The data is acquired using Inspeck Mega Capturor II 3D which is a commercial structured-light based 3D digitizer device. The Bosphorus Database contains 24 facial landmark points; provided that they are visible in the given scan (i.e., the right and left ear lobe cannot be seen from frontal pose). It provides a rich set of expressions, systematic variation of poses and different types of realistic occlusions. Each scan is intended to cover one pose and/or one expression type. Thirty-four facial expressions are composed of a wisely chosen subset of Facial Action Units (FAU) as well as the six basic emotions. Besides the facial expression data, this database contains different occlusion and head poses data.

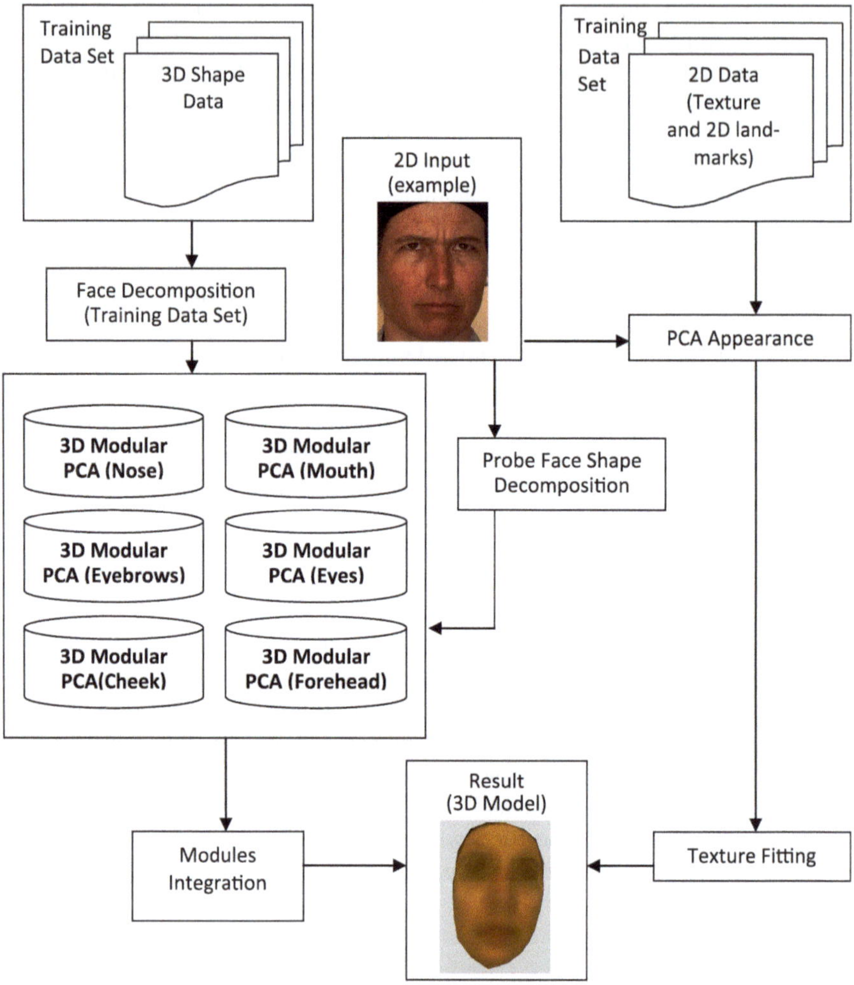

Fig. 3 3D modular morphable model framework

In this work, our 3DMMM is derived from statistics computed on 54 subjects with 6 different expressions which are anger, disgust, fear, happy, sad and surprise. Figure 4 shows a subject with six different facial expressions. Extra work need to be done as we decided to add 6 more facial landmarks which are the centre of pupils, the highest and lowest point on both eyes. These 6 extra facial landmarks are needed as it involve in the selected FAPs list.

We are dealing with two types of information, 2D and 3D data, and both data need to go under a few processes before they are ready to be used in modular PCA computation as well as the fitting procedure. The 3D points of every faces are aligned to each other and 115 of 3D points and 210 meshes are used to represent one whole face. The aligned 3D points are then divided into six modules. For each

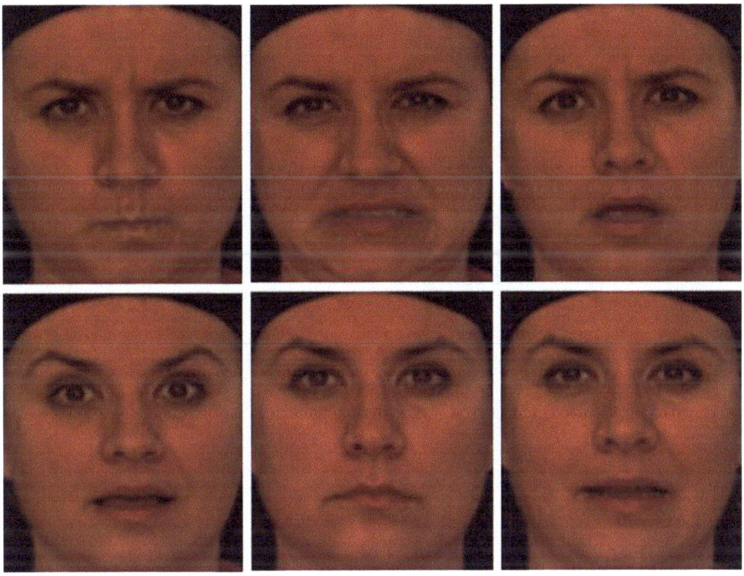

Fig. 4 Six different emotions of a subject. *Top row* anger, disgust, fear. *Bottom row* surprise, neutral and few combinations of deformation

module, the eigenvalues and its corresponding eigenvectors are computed. Out of certain amount of eigenvalues, only 97 % of the eigenvalues of the whole training data are kept and used in the next step which is fitting.

In two dimensional data, two important data are needed: (1) 2D-points that mark the facial features on a texture and (2) texture (RGB values) with a size of 50 × 50 pixels are used. The 2D points are warped using Thin Plate Spline (TPS) algorithm to ensure the colour profiles are obtained cross a free shape patch. All training texture are also normalized, this way all training texture have the same brightness and contrast. The RGB values of the texture are extracted from the normalized texture and eigenvalues and its corresponding eigenvectors are computed.

We can recognize the facial expression by measuring the similarity (mean square error) between input image and the reconstructed 3D face model. Following Blanz et al. [11] works', rigid transformation and perspective projective are implemented in the fitting process. A further discussion of fitting a new 2D image can be found in Blanz et al. [11].

5 Results and Analysis

To assess the viability of this approach, we have performed the experiments to recognize six facial expressions. In the test set, there are 4 subjects and each subject shown 6 facial expressions. Our FER experiments are carried out in a

Table 2 Facial expression recognition rate (%) using MPCA

	Anger	Disgust	Fear	Happy	Sad	Surprise
Nose						
NNS	75	50	25	50	100	25
Mouth + Jaws						
NNS	25	50	50	50	50	75
Eyes						
NNS	50	25	50	75	25	25
Eyebrows						
NNS	25	50	25	25	50	50
Cheeks						
NNS	25	50	50	75	50	25
Forehead						
NNS	25	25	25	50	50	100

person-independent manner as all test subjects were not in the training set. According to Pantic and Rothrantz [17], person independent experiment in FER is more challenging than person-dependent approach. There are no rejections, only correct recognition or false recognition as no threshold is used in this experiment.

Several experiments have been carried out and each of the results can be find in the table below: (1) FER using MPCA (2) FER for using only PCA and (3) FER after integrating all modules. Table 2 shows the FER rate for each of the face modules using nearest neighbour search approach which is calculated in Euclidean distance measure. In terms of specific expressions, recognition rate of surprise is the best and anger and fear are the worst. Nose module gives the best result and the worst is eyebrows module. The eyebrows module is the smallest region on face. We believed that the global information is lost because of the small region size and therefore affecting the FER rate.

Table 3 shows the FER rate for non-modular PCA while Table 4 shows the FER rate for combined modules. We can see that the latter one improves the FER rate compared to the former one. However, the FER rate for surprise is similar for both approaches. Although each module give a quite promising output (refer Table 2) but when they were all combined, the result is not sustained. We believed the assigned weighting factor has affected each module in the fitting process.

Table 3 Facial expression recognition rate (%) for non-moduler PCA

	Anger	Disgust	Fear	Happy	Sad	Surprise
NNS	25	25	25	50	25	50

Table 4 Facial expression recognition rate (%) for combined modules

	Anger	Disgust	Fear	Happy	Sad	Surprise
NNS	50	50	50	100	50	50

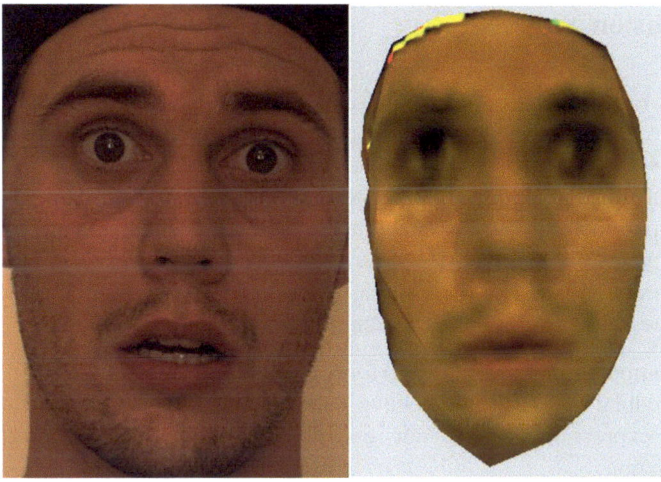

Fig. 5 Input image with anger expression (*left*). 3D model with anger appearance (*right*)

Figure 5 shows a test image with anger expression (left) and the generated 3D model (right) while Fig. 6 shows the fear expression. Another noticeable outcome from the experiment is the wrinkle and dimple feature. In real life, these two features are the two keys that help in identifying people and it also become one of the important feature that project certain facial expression. For example, in Fig. 6, lines of wrinkles on the forehead and a line from inner eyes to the outer cheek are part of the fear expression. However, this cannot be seen in the 3D model generated.

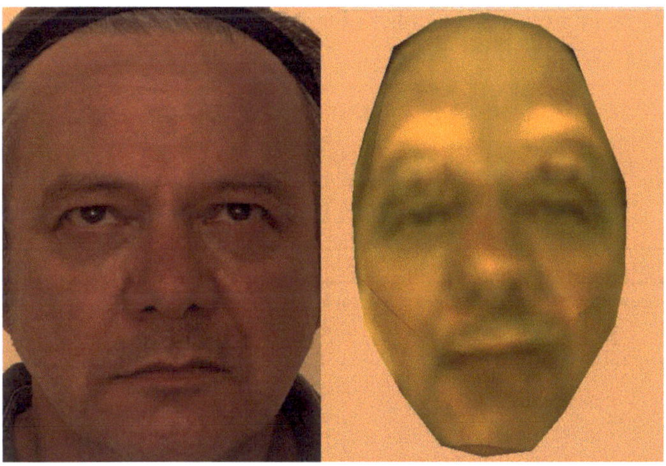

Fig. 6 Input image with fear expression (*left*). 3D model with fear appearance (*right*)

6 Conclusion

This paper explores the potential of facial expression recognition using modular approach. A face is divided into six modules and each module will have their own eigenvalues as well as eigenvector. A test image is divided into the six modules. Each module is assigned a weighting factor based on their position in priority list. The weighting factor is used to integrate the modules and then give us a new face. The system developed also yields various facial expressions even though that certain expression is not in the training set.

There are some limitations in the current work:

(1) The combined modules only perform more than average but still better than non-modular approach. We believe using only 3D facial landmarks to measure facial expression is just not enough to capture the facial expression information.
(2) The weighting factors assigned give a rather high impact on each module when combined. For instance, though the eyebrows module is put on the second last position in the priority list, it does affect the facial landmarks in forehead and eyes modules in the fitting process.
(3) Only 4 subjects with 6 facial expressions are tested in this work due to the limited data.
(4) No appearance features like wrinkle and dimple is generated in this work.
(5) The texture computation component in this work is rather time-consuming compared to the shape. This is due non-modular PCA approach used in texture component as the number of PCs that need to be calculated is quite large. Our future work will emphasize in finding a purely 3D shape feature to be used in FER as the 3D facial landmarks are not enough to measure facial expression. In order to have an effective classification system, the modules fitting process needs to be improved and number of test image will be added. We will pursue these three aspects in the future.

Appendix 1

AU	Description	FAP number	FAP name	Module
1	Inner brow raiser	31	raise_l_i_eyebrow	5
		32	raise_r_i_eyebrow	
2	Outbrow raiser	35	raise_l_o_eyebrow	5
		36	raise_l_o_eyebrow	
4	Brow lower	31_	raise_l_i_eyebrow	5
		32_	raise_r_i_eyebrow	
		37	squeeze_l_eyebrow	
		38	squeeze_r_eyebrow	

(continued)

(continued)

AU	Description	FAP number	FAP name	Module
5	Upper lid raiser	19_	open_t_l_eyelid (close_t_l_eyelid)	4
		20_	open_t_r_eyelid (open_t_r_eyelid)	
6	Cheek raiser	19	close_t_l_eyelid	5
		20	close_t_r_eyelid	
		41	lift_l_cheek	
		42	lift_r_cheek	
7	Lid tighter	21	close_b_l_eyelid	4
		22	close_b_r_eyelid	
9	Nose wrinkler	61	stretch_l_nose	1
		62	stretch_r_nose	
10	Upper lip raiser	59	raise_l_cornerlip_o	3
		60	raise_r_cornerlip_o	
12	Lip corner puller	59	raise_l_cornerlip_o	3
		60	raise_r_cornerlip_o	
		53	stretch_l_cornerlip_o	
		54	stretch_r_cornerlip_o	
15	Lip corner depressor	59_	lower_l_cornerlip (raise_l_cornerlip_o)	3
		60_	lower_r_cornerlip (raise_r_cornerlip_o)	
16	Lower lip depressor	5	raise_b_midlip	3
		16	push_b_lip	
17	Chin raiser	18	depress_chin	3
20	Lip stretcher	53	stretch_l_cornerlip	3
		54	stretch_r_cornerlip	
		5	raise_b_midlip	
23	Lip tighter	53_	tight_l_cornerlip	3
		54_	tight_r_cornerlip	
24	Lip pressor	4	lower_t_midlip	3
		16	push_b_lip	
		17	push_t_lip	
25	Lip apart	3	open_jaw(slight)	3
		5_	lower_b_midlip(slight)	
26	Jaw drop	3	open_jaw(middle)	3
		5_	lower_b_midlip(middle)	
27	Mouth stretch	3_	open_jaw(large)	3
		5_	lower_b_midlip(large	

Appendix 2

	Ekman and Friesen [7]	Raouzaiou et al. [12]	Zhang et al. [8]		Deng and Noh [13]	Lucey et al. [16]	Velusamy et al. [19]
			Primary	Auxiliary			
Anger	4 + 5 + 7 + 23	2 + 4 + 5 + 7 + 17	2 + 4 + 7 + 23 + 24	17 + 25 + 26 + 16	2 + 4 + 7 + 9 + 10 + 20 + 26	4 + 5 + 15 + 17	23 + 7 + 17 + 4 + 2
Disgust	9 + 15 + 16	5 + 7 + 10 + 25	9 + 10	17 + 25 + 26	NIL	1 + 4 + 15 + 17	9 + 7 + 4 + 17 + 6
Fear	1 + 2 + 4 + 5 + 20 + 26	4 + 5 + 7 + 24 + 26	20 + (1 + 5) + (5 + 7)	4 + 5 + 7 + 25 + 26	1 + 2 + 4 + 5 + 15 + 20 + 26	1 + 4 + 7 + 20	20 + 4 + 1 + 5 + 7
Happiness	6 + 12	26 + 12 + 7 + 6 + 20	6 + 12	16 + 25 + 26	1 + 6 + 12 + 14	6 + 12 + 25	12 + 6 + 26 + 10 + 23
Sadness	1 + 4 + 15	7 + 5 + 12	1 + 15 + 17	4 + 7 + 25 + 26	1 + 4 + 15 + 23	1 + 2 + 4 + 15 + 17	15 + 1 + 4 + 17 + 10
Surprise	1 + 2 + 5B + 26	26 + 5 + 7 + 4 + 2 + 15	5 + 26 + 27 + (1 + 2)	NIL	1 + 2+5 + 15 + 16 + 20 + 26	1 + 2 + 5 + 25 + 27	27 + 2 + 1 + 5 + 26

References

1. Fasel B, Luettin J (2003) Automatic facial expression analysis: a survey. Pattern Recogn 36(1):259–275
2. Mao X, Xue Y, Li Z, Huang K, Lv S (2009) Robust facial expression recognition based on RPCA and AdaBoost. In: 10th workshop on image analysis for multimedia interactive services
3. Tena R, De la Torre F, Matthews I (2011) Interactive region-based linear 3D face models. ACM Trans Graph 30(4):76
4. Zhao W, Chellappa R, Phillips PJ, Rosenfeld A (2003) Face recognition: a literature survey. ACM Comput Surv 35(4):399–458
5. King I, Xu L (1997) Localized principal module analysis learning for face feature extraction and recognition. In: Proceedings of workshop 3D computer vision, p 124
6. Chiang C-C, Chen Z-W, Yang C-N (2009) A module-based face synthesizing method. In: APSIPA annual summit and conference, p 24
7. Ekman P, Friesen W (1978) Facial action coding system: a technique for the measurement of facial movement. Consulting Psychologists Press, Palo Alto
8. Zhang Y, Ji Q, Zhu Z, Yi B (2008) Dynamic facial expression analysis and synthesis with MPEG-4 facial animation parameters. IEEE Trans. Circuits Syst Video Technol 18(10): 1383–1396
9. Romdhani S, Pierrard J-S, Vetter T (2005) 3D morphable face model, a unified approach for analysis and synthesis of images. In: Wenyi Zhao RC (ed) Face processing: advanced modeling and methods. Elsevier
10. Lavagetto F, Pockaj R (1999) The facial animation engine: towards a high-level interface for the design of MPEG-4 compliant animated faces. IEEE Trans Circuits Syst Video Technol 9(2):277–289
11. Blanz V, Scherbaum K, Seidel H (2007) Fitting a morphable model to 3D scans of faces. Comput Vis IEEE Int Conf 0:1–8
12. Raouzaiou A, Tsapatsoulis N, Karpouzis K (2002) Kollias S (2002) Parameterized facial expression synthesis based on MPEG-4. EURASIP J Appl Sig Proc 1:1021–1038
13. Deng Z, Noh J (2008) Computer facial animation: a survey. In: Deng Z, Neumann U (eds) Data driven 3D facial animation. Springer, pp 1–28
14. Gottumukkal R, Asari VK (2003) An improved face recognition technique based on modular PCA approach. Pattern Recognit Lett 25(4):429–436
15. ISO/IEC IS 14496-2 Visual (1999) http://kazus.ru/nuke/modules/Downloads/pub/144/0/ISO-IEC-14496-2-2001.pdf. Assessed 13 Feb 2012
16. Lucey P, Cohn JF, Kanade T, Saragih J, Ambadar Z, Matthews I (2002). The extended Cohn-Kanade dataset (CK +): a complete dataset for action unit and emotion-specified expression. In: IEEE computer society conference on computer vision and pattern recognition workshops (CVPRW), pp 94–101
17. Pantic M, Rothkrantz L (2000) Automatic analysis of facial expressions: the state of the art. IEEE Trans PAMI 22:1424–1445
18. Savran A, Alyüz N, Dibeklioğlu H, Çeliktutan O, Gökberk B, Sankur B, Akarun L (2008) Biometrics and identity management. In: Schouten B, Juul NC, Drygajlo A, Tistarelli M (eds) Bosphorus database for 3D face analysis. Springer, Berlin, pp 47–56
19. Velusamy S, Kannan H, Anand B, Sharma A, Navathe B (2011) A method to infer emotions from facial action units. In: IEEE international conference on acoustics, speech and signal processing (ICASSP), pp 2028–2031

SVM Framework for Incorporating Content-Based Image Retrieval and Data Mining into the SBIM Image Manager

Luiz A. P. Neves and Gilson A. Giraldi

Abstract With the Internet evolution, there has been a huge increase in the amount of images stored in electronic format particularly in the case of biological and medical image applications. Nowadays, hospitals and research centers can acquire large image databases which poses fundamental requirements for storage, processing and sharing data. In order to fulfill these requirements we have proposed the Shared Biological Image Manager (SBIM) system which has been developed using the programming languages PHP and Javascript as well as the Database Management System PostgreSQL. In this chapter, we propose an extension of the SBIM functionalities by incorporating data mining and image retrieval facilities. We describe an unified solution for both these services inside the Shared Biological Image Manager (SBIM) through Support Vector Machine (SVM) frameworks. Data mining is implemented using discriminant weights given by SVM separating hyperplanes to select the most discriminant features for two-class classification problems. For image retrieval, we consider an SVM ensemble based on the "one-against-all" SVM multi-class approach. The user specifics an initial feature space, the training set and the SVM (ensemble) configuration. After training, the SVM ensemble can be used to retrieve relevant data once given a query image. Finally, we discuss some details about the implementation of the content-based image retrieval (CBIR) and discriminant features discovery approaches inside the SBIM system.

L. A. P. Neves (✉)
UFPR—Federal University of Paraná, Rua Dr. Alcides Vieira Arcoverde, 1225, Curitiba, PR 81520-260, Brazil
e-mail: lapneves@gmail.com

G. A. Giraldi
LNCC—National Laboratory for Scientific Computing, Av. Getulio Vargas, 333, Petrópolis, RJ 25651-070, Brazil
e-mail: gilson@lncc.br

J. M. R. S. Tavares and R. M. Natal Jorge (eds.), *Topics in Medical Image Processing and Computational Vision*, Lecture Notes in Computational Vision and Biomechanics 8,
DOI: 10.1007/978-94-007-0726-9_3,

1 Introduction

In the last decades, the spread of web applications has improved the Internet flexibility in accessing computing resources for data processing and storage. These applications are usually formed by three tiers. For [1], the first tier is the Web browser, used to visualize Web pages. In the middle tier are programming languages used to generate dynamic content, like PHP (Hypertext Preprocessor) and ASP (Active Server Pages). The last tier is the database that will store useful information for the Website. The Web browser, in the client side, sends requests to the second tier that will retrieve and insert data into the database.

Web applications are particularly important for manipulating, searching and sharing images over the Internet. In the specific case of medical imaging Web systems have been developed to support collaborative work and information share between members of health care teams. The field of medical imaging analysis had a fast development in the past decades. It is an important tool for diagnosis and planning procedures in almost all areas in the medicine. Besides, and more important for this work, application of computational methods to study complex physiological systems need a cooperative work between research groups which may be geographically and institutionally dispersed. In Brazil, such need motivates the development of the INCT-MACC (National Institute of Science and Technology in Scientific Computing Aided Medicine) (http://macc.lncc.br/), a virtual organization working in the thematic of medicine assisted by scientific computing. In the context of the INCT-MACC, the medical imaging analysis has specific requirements that involve algorithms for processing, feature extraction, classification and image retrieval. Bioinformatic researchers, like the ones in the Brazilian Genome Project, need also services to store, discuss and share detailed images using the Internet. Such services may be implemented through a suitable image manager.

Image Managers, like Morphbank [2], Biology Image Library [3] and JCB Data Viewer [4], to name a few, compose a class of Web applications. Basically, these computer systems include facilities to store, discuss and share images from all over the world which improves scientist collaboration and education activities. In recent works we focused on image managers for medical and biological image databases because there is a lack of Web applications in these areas that allow researchers to share and manipulate images in an environment that integrates data and analysis facilities. We claim that we should consider image managers from an integrated global view of data and processing programs, putting together tools for image storage and manipulation, as well as offering functional ways to share and mining information. In order to fulfill this requirement, the Shared Biological Image Manager (SBIM) has been developed. The system allows users to have great control over the content, giving them the possibility to group images by category, search images by size, format, compression and color channel. It also has a message manager, to allow the communication among researchers.

In this chapter we propose an extension of the SBIM functionalities by incorporating data mining and image retrieval facilities. We propose solutions for both these services through Support Vector Machine (SVM) frameworks. Data mining will be implemented using discriminant weights given by the SVM separating hyperplane to select the most discriminant features for two-class classification problems [5].

For image retrieval, we consider an SVM ensemble based on the "one-against-all" SVM multi-class approach proposed in [6]. The user specifies an initial feature space, the training set and the SVM (ensemble) configuration. After training, the system uses two SVM ensembles: one for dimensionality reduction and another one for classification. Then, given a query image, the system computes reduced feature vector and the second SVM ensemble performs its classification. Finally, the Euclidean distances from the query image to the class images is used as a similarity measure for image retrieval. The SVM configuration and parameters are stored by the system for further instantiations of the framework.

The chapter is organized as follows. The Sect. 2 performs a review in related topics. In Sect. 3 we review the basic elements of SVM model. The discriminant feature analysis (DFA) is presented on Sect. 4. The SVM ensemble framework for image retrieval is discussed on Sect. 5. Section 6 discusses some details about the incorporation of the proposed approaches inside the SBIM system. Finally, we offer some perspectives for this work in Sect. 7.

2 Related Works

In this section we survey image manager systems trying to identify basic requirements and challenges related to user interface, search engines, such as Content-Based Image Retrieval (CBIR) algorithms and processing resources.

In a wide sense, image managers are part of the kernel of any image-based information system. Therefore, Web-based systems for image collections and visualization, Web applications for training and education, CBIR and hospital information systems (HIS) incorporate some kind of image manager in their engines. For instance, the Biology Image Library [3] is basically an online collection of images, movies, illustrations and animations from biology and biomedicine areas including Histology, Pathology, Microbiology, Molecular and Cellular Biology. The library aims to allow users to look for visually striking and scientifically reliable material without tools for image analysis and processing. The JCB Data Viewer [4] is a web-based tool for visualization of multi-dimensional image data files. The system has simple tools for image analysis (zoon, pan, etc.), but its main goal is to handle supplement material associated with manuscripts submitted to the Journal of Cell Biology (JCB). In the same class of systems, we find the Morphbank [2] which is a continuously growing image database focused on increasing knowledge of scientists and students about biodiversity. The images deposited in the Morphbank repositories include data from comparative anatomy, morphological phylogenetics, taxonomy among others.

Nowadays, the traditional medical teaching and training has been complemented with web based education systems. In Guliato et al. [7] it is described a Web teaching system for training the interpretation of mammograms. In this system, users can obtain texts about specific subjects, access bibliographic references and retrieve cases from a database. Also, this system has image processing tools for drawing markings on the image to identify the contour of the breast or the lesson. Afterwards, the contours are submitted to the system and evaluated.

Wangenheim et al. [8] proposes a methodology to interconnect DICOM workstations, allowing real-time meetings over the Internet for discussion about the images. The main goal of that work is to present a collaborative system that enables recording, sharing, and reenacting teleradiological collaborative discussions as well as diagnosis sessions for documentation and teaching purposes. The whole process to create a collaborative section involves its initialization, data exchange and closing procedures. All these steps are implemented through the CycAppDCM [8], an Application Layer Protocol that is layered right on top of the Transmission Control Protocol/Internet Protocol (TCP/IP).

On the other paper, Pires et al. [9] present a Mammographic image manager that is very useful for image diagnostic training by allowing simulated appraisals. CBIR is a class of techniques which uses visual contents (features) to search images from a database following a query image given by the users. Therefore, when designing a CBIR system we must be careful about interfaces to driven the query image definition, utilization of feedback, feature space specification, feature matching and output presentation. Therefore, the application of CBIR for computer-aided diagnosis involves aspects from user interfaces, system design and image processing techniques.

Such complexity is in the heart of the problem described in Welter et al. [10]. This work pointed out that despite of their potential, CBIR techniques have not yet been established in clinical practice due to the lack of an unified data concept integrating CBIR with picture archiving and communication systems (PACS). Therefore, authors suggest that CBIR systems applied to computer-aided diagnosis should integrate their results in a DICOM reporting document. On the other hand, there are many image processing issues to improve CBIR efficiency. For instance, [11] presents a CBIR system with focus on classification of breast tissue density. Texture features are defined using singular value decomposition (SVD) and a support vector machine (SVM) is applied for image retrieval.

The hospital is itself a system in which human beings and machines carry out specific actions following established rules to achieve an integrated care. Therefore, HIS must provide communication and processing information to allow the suitable degree interoperability. In this context, medical image storage, processing and mining become central issues not only due to the huge data volume to be considered but also because image analysis is fundamental for diagnosis and treatment procedures. For instance, Azevedo-Marques et al. [12, 13] describe a system that integrates the radiology information system (RIS) and the PACS of the Radiodiagnosis

Service of the Hospital das Clínicas de Ribeirão Preto (Brazil). The proposed solution has a fast distribution system and friendly interface because it uses Internet technologies, such as HTML (Hypertext Markup Language) and ASP.

Basically, the mentioned systems include resources to store, discuss and share detailed images from all over the web, training and education as well as search engines in an image database. We observe a lack of Web applications in medical and biological image that allow researchers to share and manipulate images in an environment that integrates data and analysis facilities. This is the main motivation for the development of the SBIM system, presented in [14]. Basic services provided by the older version of SBIM are:

- Image storage: Provide a standardized way to store images, allowing easy access to them.
- Image sharing: Allow researchers to share images in the Internet using a Web Browser.
- Algorithms for image analysis: Implement tools to improve the image analysis, like zoom and marking tools.
- Algorithms for image processing: Implement algorithms for digital image processing, aiming to integrate several tools in a single system.
- Communication: Provide ways for researchers to communicate without the need to use tools from outside the proposed system.

The SBIM is developed using portable softwares (PHP, Javascript and PostgreSQL). That is way the compatibility test verifies that the system properly behaves in a variety of operating systems and browsers. SBIM is clearly organized into packages and its classes relying mostly on composition to build new classes which simplifies its maintenance and extensibility.

The goal of this chapter is to propose SVM frameworks to incorporate data mining and image retrieval resources in the SBIM system. The SVM model is the main tool of our proposal, which is based on the discriminant principal component analysis technique and the CBIR methodology proposed in [5, 6], respectively.

3 Support Vector Machines

In [15] we discuss the importance of separating hyperplanes methods for learning algorithms. In this section we will present a special type of separating hyperplanes with optimality properties. So, given a training set:

$$S = \{(y_1, x_1), \ldots, (y_m, x_m)\}, \quad x \in \Re^n, \quad y \in \{-1, 1\}, \tag{1}$$

we say that the subset I for which $y = 1$ and the subset II for which $y = -1$ are separable by the hyperplane:

$$x * \phi = c, \tag{2}$$

if there exists both a unit vector ϕ ($|\phi| = 1$) and a constant c such that the inequalities:

$$x_i * \phi > c, \quad x_i \in I, \tag{3}$$

$$x_j * \phi < c, \quad x_j \in II, \tag{4}$$

hold true ("$*$" denotes the usual inner product in $\Re^m$). Besides, let us define for any unit vector ϕ the two values:

$$c_1(\phi) = \min_{x_i \in I}(x_i * \phi), \tag{5}$$

$$c_2(\phi) = \max_{x_j \in II}(x_j * \phi). \tag{6}$$

Figure 1 represents the dataset and the hyperplanes defined by ϕ and the values c_1, c_2 defined in expressions (5)–(6):

In this figure the points P_1 and P_2 gives the solutions of problems (5)–(6), respectively, and the planes π_1 and π_2 are defined by:

$$x * \phi = c_1, \tag{7}$$

$$x * \phi = c_2. \tag{8}$$

Now, let us consider the plane π, parallel to π_1, π_2, with the property:

$$d_\pi(P_1) = d_\pi(P_2), \tag{9}$$

where $d_\pi(P)$ means the Euclidean distance from a point P to a plane π. This plane is the hyperplane that separates the subsets with maximal margin. Expression (9) can be written as:

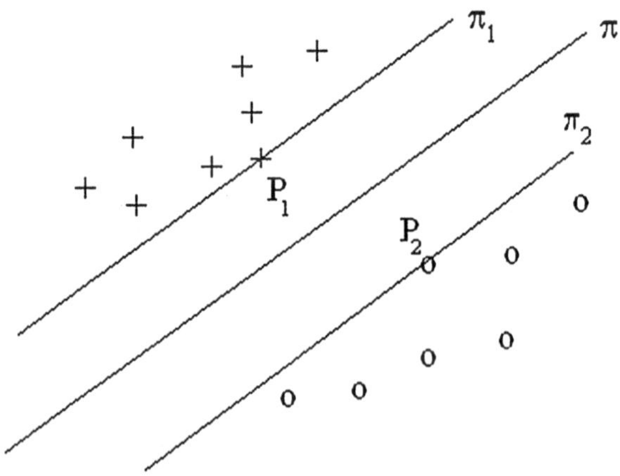

Fig. 1 Separating hyperplane π and its offsets π_1, π_2

$$\left|\frac{P_1 * \phi - c}{|\phi|}\right| = \left|\frac{P_2 * \phi - c}{|\phi|}\right|. \tag{10}$$

If we suppose $P_1 * \phi - c \geq 0$ then we have $P_2 * \phi - c \leq 0$. So, by remembering that $|\phi| = 1$, the expression (10) becomes:

$$(P_1 * \phi - c) + (P_2 * \phi - c) = 0,$$

then, by using expressions (7)–(8) we finally obtain:

$$c = \frac{c_1(\phi) + c_2(\phi)}{2}. \tag{11}$$

Besides, let us call the $d_{\pi_1}(\pi_2)$ the distance between the planes π_1 and π_2, which can be computed through the distance between the point P_1 and the plane π_2, given by:

$$d_{\pi_1}(\pi_2) \equiv d_{\pi_2}(P_1) = \frac{(P_1 * \phi - c_2)}{|\phi|}. \tag{12}$$

By using expression (7), this equation becomes:

$$d_{\pi_1}(\pi_2) = c_1 - c_2. \tag{13}$$

We call the *maximum marging hyperplane* or the *optimal hyperplane* the one, define by the unit vector ϕ_0 that maximizes the function:

$$\rho(\phi) = \frac{c_1(\phi) - c_2(\phi)}{2}, \tag{14}$$

$$|\phi| = 1. \tag{15}$$

The corresponding separating plane π has a constant c given by Eq. (11).

Now let us consider another version of the optimization problem above. Let us consider a vector ψ such that $\psi/|\psi| = \phi$. So, Eqs. (7)–(8) become:

$$x_i * \psi > |\psi|c_1, \quad x_i \in I, \tag{16}$$

$$x_j * \psi < |\psi|c_2, \quad x_j \in II. \tag{17}$$

Let us suppose that there is a constant b_0 such that $|\psi|c_1 \geq 1 - b_0$ and $|\psi|c_2 \leq -1 - b_0$. Then, we can rewrite expressions (16)–(17) as:

$$x_i * \psi + b_0 \geq 1, \quad y_i = 1, \tag{18}$$

$$x_j * \psi + b_0 \leq -1, \quad y_j = -1. \tag{19}$$

To understand the meaning of b_0 it is just a matter of using the fact that the equality in (18) holds true for P_1 and the equality in (19) is true for P_2. Therefore, it is straightforward to show that:

$$b_0 = -|\psi|\left(\frac{c_1(\phi) + c_2(\phi)}{2}\right) = -|\psi|c. \tag{20}$$

So, by substituting this equation in expressions (18)–(19) one obtains:

$$x_i * \phi \geq c + \frac{1}{|\psi|}, \quad y_i = 1, \tag{21}$$

$$x_i * \phi \leq c - \frac{1}{|\psi|}, \quad y_j = -1. \tag{22}$$

These expressions mean that we suppose that we can relax the constant c through the value $(1/|\psi|)$ without loosing the separating property. But, the vector ψ is not an unit one. Therefore the distance (12) can be obtained by:

$$d_{\pi_1}(\pi_2) = \frac{(1 - b_0) - (-b_0 - 1)}{|\psi|} = \frac{2}{|\psi|}. \tag{23}$$

In order to maximize this distance (and also maximize the function $\rho(\phi)$ in Eq. (14)) we must minimize the denominator in expression (23). So, we get an equivalent statement to define the optimal hyperplane: Find a vector ψ_0 and a constant (threshold) b_0 such that they satisfy the constraints:

$$x_i * \psi_0 + b_0 \geq 1, \quad y_i = 1, \tag{24}$$

$$x_j * \psi_0 + b_0 \leq -1, \quad y_j = -1. \tag{25}$$

and the vector ψ_0 has the smallest norm:

$$|\psi| = \psi * \psi. \tag{26}$$

We shall simplify the notation by rewriting the constraints (24)–(25) in the equivalent form:

$$y_i(x_i * \psi_0 + b_0) \geq 1, \quad i = 1, 2, \ldots, m. \tag{27}$$

In order to solve the quadratic optimization problem stated above, it is used in [16] the Kühn-Tucker Theorem, which generalizes the Lagrange multipliers for convex optimization. The corresponding Lagrange function is:

$$L(\psi, b, \alpha) = \frac{1}{2}\psi * \psi - \sum_{i=1}^{m} \alpha_i(y_i((x_i * \psi_0) + b_0) - 1), \tag{28}$$

where α_i are the Lagrange multipliers. Following the usual theory, the minimum points of this functional must satisfy the conditions:

$$\frac{\partial L}{\partial \psi} = \psi - \sum_{i=1}^{m} y_i \alpha_i x_i = 0, \tag{29}$$

$$\frac{\partial L}{\partial b} = \sum_{i=1}^{m} y_i \alpha_i = 0. \tag{30}$$

If we substitute (29) into the functional (28) and take into account the result (30) we finally render the following objective function:

$$W(\alpha) = \sum_{i=1}^{m} \alpha_i - \frac{1}{2} \sum_{i,j=1}^{m} y_i y_j \alpha_i \alpha_j (x_i * x_j). \tag{31}$$

We must maximize this expression in the nonnegative quadrant $\alpha_i \geq 0$, $i = 1, 2, \ldots, m$, under the constraint (30). In [16] it is demonstrate that the desired solution is given by:

$$\psi_0 = \sum_{i=1}^{m} y_i \alpha_i x_i, \tag{32}$$

$$b_0 = \max_{|\phi|=1} \rho(\phi), \tag{33}$$

subject to:

$$\sum_{i=1}^{m} y_i \alpha_i = 0, \tag{34}$$

$$\alpha_i (y_i ((x_i * \psi_0) + b_0) - 1) = 0, \quad i = 1, 2, \ldots, m, \tag{35}$$

$$\alpha_i \geq 0. \tag{36}$$

The expression (35) states the Kuhn-Tucker conditions. By observing these conditions one concludes that the nonzero values of α_i, $i = 1, 2, \ldots, m$, correspond only to the vectors x_i that satisfy the equality:

$$y_i ((x_i * \psi_0) + b_0) = 1. \tag{37}$$

These vectors are the closest to the optimal hyperplane. They are called *support vectors*. The separating hyperplane can be written as:

$$f(x, \alpha_0) = \sum_{i=1}^{m} y_i \alpha_i^0 (x_i * x) + b_0, \tag{38}$$

where α_i^0, $i = 1, 2, \ldots, m$, satisfy the constraints (34)–(36). So, we can construct a decision function that is nonlinear in the input space:

$$f(x, \alpha) = sign\left(\sum_{i=1}^{m} y_i \alpha_i^0 (x_i * x) + b \right), \tag{39}$$

Now we describe two generalizations for the above approach.

3.1 Generalizing the SVMs

According to Vapnik [16], a *support vector machine* implement the following idea: "It maps the input vectors x into a high-dimensional *feature space* Z through some nonlinear mapping, chosen a priori. In the space Z an optimal separating hyperplane is constructed."

The key idea behind this proposal comes from the inner product "$*$" in Eq. (38). Firstly, if we map a vector $x \in \Re^n$ into a Hilbert space Z with coordinates $(z_1, z_2, \ldots)$ we get another representation for the feature space given by:

$$z_1(x), z_2(x), \ldots, z_n(x), \ldots \tag{40}$$

Then, taking the usual inner product in the Hilbert space we get an equivalent representation for the inner product in the $\Re^n$:

$$z^1 * z^2 = \sum_{i=1}^{\infty} a_i z_i^1(x^1) z_i^2(x^2) \Longleftrightarrow K(x^1, x^2), \quad a_i \geq 0, \tag{41}$$

where $K(x^1, x^2)$ is a symmetric function satisfying the condition:

$$\int_C \int_C K(u, v) g(u) g(v) du dv \geq 0,$$

for all $g \in L^2(C)$, C being a compact subset of $\Re^n$. In this case we say that $K(u, v)$ is the kernel that generates the inner product for the feature space.

Therefore, we can generalize expression (39) by using the inner product defined by the kernel K:

$$f(x, \alpha) = sign\left(\sum_{support \quad vectors} y_i \alpha_i^0 K(x_i * x) + b \right), \tag{42}$$

or, equivalently, we can use the linear decision function in the feature space Z:

$$f(x, \alpha) = sign\left[\sum_{support \quad vectors} y_i \alpha_i^0 \left(\sum_{r=1}^{\infty} a_r z_r(x^i) z_r(x) \right) + b \right], \tag{43}$$

These expressions define the SVM method [16, 17]. In summary, SVM seeks to find the hyperplane defined by Eq. (43) which separates positive and negative observations with the maximum margin.

3.2 General Nonseparable Case

Sometimes the subsets may be nonseparables, that means, we can not find a constant b_0 such that conditions (18)–(19) hold true. In this case, one solution is to work with a more convenient optimization problem. Following [16], we will generalize the optimal hyperplane definition by using a linear optimization procedure. We must observe that the heart of the quadratic optimization problem of Sect. 3 is that $\alpha_i \geq 0$, $i = 1, 2, \ldots, m$, and conditions (27), in the sense that they define a separator with good properties. So, we can relax the later constraints by using the following idea.

Minimize the functional:

$$L = \sum_{i=1}^{m} \alpha_i + C \sum_{i=1}^{m} \xi_i, \tag{44}$$

subject to:

$$\alpha_i \geq 0, \quad \xi_i \geq 0, \quad i = 1, 2, \ldots, m, \tag{45}$$

$$y_i((x_i * \psi_0) + b_0) \geq 1 - \xi_i, \quad i = 1, 2, \ldots, m. \tag{46}$$

The constant C is a given value. Besides we can also apply an equivalent technique when using a generalized inner product defined by the kernel K in Eq. (42). In this case, the decision rule has the form given by expression (42). We can solve an optimization problem defined by the minimization of the functional (44) subject to the constraints:

$$\alpha_i \geq 0, \quad \xi_i \geq 0, \quad i = 1, 2, \ldots, m, \tag{47}$$

$$y_i \left(\sum_{j=1}^{m} y_j \alpha_j K\left(x_i * x_j\right) + b \right) \geq 1 - \xi_i. \tag{48}$$

However, we can not guarantee that these SV machines possess all the nice properties of the machines defined on the basis of the optimal hyperplane.

4 Discriminant Features Analysis

Classification is a very relevant task for image analysis. In the field of statistical learning, classification algorithms rely on a feature space and on some procedure to compute a separating hypersurface that cuts the feature space in regions that host the classes of the problem. One fundamental point in this field is to find out an efficient feature space. In general the features are specified by the knowledge of an human expert. However, once a feature space has been defined, a fundamental question is how we can determine the most discriminant features. In [5] it is proposed an approach, here called Discriminant Features Analysis (DFA), to perform this task.

In order to determine the most discriminant features, the technique presented in [5] firstly estimates the separating hyperplane. In this paper we have used the SVM classifier to perform this task. However, any separating hyperplane can be used here.

Once a n-dimensional feature space $\{x_1, x_2, \ldots, x_n\}$ is defined and a training set is selected, we apply the linear SVM framework to calculate the classification hyperplane. Then, since we are assuming only two classes to separate, the initial training set consisting of N measurements on n variables is reduced to a data set consisting of N measurements on only 1 discriminant feature given by:

$$\begin{aligned} y_1 &= x_{11}w_1 + x_{21}w_2 + \cdots + x_{n1}w_n, \\ y_2 &= x_{12}w_1 + x_{22}w_2 + \cdots + x_{n2}w_n, \\ &\ldots \\ y_N &= x_{1N}w_1 + x_{2N}w_2 + \cdots + x_{nN}w_n, \end{aligned} \tag{49}$$

where $[w_1, w_2, \ldots, w_n]^T$ are the weights corresponding to the original features calculated by the SVM approach, and $[x_{1i}, x_{2i}, \ldots, x_{ni}]$, $i = 1, \ldots, N$ are the features of each sample.

Once SVM classifier has been constructed, we can determine the discriminant contribution of each feature by investigating the weights $[w_1, w_2, \ldots, w_n]^T$ of the respective most discriminant directions. Weights that are estimated to be 0 or approximately 0 by the SVM approach have negligible contribution on the discriminant scores y_i described in Eq. (49), indicating that the corresponding features are not significant to separate the sample groups. In contrast, largest weights (in absolute values) indicate that the corresponding features contribute more to the discriminant score and consequently are important to characterise the differences between the groups.

Therefore, we select as the most important features for classification the ones with the highest discriminant weights, that is, $|w_1| \geq |w_2| \geq \cdots \geq |w_n|$. The subset of features with $w_i \neq 0$ are called the *discriminant* ones and the features with the highest weights are the most discriminant ones. Certainly, these highest weights might vary depending on the separating hyperplane used.

In addition to finding the most discriminant features between the groups, such discriminant features analysis highlights how relatively relevant the most characteristic changes are between the groups. That is, assuming that the clouds of the groups follow a multidimensional Gaussian distribution and applying limits to the variance of each cloud, such as standard deviations, we can move along this most discriminant feature and map the result back into the original domain [18]. We can understand this mapping procedure as a way of defining changes that come from "definitely group 1" and "definitely group 2" samples, and consequently investigating differences captured by the classifier that are beyond the average change described by each sample group [15].

5 SVM Ensemble for Image Retrieval

In this section we follow the methodology for image retrieval described in [6] which includes feature extraction, dimensionality reduction, construction of the SVR-based classification model and, finally, the query phase. All these steps are pictured on Fig. 2.

Feature extraction can be implemented by computing geometric, color, or texture features from the images. The simplest possibility is consider each image as a point in a n-dimensional space, where n is the number of pixels of the image. However, such idea is (in general) not efficient due to redundancies as well as invariance problems if the target application is pattern recognition. In order to discard redundancy the Principal Components Analysis (PCA) [19] may be applied to perform dimensionality reduction; that is, to get a low dimensional feature space for data representation. The efficiency of PCA approach depends on image normalizations that can not be applied for the general case.

Therefore, in [6] it is proposed a dimensionality reduction framework based on a "one-against-all" SVM multi-class approach. So, let N be the total number of classes. We firstly construct N support vector machines using the initial feature vectors.

For each SVM model i, we take all k images from class i and label them as 1. Then, using random sampling we choose $(2k)/(N-1)$ images from classes other than i and label them as -1. The obtained set of feature vectors x_m and corresponding labels l_m:

$$S = \{(l_1, x_1), (l_2, x_2), \ldots\}, \quad x_m \in \Re^n, \quad l_m \in \{-1, 1\}, \tag{50}$$

is the training set for SVM model i.

After training, given an image j, we can find the estimated labels y_i^j, $i = 1, 2, \ldots, N$, using the SVM models already constructed:

$$\begin{aligned} y_1^j &= x_{1j}w_1^1 + x_{2j}w_1^2 + \cdots + x_{nj}w_1^n, \\ y_2^j &= x_{1j}w_2^1 + x_{2j}w_2^2 + \cdots + x_{nj}w_2^n, \\ &\cdots \\ y_N^j &= x_{1j}w_N^1 + x_{2j}w_N^2 + \cdots + x_{nj}w_N^n, \end{aligned} \tag{51}$$

Each label y_i^j can be normalized and interpreted as the probability that image j belongs to class i. In [6] it is reported that the vector of estimated labels, computed by expression (51) offers a feature space that increases classification rates and performance. In what follows, we call SVM feature space, or SVM feature vector, the corresponding low dimensional space for data representation. The whole process to compute the SVM feature space is pictured on Fig. 3. Each database image has a feature vector in the initial feature space. The "one-against-all" strategy is used to construct each one of the N SVM models. In the classification

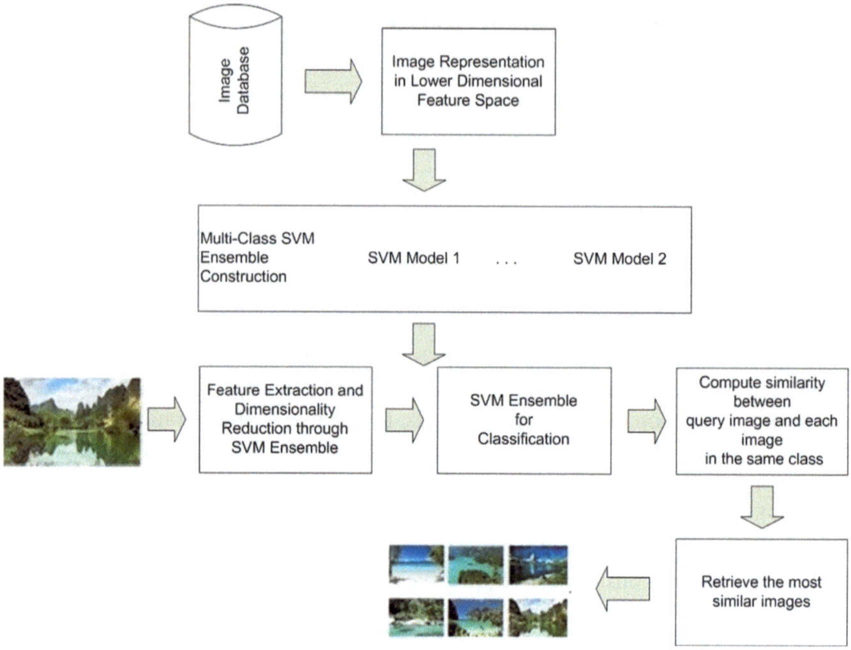

Fig. 2 Overview of the image retrieval process (Adapted from [6])

phase, each SVM model i generates an estimated label y_i^j which compose an entry of the corresponding SVM feature vector.

Using the SVM feature vectors, we construct N new SVM models using the same method described before. Then we find the class label for each database images j according to the highest estimate y_i^j, $i = 1, 2, \ldots, N$ obtained using the new feature space.

In the query phase, we firstly extract the initial feature vector of the query image. Then the SVM feature vector is computed using the SVM models constructed to define the new feature space. Finally, the class of the query image is obtained through the "one-against-all" multi-class strategy. Then it is calculated and sorted the Euclidean distance between the query image and all the images that belong to the same class. Images with the lowest Euclidean distances are considered similar images and returned by the system.

6 SVM Framework Inside SBIM

In order to incorporate data mining and image retrieval facilities in the SBIM system we must consider that, at the set up, both the proposed frameworks need that the user specifies an initial feature space, the training set and the SVM configuration.

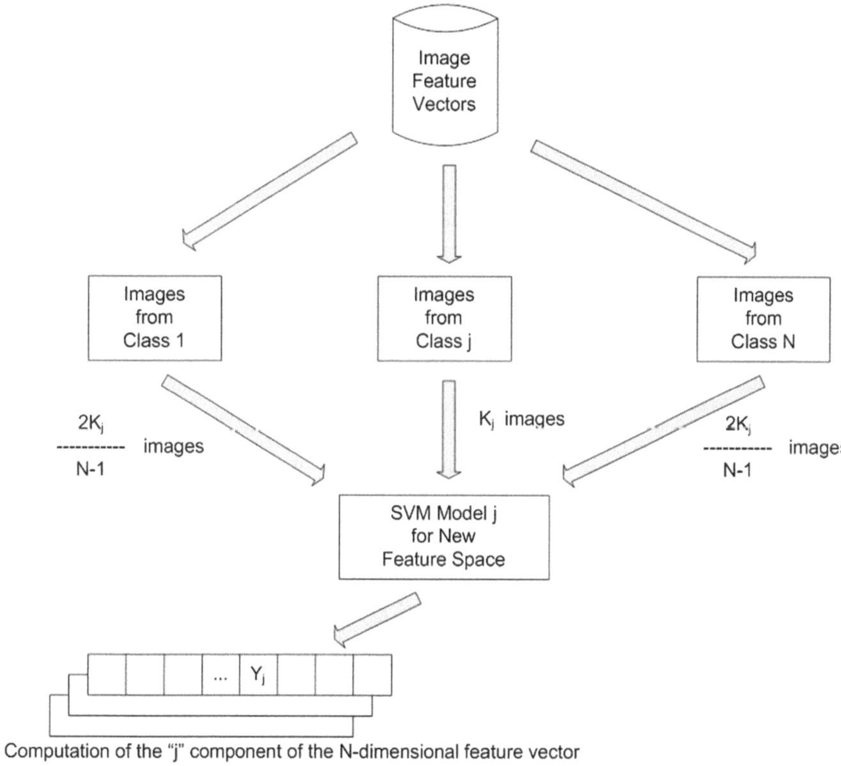

Fig. 3 Construction of the SVM feature space (Adapted from [6])

The feature space definition depends on a library for features computation. This is the main issue of this proposal because there is a huge amount of features commonly used for image analysis.

The methodology to steer the solution for this problem inside SBIM is to consider region-based features; that is, to represent images at the object level. The Fig. 4 shows the flowchart that we are going to follow, proposed in proposed [20], which uses region-based features as input for an image analysis system.

Up to know, dental X-Ray images are the main target of SBIM system due to a project involving the Federal University of Rio de Janeiro. In this context, we have developed segmentation approach based on mathematical morphology, quadtree decomposition for mask generation, thresholding and deformable models [21]. The corresponding pipeline will be incorporated in the SBIM system.

Once performed the segmentation we start the feature extraction stage. Texture features based on moments have been tested in recent works for panoramic X-Ray images. Besides, geometric features based on area and the contour geometry as well as histogram features must be considered [22]. The obtained feature space may be a high dimensional one and full of redundancies. In this case, principal component analysis (PCA) is applied for dimensionality reduction by discarding

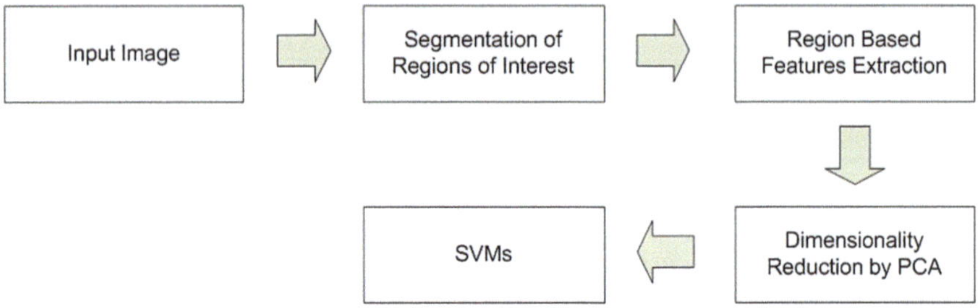

Fig. 4 Feature space and dimensionality reduction by PCA (Adapted from [20])

components with null variances. However, before this step, we must specify a training set.

The user must specify a suitable training set, like in expression (1). Each image of this set will be represented by a feature vector and the corresponding set of vectors (or their PCA transformation) will be used for SVM training. We will use the already implemented SBIM facilities to allow the user to select a set of images for this step.

The SVM configuration must be defined by the user through the Kernel definition (Sect. 3.1) and the specification of the parameter C in expression (44). SVM machines are available in the library LIBSVM (www.csie.ntu.edu.tw/~cjlin/libsvm) which will be used to implement machine learning procedures.

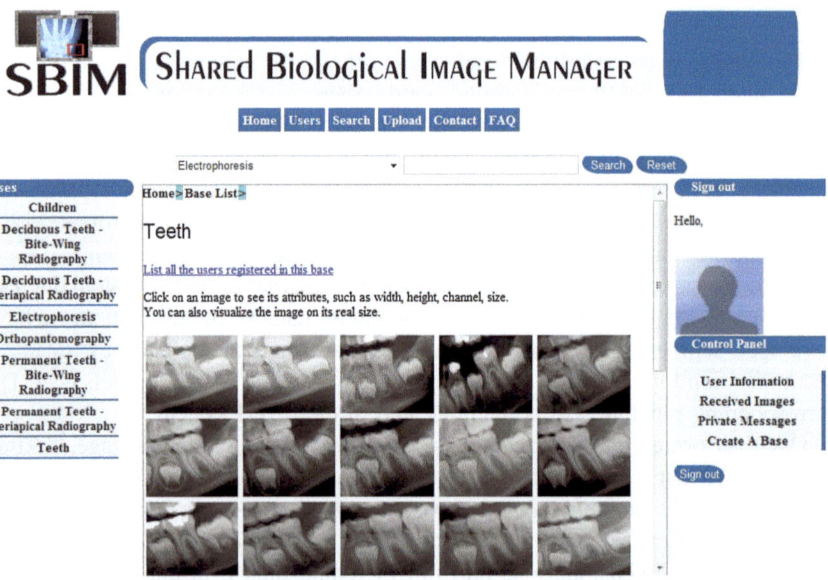

Fig. 5 SBIM overview

Figure 5 shows the current state of SBIM main user interface. Besides the usual information that can be displayed (image information, statistics, etc.) we can also present the output of the CBIR, as well as the query image, and DFA algorithm result by incorporating specific interfaces.

7 Final Comments and Perspectives

The SBIM system provides interactive tools to share and analyze the images stored in its databases. In the actual version, this is implemented through algorithms for zooming, marking and a message system.

This chapter proposes to add CBIR and data mining facilities because it is expected that the system will acquire large numbers of images and it has been very important to retrieve relevant information as well as to mine discriminant features. The DFA selects discriminant features for two-class problems by seeking for the ones that most characterize the differences between the samples of each group, no matter if the distributions of each class are well separated or not. This is an important point that must be explored for multi-class classification problems in the future.

Behind the proposal of this chapter is the idea that we should consider image managers from an integrated global view of data and processing programs, putting together tools for image storage and analysis, as well as offering functional ways to retrieve and mine information. We do believe that SBIM system will achieve this goal with the implementation of the SVM frameworks described.

Acknowledgments We would like to tank Dr. Carlos Eduardo Thomaz, from Department of Electrical Engineering, FEI, Sao Paulo, Brazil, due to the valuable discussions during the preparation of this work.

References

1. Bouchiha B, Malki M, Mostefai A, El K (2008) A framework for reegineering Web applications to Web services. INFOCOMP J Comput Sci 7(1):19–26
2. Morphbank, 2011
3. Biology Image Library, 2011
4. JCB Data Viewer, 2011
5. Thomaz CE, Giraldi GA (2010) A new ranking method for principal components analysis and its application to face image analysis. Image Vis Comput 28(6):902–913
6. Yildizer E, Balci AM, Hassan M, Alhajj R (2012) Efficient content-based image retrieval using multiple support vector machines ensemble. Expert Syst Appl 39:2385–2396
7. Macedo TAA, INDIAM, Guliato D, Bôaventura RS, Maia MA, Rangayyan RM, Simedo MS (2009) An e-learning system for the interpretation of mammograms. J Digit Imaging 22(4):405–420
8. Regert AG, Wangenheim AV, Prüsse M, Maia RS, Abdala DD, Comunello E, Nobre LFS (2009) Recording and reenactment of collaborative diagnosis sessions using DICOM. J Digit Imaging 22(6):605–619

9. Schiabel H, Pires SR, Medeiros RB (2004) Banco de imagens mamográficas para treinamento na interpretação de imagens. Radiol Bras 1(1):239–244
10. Welter P, Riesmeier J, Fischer B, Grouls C, Kuhl C, Deserno T (2011) Bridging the integration gap between imaging and information systems: a uniform data concept for content based image retrieval in computer aided-diagnosis. JAMIA 18(4):506–510
11. Oliveira JEE, Araújo AA, Deserno TM (2011) Content-based image retrieval applied to BI-RADS tissue classification in screening mammography. World J Radiol 3(1):24–31
12. Sanches PR, Azevedo-Marques PM, Caritá EC, Benedicto AA (2005) Implantação de um RIS/PACS no Hospital das Clínicas de Ribeirão Preto: uma solução baseada em Web. Radio Bras, pp 37–43
13. Santos AC, Azevedo-Marques PM, Trad CS, Júnior JE (2001) Implantação de um Mini-PACS (Sistema de Arquivamento e Distribuição de Imagens) em Hospital Universitário. Radiol Bras 1(1):221–224
14. Porcides GM, Neves LAP, Aquino LCM, Giraldi GA (2012) An on-line system for medical and biological image sharing. In: Tavares JMRS, Natal Jorge RM (eds) Computacional vision and medical image processing, pp 23–26. Taylor & Francis, Group, 2012
15. Thomaz CE, Kitani EC, Gillies DF (2006) A maximum uncertainty lda-based approach for limited sample size problems—with application to face recognition. J Brazilian Comput Soc (JBCS) 12(2):7–18
16. Vapnik VN (1998) Statistical learning theory. Wiley, New York
17. Burges CJC (1998) A tutorial on support vector machines for pattern recognition. Data Mining Knowl Discov 2(2):121–167
18. Thomaz CE, Boardman JP, Counsell S, Hill DLG, Hajnal JV, Edwards AD, Rutherford MA, Gillies DF, Rueckert D (2007) A multivariate statistical analysis of the developing human brain in preterm infants. Image Vis Comput 25(6):981–994
19. Fukunaga K (1990) Introduction to statistical patterns recognition, vol 18, no 8. Academic Press, New York, pp 831–836
20. Chang C-Y , Wang H-J, Li C-F (2009) Semantic analysis of real-world images using support vector machine. Expert Syst Appl 36:10560–10569
21. Lira PHM, Giraldi GA, Neves LAP (2009) Panoramic dental X-Ray image segmentation and feature extraction. In: Proceedings of V workshop of computing vision, Sao Paulo, Brazil, 2009
22. Jain AK (1989) Fundamentals of digital image processing. Prentice-Hall, Inc., Upper Saddle River

Identification of Foliar Diseases in Cotton Crop

Alexandre A. Bernardes, Jonathan G. Rogeri, Roberta B. Oliveira, Norian Marranghello, Aledir S. Pereira, Alex F. Araujo and João Manuel R. S. Tavares

Abstract The manifestation of pathogens in plantations is the most important cause of losses in several crops. These usually represent less income to the farmers due to the lower product quality as well as higher prices to the consumer due to the smaller offering of goods. The sooner the disease is identified the sooner one can control it through the use of agrochemicals, avoiding great damages to the plantation. This chapter introduces a method for the automatic classification of cotton diseases based on the feature extraction of foliar symptoms from digital images. The method uses the energy of the wavelet transform for feature extraction and a Support Vector Machine for the actual classification. Five possible diagnostics are provided: (1) healthy (SA), (2) injured with Ramularia disease (RA), (3) infected with Bacterial Blight (BA), (4) infected with Ascochyta Blight (AS), or (5) possibly infected with an unknown disease.

A. A. Bernardes (✉) · J. G. Rogeri · R. B. Oliveira · N. Marranghello · A. S. Pereira
Universidade Estadual Paulista (UNESP)/Instituto de Biociências, Letras e Ciências Exata (IBILCE), São José do Rio Preto, São Paulo, Brazil
e-mail: alexandreber@gmail.com

J. G. Rogeri
e-mail: jonathan@gigafort.com.br

R. B. Oliveira
e-mail: robyoliveira1@gmail.com

N. Marranghello
e-mail: norian@ibilce.unesp.br

A. S. Pereira
e-mail: aledir@ibilce.unesp.br

A. F. Araujo · J. M. R. S. Tavares
Instituto de Engenharia Mecânica e Gestão Industrial, Faculdade de Engenharia, Universidade do Porto, Porto, Portugal
e-mail: fa.alex@gmail.com

J. M. R. S. Tavares
e-mail: tavares@fe.up.pt

J. M. R. S. Tavares and R. M. Natal Jorge (eds.), *Topics in Medical Image Processing and Computational Vision*, Lecture Notes in Computational Vision and Biomechanics 8, DOI: 10.1007/978-94-007-0726-9_4, © Springer Science+Business Media Dordrecht 2013

1 Introduction

The art of growing food is fundamental for the human subsistence. The manifestation of diseases causes many damages, either financial or in terms of the quality of the crops, causing considerable losses if the degree of infestation is high. Several agrochemicals are applied to the plantation in an effort to minimize and control pathogens. However, the agrochemicals are usually harmful to the human health, can increase production costs, and may contaminate water and soil [1].

Aiming at minimizing agrochemicals use, ensuring product quality and minimizing inherent agricultural production problems, computer applications have been developed and revealed high efficacy. The use of computers in agriculture has been subject of several scientific works, many of them focusing on the identification of diseases through foliar symptoms in various cultivars, such as: wheat [1], cotton [2], rice [3–5], apple [6], orchid [7], cucumber [8, 9], rose [10], rubber tree [11], soybean [12, 13], and grape [14].

In this work, we propose the identification of foliar diseases in cotton crop because, being a pillar of textile production, is a cultivar of great economic importance. The Brazilian textile industry consumes around a million tons of cotton fiber a year, which means that cotton is particularly important for the economy, creating thousands of job positions both in the agricultural and industrial sectors of the economy.

The main goal of the computational system developed is to identify from images the existence, or not, of pathogens in a given plantation. If no pathogens are found the plantation is classified as healthy (SA). Otherwise the image under consideration undergoes a second stage of analysis in view of the automatic classification of the disease. The pathogens that are considered in this stage are among the most frequently observed in Brazil; additionally, they usually disseminate rapidly throughout the infected plantation, and can be combatted with the use of specific chemical products. Three diseases within this category can be identified by the developed system: Ramularia (RA), Bacterial Blight (BA), and Ascochyta Blight (AS). If a pathogen is found that cannot be classified as one of these three diseases, the correspondent image is classified as being infected by an unknown disease.

In recent works [15, 16] it was concluded that the decomposition of the image to be classified in color elements, can lead to successfully classification of natural objects. Thus, we used several alternatives of color patterns, such as *RGB* (Red, Green, Blue), *HSV* (Hue, Saturation, Value), *I3a* and *I3b*, as well as the gray levels of the image under analysis in an attempt to improve the distinction of the pathogen classes. The color channels I3a and I3b are obtained by changing the original color standard *I1I2I3* [15]. One of the most widely used solutions to obtain compact feature representations of an input image is by using the energy of its wavelet transform. The result of such wavelet transform is a set of feature vectors that are usually used during the further classification phases. In the proposed method, we use a support vector machine (SVM) properly trained to identify the aforementioned diseases.

1.1 Channels I3a and I3b

Channels RGB and HSV are well known in current literature. However, channels I3a and I3b are not so. They are obtained by following the modifications proposed by Camargo [15] on the color channel *I3* of the model *I1I2I3* defined by Ohta [16], in which each component represents a intensity new and are obtained by the equations:

$$I1 = \left(I_{R(i,j)} + I_{G(i,j)} + I_{B(i,j)}\right)/3, \tag{1}$$

$$I2 = \left(I_{R(i,j)} - I_{B(i,j)}\right)/2, \tag{2}$$

$$I3 = \left(\left(2 \times I_{G(i,j)}\right) \sum I_{R(i,j)} \sum I_{R(i,j)}\right) \Big/ 4, \tag{3}$$

where $I_{R,}$ I_G *and* I_B are channels of an image defined in the color space *RGB*, *i* and *j* represent the coordinates of the Cartesian axes, and their the values are corresponding to the color channels, which can vary between 0 (zero) and 255. Such modifications on the channel are produced in constants *m* and *d* of the equation:

$$I3 = \left(\left(m \times I_{G(i,j)}\right) \sum I_{R(i,j)} \sum I_{B(i,j)}\right) \Big/ d. \tag{4}$$

The changes in the values of the constants *m* and *d* are the channels *I3a* and *I3b*, as defined by Eq. (5) for channel *I3a* and by Eq. (6) for channel *I3b*, respectively. In order to distinguish injured leave areas in several crops, including cotton, $m = 2.5$ has been used for channel *I3a*, and $d = 2$ has been used for channel I3b. These values have been defined by Camargo [15] through experimentation.

$$I3a = \left(\left(2.5 \times I_{G(i,j)}\right) \sum I_{R(i,j)} \sum I_{B(i,j)}\right) \Big/ 4, \tag{5}$$

$$I3b = \left(\left(2 \times I_{G(i,j)}\right) \sum I_{R(i,j)} \sum I_{B(i,j)}\right) \Big/ 2. \tag{6}$$

1.2 Discrete Wavelet Transform

By applying a Discrete Wavelet Transform (DWT) to an input image, such image can be decomposed into four regions, usually known as sub-bands. Figure 1 displays the scheme according to which the regions are organized in the original image after being processed by a DWT. Region *A* tends to cluster the (low-frequency) approximation coefficient of lines and columns of the image; region *DL* corresponds to the clustering of the line details and column approximations; similarly, region *DC* corresponds to the clustering of the line approximations and

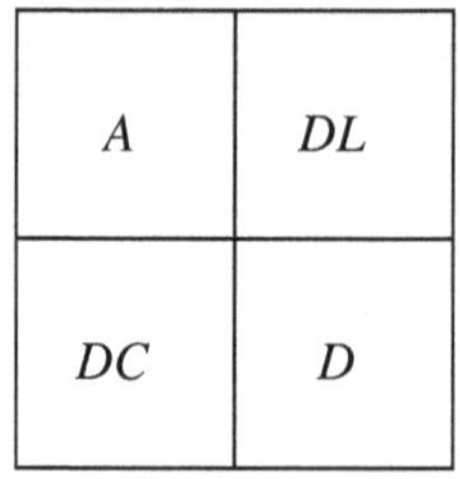

Fig. 1 Wavelet decomposition scheme

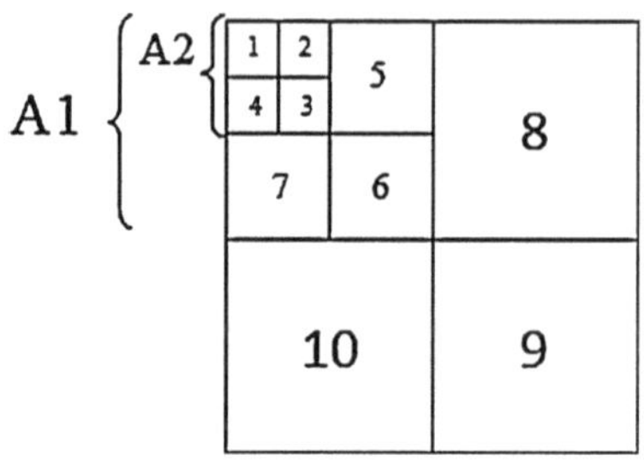

Fig. 2 Wavelet decomposition scheme through the third level

column details; and region *D* clusters (high-frequency) detail coefficients of lines and columns.

Similarly, a 2D image is a bi-dimensional signal to which successive decompositions can be applied. DWT decomposition of an image in three levels is schematically represented in Fig. 2. At the first decomposition level, the sub-bands *A1* (approximation coefficient of lines and columns of the first level—*A*), "8" (line detail coefficients—*DL*), "9" (line and column detail coefficients—*D*), and "10" (column detail coefficients—*DC*) are presented. The second level of decomposition is applied to the approximation coefficient *A1*, which is in turn decomposed into for sub-bands: *A2*(*A*), "*5*" (*DL*), "6" (*D*) e "7" (*DC*). For the third level of decomposition, region *A2* is divided into four other sub-bands: "*1*" (*A*), "2" (*DL*), "*3*" (*D*) e "4" (*DC*). It can be observed that from Fig. 2 the first level decomposition is always done with respect to the region corresponding to the approximation coefficient, and that at each decomposition step four new sub-bands are produced.

In Fig. 3b an example of decomposition of an image after the application of a DWT to the image presented in Fig. 3a is depicted. Region *A* in Fig. 3b shows the sample space corresponding to the approximation coefficients. This is a low resolution version very similar to the original image. In the other regions are shown details coefficients of the lines, in region *DL*, of the columns, in region *DC*, and of lines and columns, in region *D*.

The wavelet energy is a parameter largely used for texture feature extraction that can be computed using the DWT for each decomposed region of input the image. The computation of such energy can be applied to every sub-band of the decomposed image and calculated as:

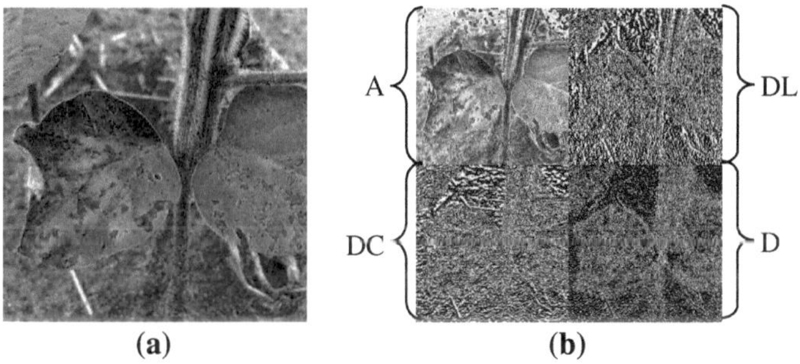

Fig. 3 Example of the decomposition of an original image (**a**) when applying DWT to the first level (**b**)

$$\text{EnergySb} = \sqrt{\frac{1}{N}\sum_{x,y}(Sb(x,y))^2}, \tag{7}$$

where *Sb(x,y)* corresponds to the sub-band coefficient for pixel *(x,y)* and *N* is the total number of pixels in the sub-band.

1.3 Support Vector Machine

For feature classification, the method presented in this work uses an Artificial Intelligence technique largely employed in binary classification, known as Support Vector Machine (SVM). This technique can achieve very interesting performances in several practical applications and, in many cases, performances superior to other learning algorithms such as Artificial Neural Networks [17]. SVMs are mainly used in pattern recognition, image processing, machine learning and bioinformatics [18]. In 1992 Vladimir Vapnik and co-workers [19] developed a strategy to separate nonlinear hyperplanes using kernel functions to modify the entry space of a higher dimensional space in which the data are linearly separable. The most usual kernels to be found in such cases are: linear, Gaussian and polynomial. In this work, the Gaussian kernel was used [17].

SVM machine learning technique is based on the structural risk minimization principle. It aims at minimizing the training set related error so as to control the empirical risk. Thus, avoiding noise to appear in place of the general features expected to provide for generalization, i.e., recognition of classes not included in the initial training of the classifier.

The dividing hyperplane is a surface that splits the feature space into two subspaces. An element is classified as belonging to class −1 if it is closer to the negative margin, and is classified to class +1 if it is closer to the positive margin. Be $\{(\vec{x}_1, y_1); (\vec{x}_2, y_2); \cdots (\vec{x}_n, y_n)\}$ a training vector set belonging to the two linearly separable classes *W1*, defined by the output $y_i = +1$, and *W2*, defined by the output

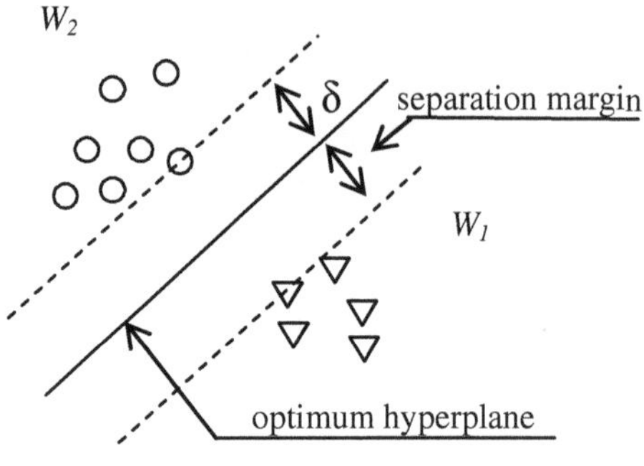

Fig. 4 Linear separation of classes *W1* and *W2* in terms of a hyperplane

$y_i = -1$. The goal of the SVM is to search for the hyperplane with the largest possible separation margin between the vectors of the two classes. This principle is illustrated in Fig. 4, being class *W1* represented by the set of triangles and class *W2* by the set of circles. These two classes are linearly separable by the maximum separation margin δ, defined as the summation of the distances from the hyperplane to the closest class separation point corresponding to the optimum separation. It is worth noting that the vectors defining the limits of the hyperplane are known as support vectors.

There are various possibilities to categorize an element into one of several classes. For instance, if one needs to classify an element into one of two classes, a classification system should be created to embed one net for each class, being each net trained independently. Figure 5 exemplifies this classification process: *R1* is trained as belonging to *class 1*, and net *R2* is trained as belonging to *class 2*. During the classification process, an element is submitted to both nets producing values *n1* from *R1* and *n2* from *R2*. If *n1* is closer to 1 (one) than *n2*, then the element is considered as belonging to *class 1*, otherwise it is sorted to *class 2*. Thus, the element under consideration is always classified as belonging to the class associated to the *n* value which is closer to 1 (one).

2 Materials and Methods

2.1 Materials

420 images of the foliar region of cotton have been obtained from two different sources and combined into one dataset. One set of images was provided by Dr. Nelson Suassuna, phytopathologist, researcher at Embrapa Cotton, in Campina Grande, Brazil [20], and the other set was obtained from the site "Forestry Images" [21] and used to complement Dr. Suassuna's image set.

The images under study are quite different in terms of dimension, bright, contrast and resolution. Such heterogeneity makes hardly the successfully classification of the dataset elements. As an example, in Fig. 6 some images of healthy

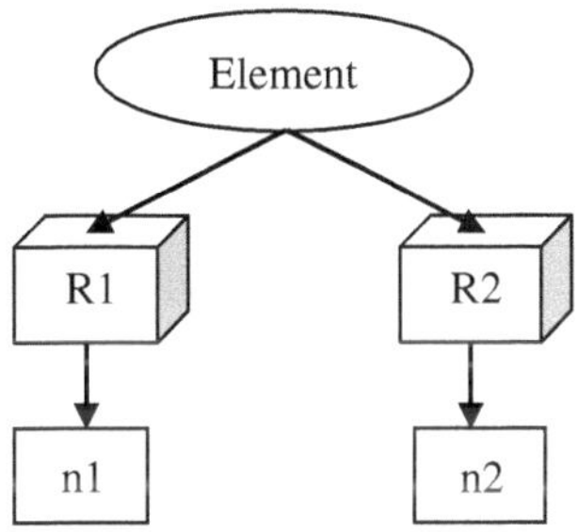

Fig. 5 Example of the SVM classification system using two classes: *R1* corresponds to net 1 trained as class 1 and *R2* corresponds to net 2 trained as class 2; *n1* and *n2* are the values obtained from the classification of the elements of the corresponding nets

regions of cotton leaves are displayed in which the differences among image features can be observed. Besides these discrepancies, the infected leaves present several degrees of severity, as can be observed in the images included in Fig. 7. In Fig. 7a it is shown the foliar region in an initial stage of BA (Bacterial Blight) pathogen infection, which is characterized by wet-like spots with a dark-green color. In Fig. 7b, the infected leaf is presented in an intermediate stage of the disease that is characterized by small brown spots with tinny yellowish regions. In Fig. 7c, the disease can be observed in an advanced stage in which the injured region is brown and yellow and is spread almost all over the leaf.

2.2 Proposed Method

In this section, we describe how the proposed system was implemented to sort the images under analysis into one of five classes. The Bloodshed Dev-C++ integrated development environment, version 4.9.9.2, was used for the implementation of the system in C and C++, while for image processing and analysis the OpenCV, version 1.0 cr, was used.

The classification process was divided into two phases:

Phase 1: Find the best feature vector for each class; and
Phase 2: Produce the final classification from the best results obtained in phase 1.

2.2.1 Phase 1: Find the Best Feature Vectors

The goal of this phase is to find the best feature vector representing each class. In order to achieve it, the following steps were adopted:

(a) The input image is decomposed in various color channels (*R*, *G*, *B*, *H*, *S*, *V*, *I3a*, *I3b*, and grey levels);
(b) Apply the DWT to the third level to each color channel;

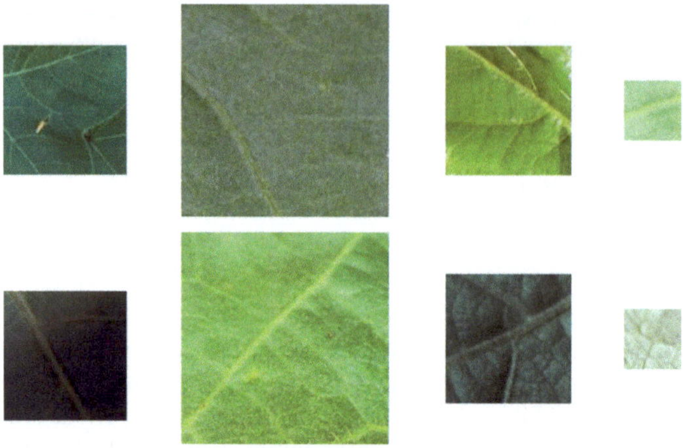

Fig. 6 Some images of healthy foliar regions of cotton leaves

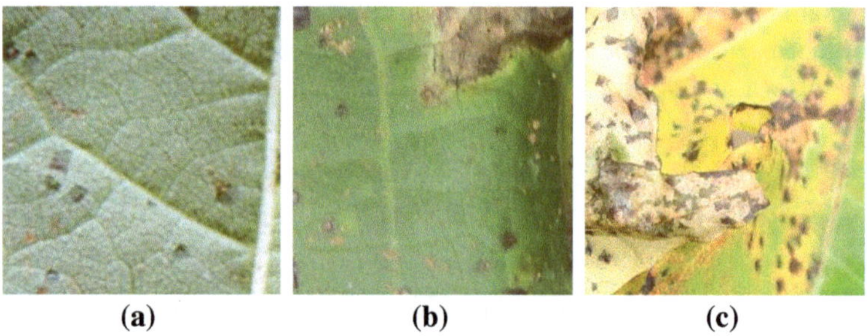

Fig. 7 Degrees of severity of BA disease in cotton crop: initial stage (**a**), intermediate stage (**b**) and advanced stage (**c**)

(c) Compute the wavelet energy for each sub-band and compose the feature vectors;
(d) Develop the SVM classification environment;
(e) Undergo the SVM training and testing;
(f) Select the best feature vectors.

(a) *Image Decomposition*
Image decomposition is the first step of the proposed method. Each image of the data bank is read in the *RGB* color model, and decomposed into the R, G, and B channels. From this decomposition, the input image is transformed to the *HSV* color space, to channels *I3a* and *I3b*, and to grey levels.

(b) *DWT down to the third level*
Decomposition using the DWT to the third level is applied to each of the nine color channels. When an image is decomposed into three levels ten sub-bands are obtained (Fig. 2). It should be noted that each sub-band is identified by a number

Fig. 8 Example of a feature vector used in our system

Feature Vector	1	2	3	4	5	6	7	8	9	10

between 1 (one) and 10. Region *A1* and the sub-bands identified by *8*, *9*, and *10*, are produced by the first level of DWT decomposition. Region *A2* and the sub-bands *5*, *6*, and *7*, correspond to the second level of DWT decomposition. Finally, the third level is composed by sub-bands *1*, *2*, *3*, and *4*, respectively.

(c) *Energy of each sub-band*

The wavelet energy for each sub-band is computed after applying DWT to the third level. The resulting values are inserted into the corresponding feature vector. It can be noted from Fig. 8 that such vectors are composed by ten elements, in each of which the related sub-band energy value is stored. Each vector element is identified by an integer number.

(d) *SVM Classification Environment*

The used net architecture of the system developed is displayed in Fig. 9. From this figure, it can be noted that 10 input elements are used. The corresponding feature vector value is assigned to each input. The intermediate, or hidden, layer presents a number of neurons equal to the number *N* of training examples. This choice for the number of neurons of the hidden layer improves the net convergence characteristics [17]. The chosen net mapping function, known as kernel, has been the Gaussian one.

In order to assess the proposed system, a sub-set of the images (feature vectors) was used in the system training. The remaining set was afterwards used for testing. It is worth noting that during the training phase, there is a corresponding output for each input, known as supervised training approach. The output *1* indicates that the element belongs to a class, and output -1 indicates that the element is not a member of the associated class.

(e) *SVM Training and Testing*

The classification process of the system developed has been divided into two stages:

Stage 1: The leaf image is labeled as healthy (SA) or injured (LE);
Stage 2: Only for injured images that have been associated to one of the three possible pathogens (RA, BA, or AS).

As such, it has been possible to choose the best descriptor, i.e., the feature vector to represent each class.

To find the best descriptor for each class in each stage, twelve different wavelet coefficients were computed for each color channel, resulting in twelve feature vectors. In Table 1 each wavelet coefficient used is indicated and associated to the corresponding support numbers as well as to the abbreviations used, namely:

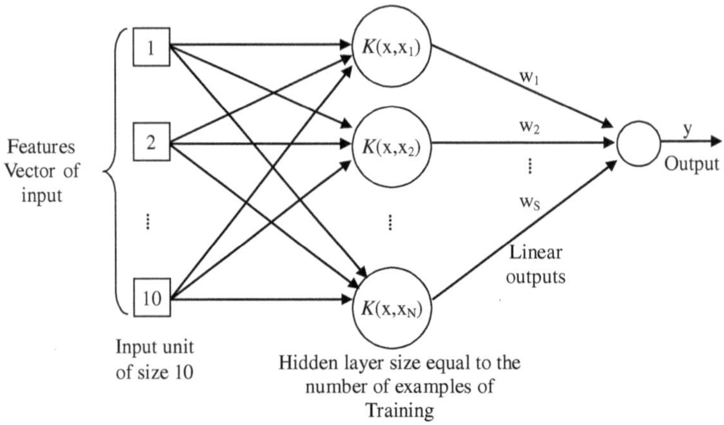

Fig. 9 SVM architecture used in our system

Table 1 Coefficients/support numbers used in the system developed

Coefficient	Support number	Abbreviation
Beylkin	18	*Bey18*
Coiflets	12 e 30	*Coi12 e Coi30*
Daubechies	4, 14, 34, 64 e 74	*Dau4, Dau14, Dau34, Dau64 e Dau74*
Haar	1	*Haar*
Symmlets	8 e 16	*Sym8 e Sym16*
Vaidyanathan	24	*Vai24*

Table 2 Images used as inputs to the SVM sorting system for classes SA and LE

Sorting stage 1			
Images	Healthy (SA)	Injured (LE)	Total
Samples	105	105	210
Test	105	105	210
Total	210	210	420

Bey18, *Coi12*, *Coi30*, *Dau4*, *Dau14*, *Dau34*, *Dau64*, *Dau76*, *Haar*, *Sym8* and *Vai24*.

Stage 1: Sorting between classes SA and LE

For this stage, a two-net SVM sorting system has been developed. One net recognizes class SA and the other one recognizes class LE. In Table 2, the image types used for training and testing during this stage are indicated. A total of 420 images was used, 210 belonging in each class. Half of these images (105) was used for training and the remainder one for testing.

Stage 2: Sorting among classes RA, BA and AS

Table 3 Images used as inputs to the SVM sorting system for classes RA, BA and AS

Sorting stage 2				
Images	RA	BA	AS	Total
Samples	35	35	35	105
Test	35	35	35	105
Total	70	70	70	210

Table 4 Best results achieve for each class

Class	Channel	Coefficient	Percentage of correct guesses (%)
SA	*H*	*Vai24*	96.2
LE	*H*	*Vai24*	100
BA	*I3b*	*Coil2* and *Sym16*	97.1
RA	*H*	*Dau4*	88.6
AS	*H*	*Bey18*	88.6

For this stage, a three-net SVM sorting system was developed. One of the nets is designed to identify class RA, another net to class BA and a remainder one to class AS. The kind of images used for training and testing during this stage are indicated in Table 3. A total of 210 images was used, with 70 belonging to each class (RA, BA, and AS). Within each class, 35 images were used for training and the remainder 35 for testing.

(f) *Best Feature Vectors*
After obtaining 108 feature vectors of classes SA and LE, as well as the hit ratio for the 108 feature vectors within classes RA, BA, and AS, the best feature vectors representing each one of the aforementioned classes were chosen among the best test results, as indicated in Table 4. The associations among classes, channels, coefficients and hit ratios are indicated in this table. The best feature vector to sort between classes SA and LE was the channel *H* using the wavelet *Vai24*. This feature vector reached 96.2 % correct guesses for class AS, and 100 % right guesses for class LE. The best result for class BA was achieved with the channel *I3b* using either the coefficients *Coil2* or *Sym16*, reaching 97.1 % successfully guesses. For class RA, 88.6 % correct guesses were produced using feature vector from the channel *H* with the wavelet *Dau4*. From Table 4, one can also note that the best result for class AS was 88.6 % hit ratio, achieved using channel *H* and the wavelet coefficient Bey18.

2.2.2 Stage 2: Final Sorting System

In the previous section the best descriptors, i.e., the best feature vectors, for each class were identified. In this section, the methodology adopted for composing the final sorting system is described. It was developed using an SVM that combines the best results for each class.

Fig. 10 Architecture of the sorting system developed

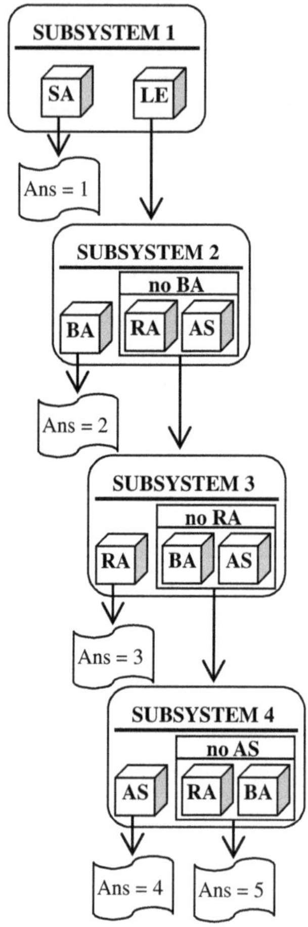

The general sorting scheme adopted is displayed in Fig. 10. It should be noted that four different sorting subsystems were built, each one devoted to the identification of one particular class. The subsystems were trained and tested with the best feature vectors from the corresponding class, as discussed in the previous section. In Fig. 10, *Res* represents the result in the classification of one image, being the number associated to it, the indication of the class to which it corresponds. Thus, *Res1* refers to class SA, *Res2* to class BA, *Res3* to class RA, *Res4* to class AS, and *Res5* represents those images that were not matched with any of the known classes.

Subsystem 1 refers to the SVM classification system that aims at separating the images of healthy leaves from those injured ones. In order to achieve this goal, two nets were built, named SA and LE. Both nets were trained and tested using channel *H* and applying the wavelet *Vai24*. During the tests, the value 1 (one) is output when an image is classified as SA, as shown in Fig. 10 by the arrow connecting the healthy net to the outputted value 1 (one). When the image is classified as LE, it is forward to the classification subsystem 2.

Subsystem 2 refers to SVM classification system aiming at distinguishing the injured leaves affected by BA from the ones not affected by this disease (RA or AS). During the tests, the value 2 is outputted when an image is classified as BA, as shown in Fig. 10 by the arrow connecting the BA net to the outputted value 2. It should be noted that this subsystem is designed to identify images of leave injured by the BA disease. Thus, when the image corresponds to the RA or AS disease is forwarded to the subsystem 3. For this classification procedure, three nets were built, each one trained for one set of feature vectors corresponding to the *BA*, *RA*, and *AS* classes, using the channel *I3a* and applying the wavelet *Coif12*.

Subsystem 3 refers to SVM classification system aiming at distinguishing between the injured leaves affected by RA from those not affected by this disease (BA or AS). Three nets were built to achieve this goal, each of which was trained with the feature vector of corresponding class (RA, BA, and AS), using the channel *H* and applying the wavelet *Dau4*. During the tests, the value 3 is outputted when an image is classified as RA, as shown in Fig. 10 by the arrow connecting the RA net to the outputted value 3. Otherwise, the image is forwarded to the last classification subsystem.

Subsystem 4 refers to the SVM classification system aiming at distinguishing between the injured leaves affected by AS from the one not affected by this disease (BA or RA). Three nets were built to achieve this goal, each of which was trained with the feature vector of corresponding class (RA, BA, and AS), using the channel *H* and applying the wavelet *Bey18*. During the tests, the value 4 is outputted when an image is classified as AS, as shown in Fig. 10 by the arrow connecting the AS net to the outputted value 4. Otherwise, value 5 is outputted, and the image is labeled as belonging to an unknown class.

2.2.3 Test Feature Vectors

After developing the SVM classification system, the feature vector sets were built for the classification tests. The characteristics of these feature vectors are depicted in Fig. 11. They are organized in 210 lines, each one representing an image descriptor. Each descriptor has 10 inputs corresponding to the energy of the ten sub-bands resultant from the wavelet decomposition of the associated image. Note that the vector is associated to 105 images of healthy leaves and to 105 leaves of injured leaves. The injured leaves are clustered according to the BA, RA, and AS pathogens, being 35 images corresponding to each one. Thus, lines 1–105 of the vector set correspond to the class SA, lines 106–140 to the descriptors for the class BA, lines 141–175 to the descriptors of class RA, and lines 176–210 to the descriptors of the class AS.

A set of vectors was generated for each classification system and named as *Vet1*, *Vet2*, *Vet3* and *Vet4*. Details on these vectors are indicated in Table 5, including the associated vector name, the classes to which they belong, the

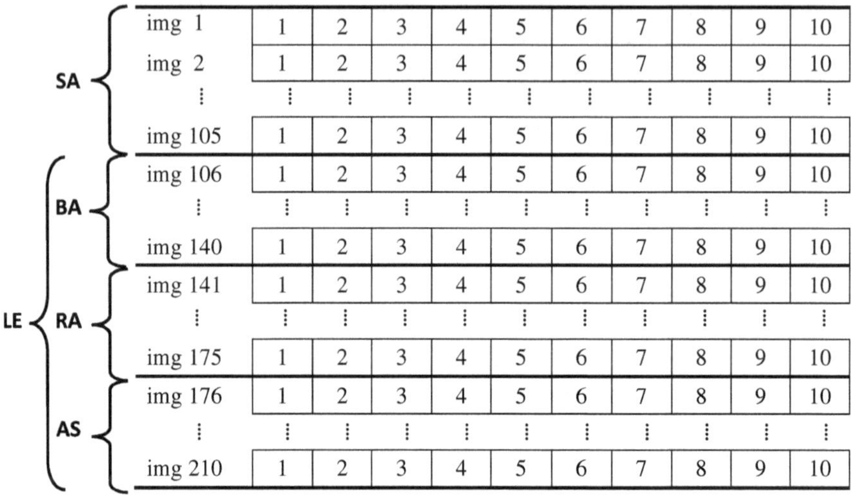

Fig. 11 Arrangement of a feature vector set used during the test phase

channels through which they were obtained, and the designation of the wavelet applied. *Vet1* was used within the scope of SVM classification *subsystem 1* to determine whether the image corresponding to each feature vector is healthy or not. Their descriptors were obtained with the same channel and wavelet as used for the SVM classification *subsystem 1*, meaning that channel *H* and wavelet *Vai24* was used. The other vectors were developed similarly. Thus, *Vet2* was used within the scope of SVM classification *subsystem 2* to determine if the image corresponding to each feature vector is from the BA class. Their descriptors were obtained using the channel *I3b* and the wavelet *Coil2*. *Vet3* on its turn was used within the scope of SVM classification *subsystem 3* to determine if the image corresponding to each feature vector is from the RA class. Their descriptors were obtained using the channel *H* and the wavelet *Dau4*. Finally, *Vet4* was used within the scope of SVM classification *subsystem 4* to determine if the input image corresponding to each feature vector is from the AS class. Their descriptors were obtained using the channel *H* and the wavelet *Bey18*.

The results obtained from the classification of each feature vector through the final classification system in which the output was: 1 (one) whenever the feature vector was considered to be within the class SA, 2 (two) whenever the feature vector was considered to be within the class BA, 3 (three) whenever the feature vector was considered to be within the class RA, 4 (four) whenever the feature vector was considered to be within the class AS, and 5 (five) whenever the feature vector could not be matched to any of the mentioned classes.

Table 5 Description of the feature vectors used

Vector	Classification subsystem	Channel	Coefficient
Vet1	*Subsystem 1*	*H*	*Vai24*
Vet2	*Subsystem 2*	*I3b*	*Coi12*
Vet3	*Subsystem 3*	*H*	*Dau4*
Vet4	*Subsystem 4*	*H*	*Bey18*

Table 6 Test results for the 105 "Healthy" images

SA	False positives			
	BA	RA	AS	None
96.2 %	1.9 %	1.9 %	0.0 %	0.0 %

Table 7 Test results for the 35 "Bacterial Blight" images

BA	False positives			
	SA	RA	AS	None
97.1 %	0.0 %	0.0 %	0.0 %	2.9 %

Table 8 Test results for the 35 "Ramularia" images

RA	False positives			
	SA	BA	AS	None
80.0 %	0.0 %	8.6 %	11.4 %	0.0 %

3 Results and Discussion

From the test set of 210 images, 188 were correctly classified. Therefore, 101 images were found to be within class SA, 34 images were classified as within class BA, 28 images were sorted to class RA, and 25 images were matched to class AS. This result amounts to a total of about 89.5 % of correct guesses.

From a total of 105 images, 101 images were properly classified as belonging to healthy class. Details about the percentage for each diagnostic of the "healthy" images are indicated in Table 6. From this table, it can be noted that 96.2 % of the images were correctly classified. Within the remaining 3.8 % of false positives, 1.9 % were identified as being affected by the Bacterial Blight (BA), and the remainder 1.9 % were identified as affected by the Ramularia (RA) disease. Moreover, any image was classified as being affected by the Ascochyta Blight (AS) disease nor as not belonging to one of the four known classes.

For the Bacterial Blight class, 34 of the 35 images were correctly classified. The percentages of classification for this class are indicated in Table 7, and it can be observed that 97.1 % of the tested images were properly classified, and that 2.9 % were matched to no known disease, being thus false positives. No image was matched to the SA, RA, or AS classes.

Table 9 Test results for the 35 "Ascochyta Blight" images

AS	False positives			
	SA	BA	RA	None
71.4 %	0.0 %	11.4 %	14.3 %	2.9 %

For the Ramularia class, 28 of the 35 input images were correctly classified. The percentages of classification for this class are indicated in Table 8. From this table, it can be realized that 80.0 % of the tested images were properly classified, and that 20.0 % were false positives. Within the set of incorrectly classified images, 8.6 % were considered as belonging to the BA class, and 11.4 % as being of the AS class. No images were classified as being part of the SA class or as being infected with an unknown disease.

For the Ascochyta Blight class, 25 of the 35 input images were correctly classified. The percentages of classification for this class are indicated in Table 9. One can note that 71.4 % of the tested images were properly classified, and that 29.6 % were false positives. In the set of images incorrectly classified, 11.4 % were considered as being part of the BA class, 14.3 % as belonging to the RA class, and 2.9 % as infected with an unknown disease. No images were classified as being of the class SA.

From the SA columns of Tables 7, 8, and 9, it is noted that no image of injured leaf has been classified as healthy. Hence, one can conclude that all 105 images of leaves affected by Bacterial Blight, Ramularia and Ascochyta Blight pathogens were classified as being injured leaves, achieving 100 % correct guesses with respect to the separation of healthy from unhealthy leaves, and therefore, no false negatives were detected. This work concerned the foliar images of cotton crops, a subject that, to the best of the authors' knowledge, is not found in the available literature. Related works considering other crops were found, some of which are described in the following paragraphs.

Haung [7] produced four diagnosis (either as healthy or one of three diseases) for rubber tree crop, achieving 97.2 % correct guesses for injured leaves and an average of 89.6 % of overall right guesses. However, the tests were conducted using only injured leave images.

Abdullah et al. [11] classified pathogens of rubber tree using test images of only one kind of pathogen. Their best reported result was 80 % of correct guesses.

Meunkaewjinda et al. [14] regarded three diagnosis (either healthy or one of two diseases) for grape crop. They used 1478 images for training the net an achieved 86.3 % of correct guesses.

Phadikar and Sil [22] concerned two classification classes (healthy or not) in their study of rice crop and achieved 92 % of correct guesses.

4 Conclusions

The identification of pathogens in crops from their images is very important. However, it is also complex and difficult to achieve, mainly when the available image dataset is heterogeneous, containing images of different dimension, bright, contrast and resolution.

During the present work, a classification system was developed to automatically identify the existence or not of pathogens or foliar organs from images of cotton crops. Whenever no pathogens were found, the images were classified as healthy (SA). Otherwise, one of three pathogens was investigated, namely Ramularia (RA), Bacterial Blight (BA) and Ascochyta Blight (AS). Every time that an image was found not to be healthy and could not be classified as one of the three previously mentioned pathogens, it was classified as being infected by an unknown disease.

The highest difficulty of this work was to attain feature vectors that properly represented each class, because the available image dataset was very heterogeneous, as already mentioned. To solve this problem, the energy of the wavelet transform was computed from each sub-band obtained from the three-level decomposition of the original image. In order to find the best descriptor for each class, 108 feature vectors were built from the input image decomposition in channels *R*, *G*, *B*, *H*, *S*, *V*, *I3A*, *I3B*, and grey levels, using the wavelets *Bey18*, *Coi12*, *Coi30*, *Dau4*, *Dau14*, *Dau34*, *Dau64*, *Dau76*, *Haar*, *Sym8*, *Sym16*, and *Vai24*. These channels and wavelets were chosen for being widely reported as presenting adequate results in several applications [1, 3, 4, 7, 8, 15].

The feature vectors obtained were used for training the classification system. A Support Vector Machine (SVM) was used for classification as this technique has presented better results than other learning algorithms, such as Artificial Neural Networks. Supervised learning was used for training the SVM and a Gaussian function was used in the net mapping.

A total of 216 feature vectors was built, being 108 of which used to identify the best vector to represent the SA and LE classes, and the remainder 108 used to find the best representatives for the BA, RA, and AS classes. The best feature vectors found were then used in the final classification system, in which the classification was achieved in a pipeline, being the original image initially classified as healthy or not, and those found to be unhealthy were then classified as BA, RA, AS, or neither of these classes. As such, the final classification achieved 96.2 % of correct guesses for the SA class, 97.1 % for the BA class, 80 % for the RA class, and 71.4 % for the AS class.

Considering the results of this work and those found in the available literature, it is possible to say that the approach developed appears to be quite promising, particularly taking into account the fact that a reduced number of samples was used in the SVM training. Besides, it can be concluded that the descriptors built properly represent each class, in spite of the heterogeneity of the presented image dataset, as they allowed an encouraging overall average of correct guesses around 89.5 %.

References

1. Moshou D, Bravo C, West J, Wahlena S, Mccartney A, Ramona H (2004) Automatic detection of 'yellow rust' in wheat using reflectance measurements and neural networks; Comput Electron Agric 44(3):173–188
2. Zhang Y-C, Mao H-P, Hu B, Li M-X (2007) Features selection of cotton disease leaves image based on fuzzy feature selection techniques. International conference on wavelet analysis, vol 1, Beijing, China. 2007 pp 124–129
3. Sanyal P, Patel SC (2008) Pattern recognition method to detect two diseases in rice plants. Imaging Sci J 56(6):319–325
4. Anthonys G, Wickramarachchf N (2009) An image recognition system for crop disease identification of paddy fields in Sri Lanka. Fourth international conference on industrial and information systems, ICIIS 2009, Sri Lanka, pp 403–407
5. Otsu N (1979) A threshold selection method from gray-level histograms. IEEE Trans Sys Man Cyber 9:62–66
6. Nakano K (1997) Application of neural networks to the color grading of apples. Faculty of Agriculture, Niigata University, 2-8050 Ikarashi, Niigata 950-21, Japan, vol 18, pp 105–116
7. Huang K (2007) Application of artificial neural network for detecting Phalaenopsis seedling diseases using color and texture features. Comput Electron Agric 57(1):3–11
8. El-Helly M, El-Beltagy S, Rafea A (2004) Image analysis based interface for diagnostic expert systems. In: Proceedings of the winter international symposium on information and communication technologies. ACM International conference proceeding series, Cancun, México, Trinity College Dublin, vol 58, pp 1–6
9. Youwen T, Tianlai L, Yan N (2008) The recognition of cucumber disease based on image processing and support vector machine; Congress on image and signal processing, 2008, vol 2, pp 262–267
10. Boissard P, Martin V, Moisan S (2008) A cognitive vision approach to early pest detection in greenhouse crops. Comput Electron Agric 62(2):81–93
11. Abdullah NE, Rahim AA, Hashim H, Kamal MM (2007) Classification of rubber tree leaf diseases using multilayer perceptron neural network; research and development. SCOReD 5th Student Conference. pp 1–6
12. Cui D, Zhang Q, Li M, Zhao Y, Hartman GL (2009) Detection of soybean rust using a multispectral image sensor, Sens Instrum Food Qual Saf 3(1):49–56, 2009
13. Weizheng S, Yachun W, Zhanliang C, Hongda W (2008) Grading method of leaf spot disease based on image processing. In: Proceedings of the 2008 international conference on computer science and software engineering, CSSE. IEEE Computer Society, Washington, DC, vol 06, pp 491–494
14. Meunkaewjinda A, Kumsawat P, Attakitmongcol K, Srikaew A (2008) Grape leaf disease detection from color imagery using hybrid intelligent system. Electrical Engineering/Electronics, Computer, Telecommunications and Information Technology, vol 1, pp 513–516
15. Camargo A, Smith JS (2009) An image-processing based algorithm to automatically identify plant disease visual symptoms. Biosyst Eng 102(1):9–21
16. Ohta Y, Kanade T, Sakai T (1980) Color information for region segmentation. Computer Graphics and Image Processing. Department of Information Science, Kyoto, Japan, vol 13, no (3), pp 222–241
17. Fonseca E, Guido RC, Scalassara PR, Maciel CD, Pereira JC (2007) *Wavelet* time-frequency analysis and least-squares support vector machine for the identification of voice disorders. Comput Biol Med 37(4) 571–578
18. Yu Z, Wong H, Wen GA (2011) Modified support vector machine and its application to image segmentation. Image Vis Comput 29:29–40
19. Vapnik V (1998) Statistical learning theory, 2nd edn. Springer, New York
20. Suassuna ND (Private Communication) Brazilian Company of Agricultural Research, Campina Grande, PB, Brazil

21. FI Forestry Images (2010) A joint project of the center for invasive species and ecosystem health, USDA forest service and international society of arboriculture. The university of Georgia—Warnell school of forestry and natural resources and college of agricultural and environmental sciences. Available at: http://www.forestryimages.org (Accessed Aug 2010)
22. Phadikar S, Sil J (2008) Rice disease identification using pattern recognition techniques. Proceedings of 11th international conference on computer and information technology (ICCIT 2008), Khulna, Bangladesh, pp 420–423

Towards Ontological Cognitive System

Carles Fernandez, Jordi Gonzàlez, João Manuel R. S. Tavares and F. Xavier Roca

Abstract The increasing ubiquitousness of digital information in our daily lives has positioned video as a favored information vehicle, and given rise to an astonishing generation of social media and surveillance footage. This raises a series of technological demands for automatic video understanding and management, which together with the compromising attentional limitations of human operators, have motivated the research community to guide its steps towards a better attainment of such capabilities. As a result, current trends on cognitive vision promise to recognize complex events and self-adapt to different environments, while managing and integrating several types of knowledge. Future directions suggest to reinforce the multi-modal fusion of information sources and the communication with end-users.

1 Introduction

The revolution of information experienced by the world in the last century, especially emphasized by the household use of computers after the 1970s, has led to what is known today as the society of knowledge. Digital technologies have converted post-modern society into an entity in which networked communication and information management have become crucial for social, political, and economic practices. The major expansion in this sense has been rendered by the global

C. Fernandez · J. Gonzàlez · F. Xavier Roca (✉)
Department of Computer Science and Computer Vision Centre, Edifici O. Universitat Autonoma de Barcelona, 08193 Bellaterra, Spain
e-mail: Xavier.Roca@uab.cat

J. M. R. S. Tavares
Instituto de Engenharia Mecânica e Gestão Industrial, Departamento de Engenharia Mecânica, Faculdade de Engenharia, Universidade do Porto, Rua Dr. Roberto Frias, Porto S/N - 4200-465, Portugal

J. M. R. S. Tavares and R. M. Natal Jorge (eds.), *Topics in Medical Image Processing and Computational Vision*, Lecture Notes in Computational Vision and Biomechanics 8, DOI: 10.1007/978-94-007-0726-9_5, effect of the Internet: since its birth, it has grown into a medium that is uniquely capable of integrating modes of communication and forms of content.

In this context, the assessment of interactive and broadcasting services has spread and generalized in the last decade—e.g., residential access to the Inter-net, video-on-demand technologies—posing video as the privileged information vehicle of our time, and promising a wide variety of applications that aim at its efficient exploitation. Today, the automated analysis of video resources is not tomorrow's duty anymore. The world produces a massive amount of digital video files every passing minute, particularly in the fields of multimedia and surveillance, which open windows of opportunity for smart systems as vast archives of recordings constantly grow.

Automatic content-based video indexing has been requested for digital multimedia databases for the last two decades [1]. This task consists of extracting high-level descriptors that help us to automatically annotate the semantic content in video sequences; the generation of reasonable semantic indexes makes it possible to create powerful engines to search and retrieve video content, which finds immediate applications in many areas: from the efficient access to digital libraries to the preservation and maintenance of digital heritage. Other usages in the multimedia domain would also include virtual commentators, which could describe, analyze, and summarize the development of sport events, for instance.

More recently, the same requirements have applied also to the field of video surveillance. Human operators have attentional limitations that discourage their involvement in a series of tasks that could compromise security or safety. In addition, surveillance systems have strong storage and computer power requirements, deal with continuous 24/7 monitoring, and manage a type of content that is susceptible to be highly compressed. Furthermore, the number of security cameras increases exponentially worldwide on a daily basis, producing huge amounts of video recordings that may require further supervision. The conjunction of these facts establishes a need to automatize the visual recognition of events and content-based forensic analysis on video footage.

We find a wide range of applications coming from the surveillance domain that point to real-life, daily problems: for example, a smart monitoring of elder or disabled people makes it possible to recognize alarming situations, and speed up reactions towards early assistance; road traffic surveillance can be useful to send alerts of congestion or automatically detects accidents or abnormal occurrences; similar usage can be directed to urban planning, optimization of resources for transportation allocations, or detection of abnormality in crowded locations such in airports or lobbies.

Such a vast spectrum of social, cultural, commercial, and technological demands have repeatedly motivated the research community to direct their steps towards a better attainment of video understanding capabilities.

1.1 Collaborative Efforts on Video Event Understanding

A notable amount of European Union (EU) research projects have been recently devoted to the unsupervised analysis of video contents, in order to automatically extract events and behaviors of interest, and interpret them in selected contexts. These projects measure the pulse of the research in this field demonstrate previous

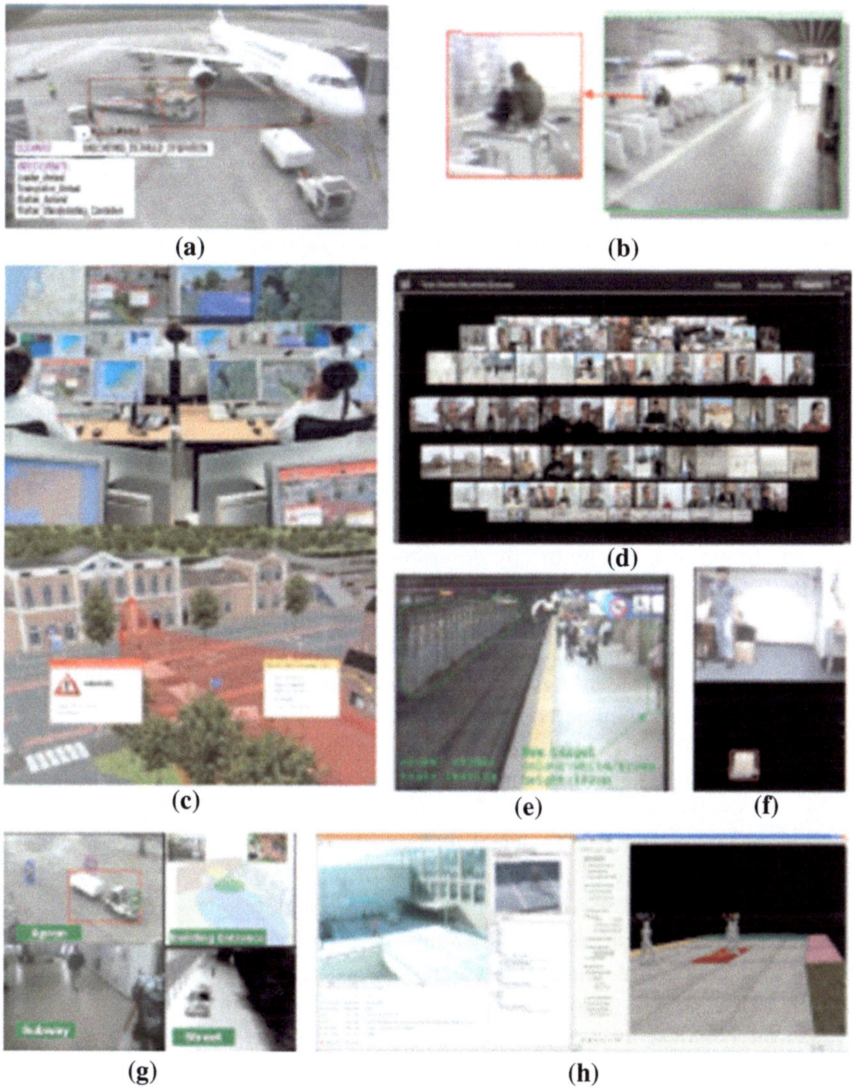

Fig. 1 Snapshots of the referred projects: **a** AVITRACK, **b** ADVISOR, **c** BEWARE, **d** VIDI-Video, **e** CARE-TAKER, **f** ICONS, **g** ETISEO and **h** HERMES

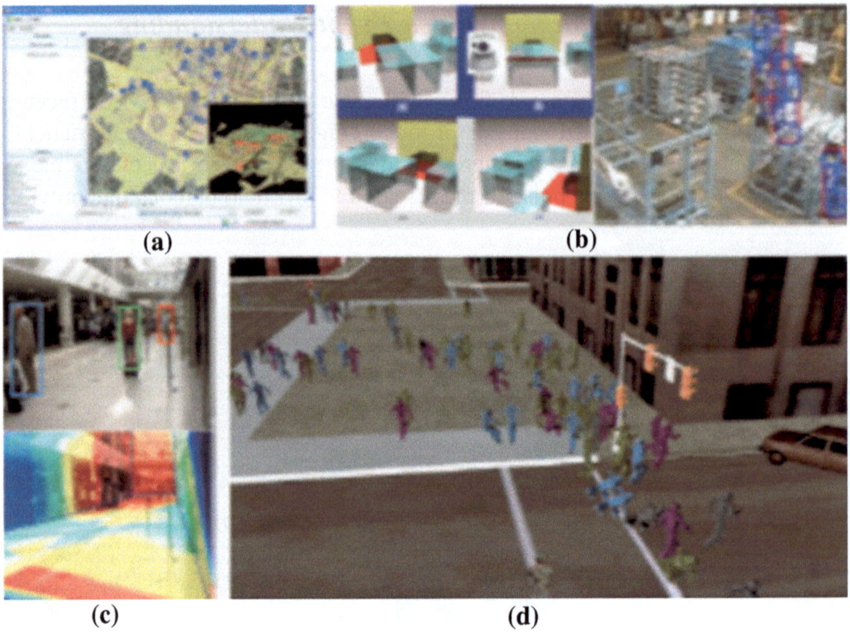

Fig. 2 Snapshots of the most recent projects in the field: **a** SHARE, **b** SCOVIS, **c** SAMURAI and **d** ViCoMo

success on particular initiatives, and propose a series of interesting applications to such techniques. And, last but not least, they motivate the continuation of this line of work. Some of them are briefly described next, and depicted in Figs. 1 and 2.

ADVISOR (IST-11287, 2000–2002): It addresses the development of management systems for networks of metro operators. It uses Closed Circuit Television (CCTV) for computer assisted automatic incident detection, content based annotation of video recordings, behavior pattern analysis of crowds and individuals, and ergonomic human computer inter-faces.

ICONS (DTI/EPSRC LINK, 2001–2003): Its aim is to advance towards (i) zero motion detection, detection of medium- to long-term visual changes in a scene, e.g., deployment of a parcel bomb, theft of a precious item, and (ii) behavior recognition –characterize and detect undesirable behavior in video data, such as thefts or violence, only from the appearance of pixels.

AVITRACK (AST-CT-502818, 2004–2006): It develops a framework for automatically supervision of commercial aircraft servicing operations from the arrival to the departure on an airport's apron. A prototype for scene understanding and simulation of the apron's activity was going to be implemented during the project on Toulouse airport.

ETISEO (Techno-Vision, 2005–2007): It seeks to work out a new structure contributing to an increase in the evaluation of video scene understanding.

ETISEO focuses on the treatment and interpretation of videos involving pedestrians and (or) vehicles, indoors or outdoors, obtained from fixed cameras.

CARETAKER 5 (IST-027231, 2006–2008): This project aims at studying, developing and assessing multimedia knowledge-based content analysis, knowledge extraction components, and metadata management sub-systems in the context of automat-ed situation awareness, diagnosis and decision sup-port.

SHARE 6 (IST-027694, 2006–2008): It offers an information and communication system to support emergency teams during large-scale rescue operations and disaster management, by exploiting multimodal data, as audio, video, texts, graphics, location. It in-corporates domain dependent ontology modules, and allows for video/voice analysis, indexing/retrieval, and multimodal dialogues.

HERMES (IST-027110, 2006–2009): Extraction of descriptions of people's behavior from videos in restricted discourse domains, such as inter-city roads, train stations, or lobbies. The project studies human movements and behaviors at several scales, addressing agents, bodies and faces, and the final communication of meaningful contents to end-users.

BEWARE (EP/E028594/1, 2007–2010): The project aims to analyze and combine data from alarm panels and systems, fence detectors, security cameras, public sources and even police files, to unravel patterns and signal anomalies, e.g., by making comparisons with historical data. BEWARE is self-learning and suggests improvements to optimize security.

VIDI-Video (IST-045547, 2007–2010): Implementation of an audio-visual semantic search engine to enhance access to video, by developing a 1000 element thesaurus to index video content. Several applications have been suggested in surveillance, conferencing, event reconstruction, diaries, and cultural heritage documentaries.

SAMURAI (IST-217899, 2008–2011): It develops an intelligent surveillance system for monitoring of critical public infrastructure sites. It is to fuse data from networked heterogeneous sensors rather than just using CCTV; to develop real-adaptative behavior profiling and abnormality detection, instead of using predefined hard rules; and to take command input from human operators and mobile sensory in-put from patrols, for hybrid context-aware behavior recognition.

SCOVIS (IST-216465, 2007–2013): It aims at automatic behavior detection and visual learning of procedures, in manufacturing and public infrastructures. Its synergistic approach based on complex camera networks also achieves model adaptation and camera network coordination. User's interaction improves behavior detection and guides the modeling process, through high-level feedback mechanisms.

ViCoMo (ITEA2-08009, 2009–2012): This project concerns advanced video interpretation algorithms on video data that are typically acquired with multiple cameras. It is focusing on the construction of realistic context models to improve the decision making of complex vision systems and to produce a faithful and meaningful behavior.

As it can be realized from the aforementioned projects, many efforts have been taken in the last decade, and are still increasing nowadays, in order to tackle the problem of video interpretation and intelligent video content management. It is clear from this selection that current trends on the field suggest a tendency to focus on the multi-modal fusion of different sources of information, and on more powerful communication with end-users. From the large amount of projects existing in the field we derive another conclusion: such a task is not trivial at all, and requires research efforts from many different areas to be joint into collaborative approaches, which success where individual efforts fail.

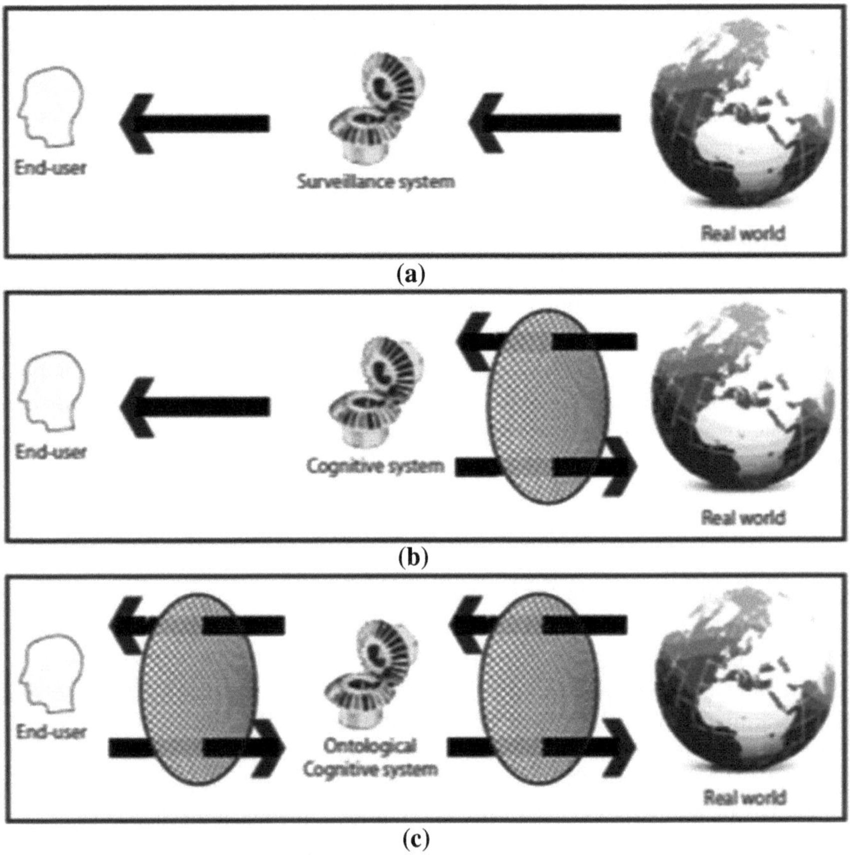

Fig. 3 Evolution of video surveillance systems, since its initial passive architecture (**a**) to the reactive, bidirectional communication scheme offered by cognitive vision systems (**b**), which highlight relevant footage contents. By incorporating ontological and interactive capabilities to this framework (**c**), the system performs like a semantic filter also to the end-users, governing the interactions with them in order to adapt to their interests and maximize the efficiency of the communication

2 Past, Present and Future of Video Surveillance

The field of video surveillance has experienced a remarkable evolution in the last decades, which can help us think of the future characteristics that would be desirable for it. In the traditional video surveillance scheme, the primary goal of the camera system was to present to human operators more and more visual information about monitored environments, see Fig. 3. First-generation systems were completely passive, thus having this information entirely processed by human operators. Nevertheless, a saturation effect appears as the information availability increases, causing a decrease in the level of attention of the operator, who is ultimately responsible of deciding about the surveilled situations.

The following generation of video surveillance systems used digital computing and communications technologies to change the design of the original architecture, customizing it according to the requirements of the end-users. A series of technical advantages allowed them to better satisfy the demands from industry, i.e., higher-resolution cameras, longer retention of recorded video, Digital Video Recorders (DVRs) replaced Video Cassette Recorders (VCRs) and video encoding standards appeared, reduction of costs and size, remote monitoring capabilities provided by network cameras, or more built-in intelligence, among others [2].

The continued increase of machine intelligence has derived into a new generation of smart surveillance systems lately. Recent trends on computer vision and artificial intelligence have deepened into the study of cognitive vision systems, which use visual information to facilitate a series of tasks on sensing, understanding, reaction, and communication, see Fig. 3b. Such systems enable traditional surveillance applications to greatly enhance their functionalities by incorporating methods for:

1. Recognition and categorization of objects, structures, and events.
2. Learning and adaptation to different environments.
3. Representation, memorization, and fusion of various types of knowledge.
4. Automatic control and attention.

As a consequence, the relation of the system with the world and the end-users is enriched by a series of sensors and actuators, e.g., distributions of static and active cameras, enhanced user interfaces; thus, establishing a bidirectional communication flow, and closing loops at a sensing and semantic level. The resulting systems provide a series of novel applications with respect to traditional systems, like automated video commentary and annotation, or image-based search engines. In the last years, European projects, like CogVis or CogViSys, have investigated these and other potential applications of cognitive vision systems, especially concerning video surveillance.

Recently, a paradigm has been specifically proposed for the design of cognitive vision systems aiming to analyze human developments recorded in image sequences. This is known as Human Sequence Evaluation (HSE) [3]. An HSE system is built upon a linear multilevel architecture, in which each module tackles a specific abstraction level. Two consecutive modules hold a bidirectional communication scheme, in order to:

1. generate higher-level descriptions based on lower-level analysis, i.e., bottom-up inference, and
2. support low-level processing with high-level guidance, i.e., top-down reactions. HSE follows as well the aforementioned characteristics of cognitive vision systems.

Nonetheless, although cognitive vision systems conduct a large number of tasks and success in a wide range of applications; in most cases, the resulting prototypes are tailored to specific needs or restricted to definite domains. Hence, current research aims to increase aspects like extensibility, personalization, adaptability, interactivity, and multi-purpose of these systems. In particular, it is becoming of especial importance to stress the role of communication with end-users in the global context, both for the fields of surveillance and multimedia: end-users should be allowed to automatize a series of tasks requiring content-mining, and should be presented the analyzed information in a suitable and efficient manner, see Fig. 3c.

As a result of these considerations, the list of objectives to be tackled and solved by a cognitive vision system has elaborated on the original approach, which aimed at the single—although still ambitious today—task of transducing images to semantics. Nowadays, the user itself has become a piece of the puzzle, and therefore has to be considered a part of the problem.

3 Mind the Gaps

The search and extraction of meaningful information from video sequences are dominated by five major challenges, all of them defined by gaps [4]. These gaps are disagreements between the real data and that one expected, intended, or retrieved by any computer-based process involved in the information flow conducted between the acquisition of data from the real world, and until its final presentation to the end-users. The five gaps are described next; see Fig. 4a.

1. Sensory gap: The gap between an object in the world and the in-formation in an image recording of that scene. All these recordings will be different due to variations in viewpoint, lighting, and other circumstantial conditions.
2. Semantic gap: The lack of coincidence between the information that one can extract from the sensory data and the interpretation that same data has for a user in a given situation. It can be understood as the difference be-tween a visual concept and its linguistic representation.
3. Model gap: The impossibility to theoretically account the amount of notions in the world, due to the limited capacity to learn them
4. Query/context gap: The gap between the specific need for information of an end-user and the possible retrieval solutions manageable by the system.

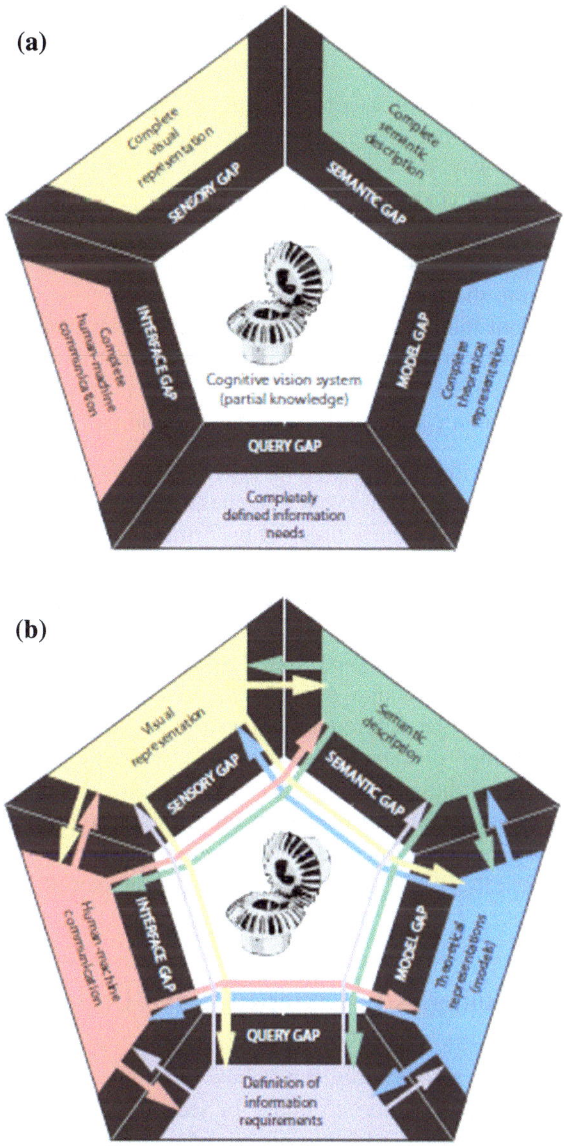

Fig. 4 **a** The five gaps that need to be bridged for the successful analysis, extraction, search, retrieval, and presentation of video content. **b** In some cases, a collaborative and integrative use of different knowledge sources allows us to achieve or enrich the accomplishment of these tasks. (*Arrows* stand for reusing ontological knowledge to enhance analyses in other areas.)

5. Interface gap: The limited scope of information that a system inter-face offers compared to the amount of data actually intended to transmit.

Although each of these challenges becomes certainly difficult to overcome by its own, a proper centralization of information sources and the wise reutilization of knowledge derived from them facilitates the overwhelming task of bridging each of these gaps. There exist multiple examples of how the multiple resources of the system can be redirected to solve problems in a different domain, let us consider three of them:

- From semantic to sensory gap: tracking errors or occlusions at a visual level can be identified by high-level modules that imply semantics oriented to that end. This way, the system can be aware of where and when a target is occluded, and predict its repartition.
- From sensory to interface gap: the reports or responses in user interfaces can become more expressive by adding selected, semantically relevant key-frames from the sensed data.
- From interface to query gap: in case of syntactic ambiguities in a query, e.g., "zoom in on any person in the group that is running", end-users can be asked about their real interests via a dialogue interface: "Did you mean 'the group that is running', or 'the person that is running?'.

Given the varied nature of types of knowledge involved in our intended system, an ontological framework becomes a sensible choice of design: such a framework integrates different sources of in-formation by means of temporal and multi-modal fusion, i.e., horizontal integration, using bottom-up or top-down approaches, i.e., vertical integration, and incorporating prior hierarchical knowledge by means of an extensible ontology.

We propose the use of ontologies to help us integrate, centralize, and relate the different knowledge representations, such as visual, semantic, linguistic, etc., implied by the different modules of the cognitive system. By doing so, the relevant knowledge or capabilities in a specific area can be used to enhance the performance of the system in other distinct areas, as represented in Fig. 4b. Ontologies will enable us to formalize, account, and redirect the semantic assets of the system in a given situation, and exploit them to empower the aforementioned capabilities, especially targeting the possibilities of interaction with end-users.

4 Ontologies to Enhance Video Understanding

It has been repeatedly stated how ontologies can be used effectively for relating semantic descriptors to image or video content, or at least use them to represent and fuse structured prior information from different sources towards that end [5]. Sever-al classical methods from artificial intelligence to represent or match ontological knowledge—e.g., Description Logics (DL), frame-based representations, semantic networks—are becoming popular again since the start of the Semantic Web initiative [6, 7]. Nevertheless, the challenge today is how to apply these approaches to highly ambiguous or uncertain information, like that coming from language and vision, respectively. For this reason, the incorporation of ontologies into cognitive vision systems has also awakened the interests of many researchers in the field [8, 9]. The use of DL to model uncertainty has been long discussed; an overview of the research in this field is presented in [10].

In the case of video surveillance, ontologies have been used to assist to the recognition of video events. Several authors have engaged initiatives to standardize taxonomies of video events, e.g., [11] proposed a formal language to describe event ontologies, VERL, and a markup language, VEML, to annotate instances of ontological events. The use of this language is exemplified in videos from the security and meeting domains. In [12] the authors present an ontology of eventive verbs for multimodal storytelling system including visual and linguistic concepts.

Regarding the field of multimedia, the automatic processing of multimedia content has been enhanced by the apparition of new multimedia standards, such as MPEG-7, which provide basic functionalities in order to manipulate and transmit objects and metadata, and measure similarity in images or video based on visual criteria. However, most of the se-mantic content of video data is out of the scope of these standards. In these cases, ontologies are often used to extend standardized multimedia annotation by means of concept hierarchies [13, 14], and also to provide meaningful query languages—e.g., RDQL or SWRL– as tools to build, annotate, integrate, and learn ontological information. An overview of such languages is presented in [15]. There have been efforts towards the generation of textual representations and summaries from ontologies [16, 17]. In fact, these approaches are general-purpose ontology verbalizers, agnostic of the class types and their properties, which result in outputs that are in general too verbose and redundant. Our contribution adapts the textual descriptions and summaries to the type of content described, regarding its organization into the modeled domain ontology.

Ontology-based approaches are also suitable for designing processes to query, report, or mine data from distributed and heterogeneous sources. These capabilities derive a series of tasks that are usually requested in the domain of multimedia semantics, such as automatic video annotation to enable query-based video retrieval. In [18] the authors have recently presented an ontology-based framework for semantic video annotation based on the learning of spatio-temporal rules. First Order Inductive Learner (FOIL) is adapted to learn rule patterns that have been then validated on some TRECVID video events. Similarly, other approaches emphasize the use of ontologies to enable forensic applications in video surveillance [19].

The understanding of linguistic events has also been approached with ontologies. For instance, [20] presented an ontology-driven approach that, based on Discourse Representation Theory from linguistics, computes conceptual relations between events extracted form a text and a referring expression representing some other event, a state or an entity. Recent large-scale endeavors like the Virtual Human Project [21] propose a complete architecture for virtual humans, including NL capabilities for generation and under-standing, speech recognition and text-to-speech synthesis, task reasoning, behavior blending, and virtual environment generation. An ontological design was chosen for flexibility and extensibility, and to deal with the many multimodal representations of knowledge considered. This work stresses the importance of ontologies especially when relating language and concepts.

5 Conclusions

Human Sequence Evaluation (HSE) concentrates on how to extract descriptions of human behaviour from videos in a restricted discourse domain, such as (i) pedestrians crossing inner-city roads where pedestrians appear approaching or waiting at stops of busses or trams, and (ii) humans in indoor worlds like an airport hall, a train station, or a lobby. These discourse domains allow exploring a coherent evaluation of human movements and facial expressions across a wide variation of scale. This general approach lends itself to various cognitive surveillance scenarios at varying degrees of resolution: from wide-field-of-view multiple-agent scenes, through to more specific inferences of emotional state that could be elicited from high resolution imagery of faces. The true challenge of the HERMES project will consist in the development of a system facility, which starts with basic knowledge about pedestrian behaviour in the chosen discourse domain, but could cluster evaluation results into semantically meaningful subsets of behaviours. The envisaged system will comprise an internal logic-based representation, which enables it to comment each individual subset, giving natural language explanations of why the system has created the subset in question.

Multiple issues will be contemplated to perform HSE, such as detection and localization; tracking; classification; prediction; concept formation and visualization; communication and expression, etc. And this is reflected in the literature: a huge number of papers confront some of the levels, but rarely all of them. Summarizing, agent motion will allow HSE to infer behavior descriptions. The term behaviour will refer to one or several actions, which acquire a meaning in a particular context.

Body motion will allow HSE to describe action descriptions. We define an action as a motion pattern, which represents the style of variation of a body posture during a predefined interval of time. Therefore, body motion will be used to recognize style parameters, such as age, gender, handicapped and identification.

Lastly, face motion will lead to emotion descriptions. The emotional characteristics of facial expressions will allow HSE to confront personality modeling, which would enable us to carry out multiple studies and researches on advanced human-computer interfaces.

So these issues will require, additionally, assessing how, and by which means, the knowledge of context and a plausible hypothesis about he internal state of the agent may influence and support the interpretation processes.

Acknowledgments The authors wish to acknowledge the support of the Spanish Research Programs Consolider-Ingenio 2010: MIPRCV (CSD200700018); Avanza I + D Di-CoMa (TSI-020400-2011-55); along with the Spanish projects TIN2009-14501-C02-01 and TIN2009-14501-C02-02; MICIN the A.I. PT2009-0023.

References

1. Foresti GL, Marcenaro L, Regazzoni CS (2002) Automatic detection and indexing of video-event shots for surveillance applications. IEEE Trans Multimedia 4(4):459–471
2. Nilsson F (2009) Intelligent network video: understanding modern video surveillance systems. CRC Press, Boca Raton
3. Gonzàlez J, Rowe D, Varona J, Roca X (2009) Understanding dynamic scenes based on human sequence evaluation. Image Vis Comput 27(10):1433–1444
4. Smeulders AWM, Worring M, Santini S, Gupta A, Jain R (2000) Contentbased image retrieval at the end of the early years. IEEE Trans Pattern Anal Mach Intell 22(12):1349–1380
5. Town C (2006) Ontological inference for image and video analysis. Mach Vis Appl 17(2):94–115
6. Kompatsiaris Y, Hobson P (2008) Semantic multimedia and ontologies: theory and applications. Springer, Heidelberg
7. Baader F, Calvanese D, McGuiness D, Nardı D, Patel-Schneider P (2003) The Description Logic handbook. Cambridge University Press, Cambridge
8. Maillot N, Thonnat M, Boucher A (2004) Towards ontology-based cognitive vision. Mach Vis Appl 16(1):33–40
9. Staab S, Studer R (2004) Handbook on ontologies. Springer, Heidelberg
10. Nevatia R, Hobbs J, Bolles B (2004) An ontology for video event representation. In: Proceedings of the international workshop on Detection and Recognition of Events in Video
11. Ma M, Mc Kevitt P (2004) Visual semantics and ontology of eventive verbs. In: Proceeding of the 1st international joint conference on natural language processing, pp. 278–285
12. Troncy R, Celma O, Little S, Garcıa R, Tsinaraki C (2007) Mpeg-7 based multimedia ontologies: interoperability support or interoperability issue. In: 1st international workshop on multimedia annotation and retrieval enabled by Shared Ontologies, pp. 2–15
13. Jaimes A, Chang S (2000) A conceptual framework for indexing visual information at multiple levels. In: Proceedings of the IS&T SPIE internet imaging
14. Zhang Z, Miller JA (2005) Ontology query languages for the semantic web: A performance evaluation. J Web Semant
15. Bontcheva K (2005) Generating tailored textual summaries from ontologies. In: Proceeding of the extended Semantic Web: Research and ApplicationsLecture Notes in Computer Science 3532, pp. 531–545
16. Wilcock G (2003) Talking OWLs: towards an ontology verbalizer. In Proceeding of the international semantic web conference
17. Bertini M, Del Bimbo A, Serra G (2008) Learning rules for semantic video event annotation. In: Proceedings of the international conference on visual information systems (VISUAL)
18. Vadakkeveedu K, Xu P, Fernandes R, Mayer RJ (2007) A content based video retrieval method for surveillance and forensic applications. In: Proceedings of SPIE, vol 6560, p. 656004
19. Cimiano P, Reyle U, Saric J (2005) Ontology driven discourse analysis for information extraction. Data Knowl Eng J 55:59–83
20. Hartholt A, Russ T, Traum D, Hovy E, Robinson S (2008) A common ground for virtual humans: using an ontology in a natural language oriented virtual human architecture. In: Language Resources and Evaluation Conference (LREC)
21. Baader F, Calvanese D, McGuinness DL, Patel-Schneider P, Nardi D (2003) The description logic handbook: theory, implementation, and applications. Cambridge University Press, Cambridge

A Novel Edge Detector Based on Discrete t-norms for Noisy Images

M. González-Hidalgo, S. Massanet and A. Mir

Abstract Image edge detection is one of the more fashionable topics in image processing and it is an important preprocessing step in many image processing techniques since its performance is crucial for the results obtained by subsequent higher-level processes. In this paper, an edge detection algorithm for noisy images, corrupted with salt and pepper noise, using a fuzzy morphology based on discrete t-norms is proposed. It is shown that this algorithm is robust when it is applied to different types of noisy images. The obtained results are objectively compared with other well-known morphological algorithms such as the ones based on the Łukasiewicz t-norm, representable and idempotent uninorms and the classical umbra approach. This comparison is addressed using some different objective measures for edge detection, such as Pratt's figure of merit, the ρ-coefficient, and noise removal like the structural similarity index and the fuzzy DI-subsethood measure. The filtered results and the edge images obtained with our approach improve the values obtained by the other approaches.

1 Introduction

Edge detection is a fundamental low-level image processing operation, which is essential to carry out several higher level operations such as image segmentation, computer vision, motion and feature analysis and recognition. Its performance is

M. González-Hidalgo (✉) · S. Massanet · A. Mir
Department of Mathematics and Computer Science, University of the Balearic Islands, 07122 Palma de Mallorca, Spain
e-mail: manuel.gonzalez@uib.es

S. Massanet
e-mail: s.massanet@uib.es

A. Mir
e-mail: arnau.mir@uib.es

J. M. R. S. Tavares and R. M. Natal Jorge (eds.), *Topics in Medical Image Processing and Computational Vision*, Lecture Notes in Computational Vision and Biomechanics 8,
DOI: 10.1007/978-94-007-0726-9_6,

crucial for the final results of the image processing techniques. A lot of edge detection algorithms have been developed over the last decades. These different approaches vary from the classical ones [18] based on a set of convolution masks, to the new techniques based on fuzzy sets [3].

The fuzzy mathematical morphology is a generalization of the binary morphology [19] using techniques of fuzzy sets (see [1, 16]). Mathematical morphology, either crisp or fuzzy, provides an alternative approach to image processing based on the shape concept represented by the so-called structuring element (see [19]). The fuzzy operators used to build a fuzzy morphology are conjunctions (usually t-norms, or recently conjunctive uninorms in [11]) and implications. As gray-scale images are not represented in practice as functions of $\mathbb{R}^{\ltimes}$ into $[0, 1]$ but as discrete functions, discrete fuzzy operators can also be used. In [7] and [8], the discrete t-norms and their residual implications which have to be used as conjunctions and implications in order to generate a "good" morphology, i.e., a morphology which satisfies the usually required algebraic properties, were fully determined.

Among the techniques used for edge detection, several have been designed based on residuals and morphological gradients obtained from the crisp or fuzzy mathematical morphology. See for example, [10] and [13] and references therein. All these works show that the morphological gradients remain relevant and useful in the analysis and image processing. In this work the feasibility of alternate filters will be studied, from opening and closing of the fuzzy morphology based on discrete t-norms (studied in detail in [8]). There, the authors used the alternate filters to reduce the noise and here we will use them in the design of an edge detection algorithm for noisy images reaching a compromise between elimination and smoothing of noise and the detection of the features of the images. In this work, we study the performance of this algorithm in presence of salt and pepper noise. Moreover, the behaviour of this algorithm is investigated depending on the amount of noise in the images. Some different objective measures are used to evaluate the filtered results, the recently defined Structural Similarity Index Measurement (SSIM) (see [20]) and the fuzzy DI-subsethood measure $EQ_{\sigma DI}$ (see [4]). In addition, Pratt's figure of merit [18] and the ρ-coefficient [12] are used as performance measures to evaluate the obtained edge images . It can be noticed that the discrete approach outperforms the other considered fuzzy morphological approaches.

2 Preliminaries

We will suppose the reader to be familiar with the basic definitions and properties of the fuzzy discrete logical operators that will be used in this work, specially those related to discrete t-norms and discrete residual implications (see [15]). From now on, the following notation will be used: $L = \{0, \ldots, n\}$ a finite chain, I will denote a discrete implication, C a discrete conjunction, N_C the only strong negation on L

which is given by $N_C(x) = n - x$ for all $x \in L$, T a discrete t-norm, I_T its residual implication, A a gray-scale image and B a gray-level structuring element that takes values on L.

Definition 1 The *fuzzy discrete dilation* $D_C(A,B)$ and *the fuzzy discrete erosion* $E_I(A,B)$ of A by B are the gray-scale images defined as

$$\begin{aligned} D_C(A,B)(y) &= \max_x C(B(x-y), A(x)), \\ E_I(A,B)(y) &= \min_x I(B(x-y), A(x)). \end{aligned}$$

Definition 2 The *fuzzy discrete closing* $C_{C,I}(A,B)$ and the *fuzzy discrete opening* $O_{C,I}(A,B)$ of A by B are the gray-scale images defined as

$$\begin{aligned} C_{C,I}(A,B)(y) &= E_I(D_C(A,B), \hat{B})(y), \\ O_{C,I}(A,B)(y) &= D_C(E_I(A,B), \hat{B})(y). \end{aligned}$$

Note that the reflection $\hat{B}$ of a N-dimensional fuzzy set B is defined by $\hat{B}(x) = B(-x)$, for all $x \in \mathbb{Z}^{\mathbb{N}}$.

Obviously a discrete t-norm is a conjunction. Thus, these operators and their residual implications can be used to define fuzzy discrete morphological operators using the previous definitions. In [7] and [8], the discrete t-norms that have to be used in order to preserve the morphological and algebraic properties that are satisfied by the classical morphological operators were fully determined. Among these properties, we highlight the following ones:

- The fuzzy dilation D_T is increasing in both arguments, the fuzzy erosion E_{I_T} is increasing in their first argument and decreasing in their second one, the fuzzy closing C_{T,I_T} and the fuzzy opening O_{T,I_T} are both increasing in their first argument.
- If $B(0) = n$ the fuzzy dilation is extensive and the fuzzy erosion is anti-extensive $E_{I_T}(A,B) \subseteq A \subseteq D_T(A,B)$. The fuzzy closing is extensive and the fuzzy opening is anti-extensive: $O_{T,I_T}(A,B) \subseteq A \subseteq C_{T,I_T}(A,B)$. Moreover, the fuzzy closing and the fuzzy opening are idempotent, i.e.,$C_{T,I_T}(C_{T,I_T}(A,B),B) = C_{T,I_T}(A,B)$, and $O_{T,I_T}(O_{T,I_T}(A,B),B) = O_{T,I_T}(A,B)$.
- Among other discrete t-norms, the nilpotent minimum that is given by

$$T_{nM}(x,y) = \begin{cases} 0 & \text{if } x+y \leq n, \\ \min\{x,y\} & \text{otherwise}, \end{cases}$$

guarantees also the duality between fuzzy morphological operators.

3 The Proposed Edge Detector Algorithm

The main goal of this work is to develop an algorithm which can detect and preserve, in presence of noise, edges in images. We will use a residual operator from fuzzy opening and closing operations in order to detect edge images and, at the same time, denoise the image. Recall that a residual operator of two morphological operations or transformations is their difference. In previous works, [7] and [8], the performance of fuzzy gradients and top-hat transformations based on discrete t-norms in order to detect edges in natural images was presented.

From the algebraic properties of the fuzzy morphology based on discrete t-norms, we can define four idempotent and increasing filters, called *alternate filters*, through combinations of the closing and opening operators (see [8]). One of them is the following one

$$F(A,B_1) = C_{T,I_T}(O_{T,I_T}(C_{T,I_T}(A,B_1),B_1),B_1),$$

where B_1 is any structuring element. Consider now another structuring element B_2 satisfying $B_2(0) = n$. Using this structuring element, the following property holds

$$E_{I_T}(F(A,B_1),B_2) \subseteq F(A,B_1) \subseteq D_T(F(A,B_1),B_2).$$

Thus we can compute the next residual operator

$$\delta^{1+}_{T,I_T}(A,B_1,B_2) = D_T(F(A,B_1),B_2) \setminus E_{I_T}(F(A,B_1),B_2). \tag{1}$$

In Eq. (1), the alternate filter and the so-called *symmetrical fuzzy gradient* are involved. The alternate filters are used to remove and to smooth noise in [8]. So, the proposed algorithm is the following one: first, we pre-process the image by an alternate filter in order to filter the noise and smooth the image, and then we apply a fuzzy gradient operator to detect edges.

At this point, the edge image on a fuzzy way is obtained, i.e., we have generated an image where each pixel value represents its membership to the edge set. However, this idea contradicts the Canny restrictions [5]. These restrictions force a representation of the edges as binary images with edges of one pixel wide. Thus, in order to satisfy the Canny's restrictions, the fuzzy edge image has to be thinned and binarized. However, these two operations can be carried out in a different order. This is the essence of the two algorithms that will be also analysed in the next section (see Fig. 1).

Algorithm 1 consists on applying non-maxima suppression (NMS) to the fuzzy edge image in order to obtain edges of one pixel wide. The fuzzy edge image will contain large values where there is a strong image gradient, but to identify edges the broad regions present in areas where the slope is large must be thinned so that only the magnitudes at those points which are local maxima remain. NMS performs this by suppressing all values along the line of the gradient that are not peak values (see [5]). NMS has been performed using P. Kovesis' implementation in

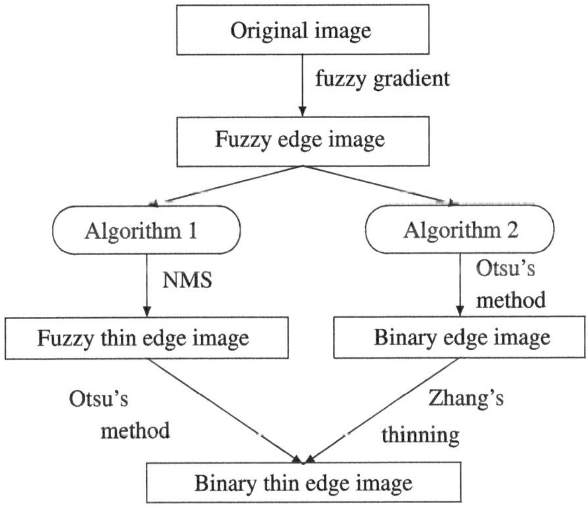

Fig. 1 Block diagrams of the two algorithms considered

Matlab [14]. After that, the well-known Otsu's thresholding method [17] is applied to binarize the fuzzy thin edges.

On the other hand, Algorithm 2 performs Otsu's thresholding method at a first stage and then, a binary thinning algorithm is applied. In this case, we will use the well-known Zhang and Suen's algorithm [21] because of its simplicity and speed. These two methods to transform the fuzzy edge image to a binary thin edge image give some of the best results according to some performance measures (see [6]).

4 Experimental Results and Analysis

In this section, some experimental results are carried out. The purpose of these experiments is twofold. First, we want to show the robustness and good behaviour of the proposed edge detector for some images with different amount of noise. Then, the edge detector based on discrete t-norms will be compared with other detectors based on fuzzy and classical techniques. This comparison, in addition of the visual observation of the obtained results with the different approaches, will be based on a more objective method: the use of performance measures.

4.1 Performance Measures

For the objective comparison of the obtained edge images, some performance measures on edge detection have been considered. These measures need, in addition to the binary thin edge image (DE) obtained, a ground truth edge image (GT) that is a binary thin edge image containing the true edges of the original image, i.e., the reference edge image. In this work, we will use the following measures to quantify the similarity between (DE) and (GT):

1. Pratt's figure of merit [18] defined as

$$FoM = \frac{1}{\max\{card\{DE\}, card\{GT\}\}} \cdot \sum_{x \in DE} \frac{1}{1 + ad^2},$$

where *card* is the number of edge points of the image, a is a scaling constant and d is the separation distance of an actual edge point to the ideal edge points. In our case, we considered $a = 1$ and the Euclidean distance d.
2. The ρ-coefficient [12], defined as

$$\rho = \frac{card(E)}{card(E) + card(E_{FN}) + card(E_{FP})},$$

where E is the set of well-detected edge pixels, E_{FN} is the set of ground truth edges missed by the edge detector and E_{FP} is the set of edge pixels detected but with no counterpart on the ground truth image. Since edges cannot always be detected at exact integer image coordinates, we consider that an edge pixel is correctly detected if a corresponding ground truth edge pixel is present in a 5×5 square neighbourhood centred at the respective pixel coordinates, as it was considered in [12].

Larger values of FoM and $\rho (0 \leq FoM, \rho \leq 1)$ are indicators of better capabilities for edge detection.

As we have already observed, the performance measures need a dataset of images with their ground truth edge images (edges specifications) in order to compare the outputs obtained by the different algorithms. So, 10 images and their edge specifications from the public dataset of the University of South Florida [2] have been used in the experiments (see Fig. 2). The salt and pepper noise in the images has been added using the standard functions of Matlab R2011a.

On the other hand, as in the case of edge detection, different objective measures can be used to evaluate the performance of a filter. Among them, we will use the SSIM (see [20]) and the fuzzy DI-subsethood measure $EQ_{\sigma DI}$ (see [4]). Recently, SSIM was introduced under the assumption that human visual perception is highly adapted for extracting structural information from a scene. The SSIM is an alternative complementary framework for quality assessment based on the degradation of structural information. Let O_1 and F_2 be two images of dimensions $M \times N$. We suppose that O_1 is the original noise-free image and F_2 is the restored image for which some filter has been applied. The two measures are defined as follows:

$$SSIM(F_2, O_1) = \frac{(2\mu_1\mu_2 + C_1)}{(\mu_1^2 + \mu_2^2 + C_1)} \cdot \frac{(2\sigma_{12} + C_2)}{(\sigma_1^2 + \sigma_2^2 + C_2)},$$

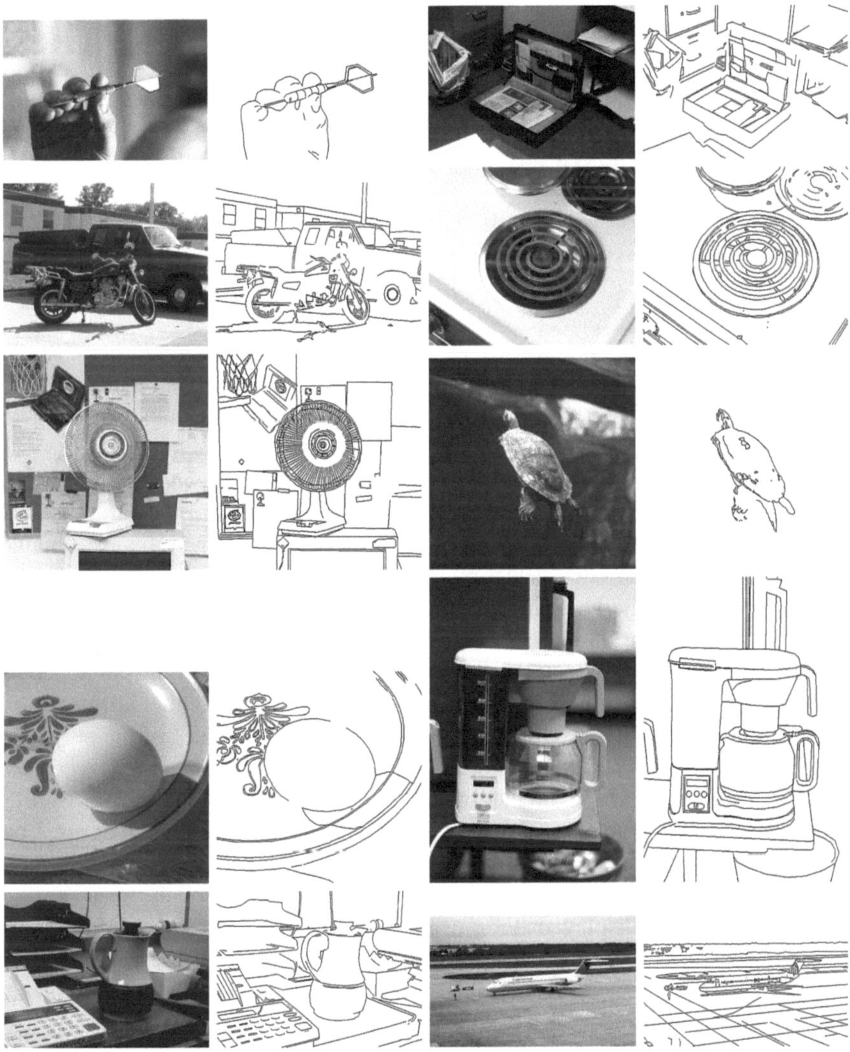

Fig. 2 Original images and their ground truth edge images

where $\mu_k, k = 1,2$ is the mean of the image O_1 and F_2 respectively, σ_k^2 is the variance of each image, σ_{12} is the covariance between the two images, $C_1 = (0.01 \cdot 255)^2$ and $C_2 = (0.03 \cdot 255)^2$ (see [20] for details),

$$EQ_{\sigma DI}(F_2, O_1) = \frac{1}{255MN} \sum_{i=1}^{M} \sum_{j=1}^{N} (255 - |O_1(i,j) - F_2(i,j)|).$$

Larger values of SSIM and $EQ_{\sigma DI}$ ($0 \leq SSIM, EQ_{\sigma DI} \leq 1$) are indicators of better capabilities for noise reduction and image recovery.

4.2 Robustness of the Method

In the following experiments, the nilpotent minimum discrete t-norm T_{nM} has been used. During these experimental results, the structuring elements B used for the fuzzy discrete morphological operators are represented by the matrices

$$B_1 = \begin{pmatrix} 0 & 255 & 0 \\ 255 & 255 & 255 \\ 0 & 255 & 0 \end{pmatrix}, \quad B_2 = \begin{pmatrix} 219 & 219 & 219 \\ 219 & 255 & 219 \\ 219 & 219 & 219 \end{pmatrix}.$$

The structuring element B_1 is a widely used 3×3 disk-shaped structuring element while B_2 has been already used in [16]. We will use the structuring element B_1 to remove salt and pepper noise and then B_2 is applied into the fuzzy gradient to detect the fuzzy edges. Note that taking into account the character and behaviour of the salt and pepper noise, a structuring element like B_1 is adequate to remove it. On the other hand, a structuring element like B_2 would expand the salt noise for noise removal purposes but it is a structuring element that obtains notable experimental results on edge detection.

In Fig. 3 we display the results obtained by the proposed fuzzy edge detection algorithm using Algorithms 1 and 2 when five different salt and pepper noise functions, of parameter 0.02, 0.04, 0.06, 0.08 and 0.1 respectively, were added to one of the images shown in Fig. 2. Note that there are also the filtered images by the proposed alternate filter. Our goal is to study the performance of the proposed algorithm when we increase the amount of noise present in the image. We can see as the edge images are little affected with the increase of noise and many features remain detected. In Table 1, we can observe that the performance measures on edge detection and noise removal remain high.

On the other hand, in Fig. 4 the evolution of the values of the measures of Fig. 3 is graphically displayed. First of all, note that the values of the measures concerning filtering performance, *SSIM* and $EQ_{\sigma DI}$, follow a descending progression. This behaviour is related to the fact that as higher is the amount of noise, more difficult is to reduce the noise without affecting the image substantially and consequently, the filtered image differs more from the original non-corrupted one. However, the alternate filter achieves quite remarkable results since all the performance values are over 0.99. Focusing now on edge detection performance measures, a more complex behaviour can be observed. The graphs are not strictly decreasing and contrary to what it would be expected, sometimes better results can be obtained with a higher amount of noise. For example, for the image with added salt and pepper noise of parameter 0.04, we obtain a value of *FoM* of 0.5057 with Algorithm 1, but a higher value of 0.5202 is obtained for the image with added salt and pepper noise of parameter 0.06. This unexpected phenomenon may be due to:

1. the small range of the obtained values for the different amounts of noise (a maximum of 0.5202 and a minimum of 0.4944 for values of *FoM* with Algorithm 1),

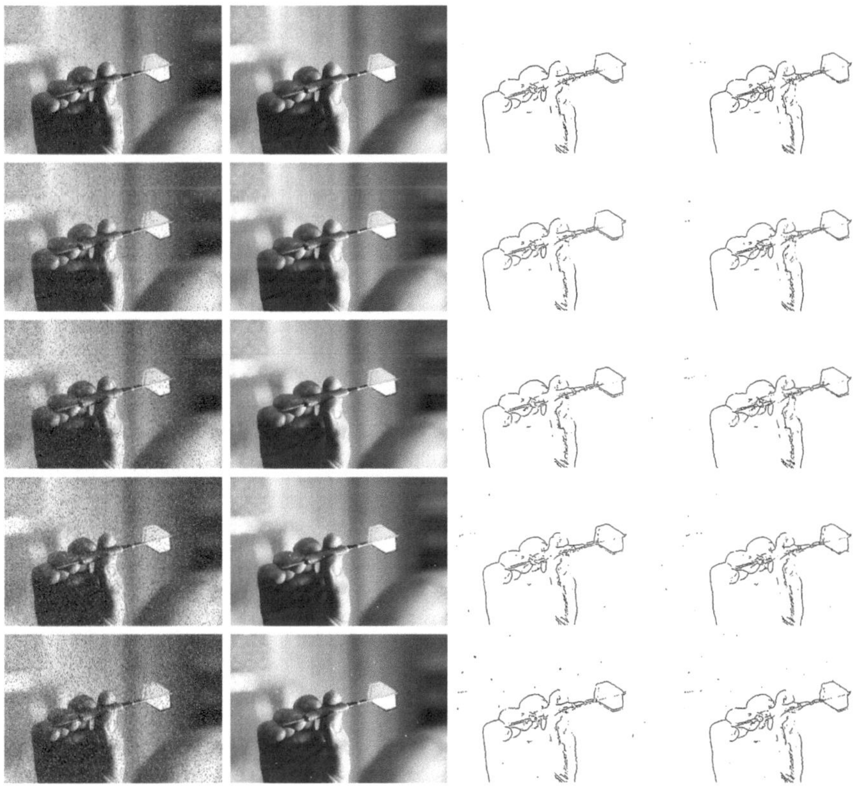

Fig. 3 From top to down, corrupted image with salt and pepper noise with 0.02, 0.04, 0.06, 0.08 and 0.1 (column 1), filtered image (column 2) and binary thin edge image with Algorithm 1 (column 3) and Algorithm 2 (column 4) using T_{nM} with B_1 and B_2, respectively

Table 1 Measures from the results of Fig. 3

Noise	Filtered image		Edge image			
			Algorithm 1		Algorithm 2	
	SSIM	$EQ_{\sigma DI}$	*FoM*	ρ	*FoM*	ρ
0.02	0.9974	0.9936	0.5105	0.6174	0.5104	0.6289
0.04	0.9971	0.9933	0.5057	0.6267	0.5041	0.6304
0.06	0.9967	0.9930	0.5202	0.6172	0.4913	0.6240
0.08	0.9954	0.9925	0.5165	0.6218	0.4982	0.6207
0.10	0.9947	0.9920	0.4944	0.6023	0.4784	0.6098

2. some possible defects in the ground truth edge images (recall that they are generated by humans and therefore, they are not infallible),
3. the possibility of transformation of a noisy pixel into a true edge pixel.

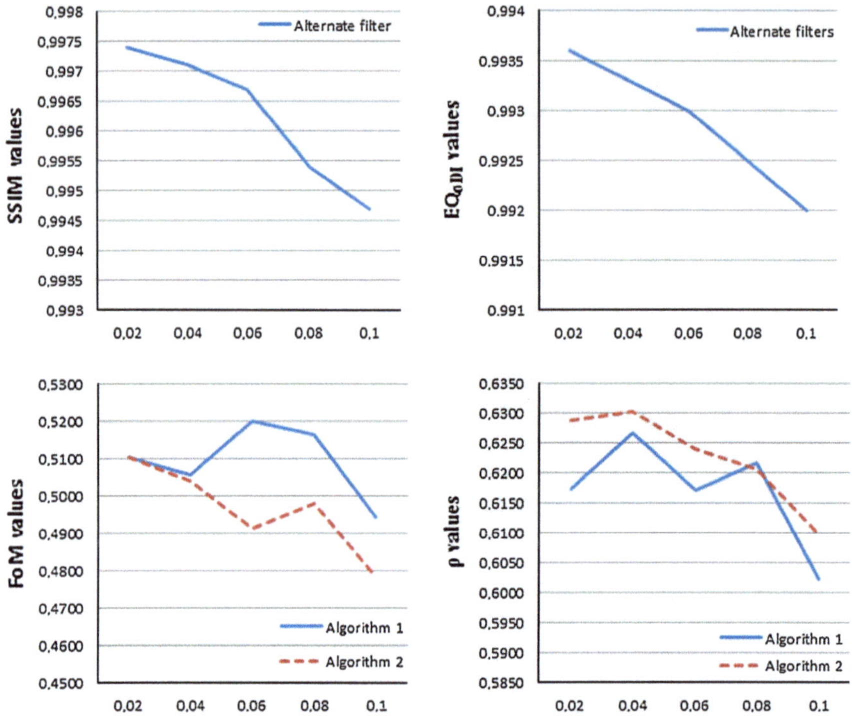

Fig. 4 Evolution of the values of the measures from the images of Fig. 3 depending on the amount of salt and pepper noise

Finally, it is worth mentioning that the two considered performance measures on edge detection do not point to the same algorithm as the best method to transform the fuzzy edge image to the binary thin edge image. While Algorithm 1 outperforms Algorithm 2 according to *FoM*, the ρ-measure gives better marks to the latter. Thus, a visual observation of the results is needed. In this case, we think that Algorithm 1 obtains images more pleasing to look at because it preserves better the geometry of the original image (see Fig. 5).

4.3 Comparison with Other Fuzzy Based Edge Detectors

In this section, we compare the edge images obtained with our edge detector based on discrete t-norms with those obtained using an analogous edge detector using now the classical gray-scale morphology based on the umbra approach, and those obtained using the fuzzy approach based on the Łukasiewicz continuous t-norm, $T_{LK}(x,y) = \max\{0, x+y-1\}$ for all $x, y \in [0,1]$. Recall that the pair $(T_{LK}, I_{T_{LK}})$ is the representative of the only class of t-norms (nilpotent ones) that guarantees the fulfilment of all the properties in order to have a good fuzzy mathematical

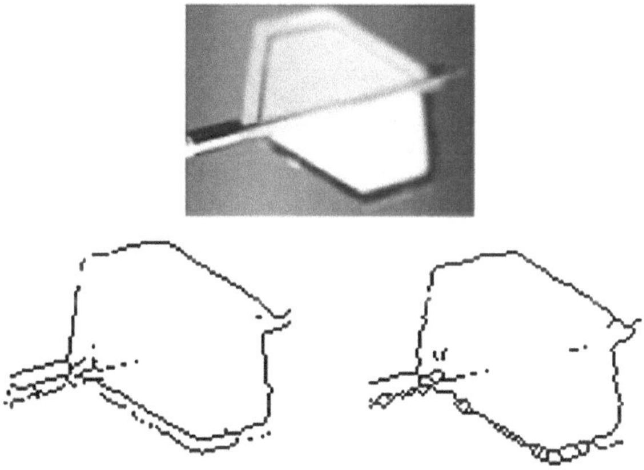

Fig. 5 Comparison of the details of the original image with the results obtained with Algorithms 1 (*left*) and 2 (*right*) for the corrupted image with added salt and pepper noise of parameter 0.04 of Fig. 3

morphology, including duality and generalized idempotence (see [16]). On the other hand, the results are also compared to the ones obtained using an idempotent or a representable uninorm. This approach, developed for edge detection purposes in [10] and [9], obtains the best marks in all the comparisons made until now with edge detectors obtained from usual fuzzy morphologies based on t-norms. In this approach, two types of left-continuous conjunctive uninorms and their residual implications are used. Specifically, they are defined as follows:

- *Representable uninorms*: Let $e \in (0,1)$ and let $h : [0,1] \to [-\infty, \infty]$ be a strictly increasing continuous function with $h(0) = -\infty, h(e) = 0$ and $h(1) = \infty$. Then

$$U_h(x,y) = \begin{cases} h^{-1}(h(x)+h(y)) & \text{if}(x,y) \notin \{(1,0),(0,1)\}, \\ 0 & \text{otherwise,} \end{cases}$$

is a conjunctive representable uninorm with neutral element e, and its residual implicator I_{U_h} is given by

$$I_{U_h}(x,y) = \begin{cases} h^{-1}(h(y)-h(x)) & \text{if}(x,y) \notin \{(0,0),(1,1)\}, \\ 1 & \text{otherwise.} \end{cases}$$

- A specific type of *idempotent uninorms*. Let N be a strong negation. The function given by

$$U^N(x,y) = \begin{cases} \min\{x,y\} & \text{if} y \leq N(x), \\ \max\{x,y\} & \text{otherwise,} \end{cases}$$

is a conjunctive idempotent uninorm. Its residual implicator is given by

$$I_{U^N}(x,y) = \begin{cases} \min\{N(x),y\} & \text{if} y < x, \\ \max\{N(x),y\} & \text{if} y \geq x. \end{cases}$$

Table 2 Means of the performance measures on edge detection obtained by the different edge detectors

Noise	Measure	T_{nM}		T_{LK}		U_h		U^N		Umbra	
		Alg. 1	Alg. 2	Alg. 1	Alg. 2	Alg. 1	Alg. 2	Alg. 1	Alg. 2	Alg. 1	Alg. 2
0.02	*FoM*	0.4057	0.4063	0.2013	0.1951	0.3044	0.3234	0.3970	0.4013	0.2024	.1884
	ρ	0.5650	0.5715	0.3093	0.2980	0.4602	0.4875	0.5582	0.5630	0.3079	0.2830
0.04	*FoM*	0.4050	0.4037	0.2045	0.1995	0.3051	0.3215	0.3981	0.4008	0.2192	0.1923
	ρ	0.5687	0.5733	0.3200	0.3077	0.4674	0.4896	0.5624	0.5662	0.3425	0.2913
0.06	*FoM*	0.4075	0.4021	0.2078	0.1986	0.3038	0.3197	0.3960	0.3976	0.2203	0.1855
	ρ	0.5708	0.5748	0.3283	0.3115	0.4655	0.4893	0.5634	0.5650	0.3483	0.2843
0.08	*FoM*	0.4066	0.4013	0.2100	0.1931	0.2956	0.3120	0.4004	0.4032	0.2133	0.1942
	ρ	0.5729	0.5760	0.3331	0.3038	0.4551	0.4845	0.5700	0.5732	0.3377	0.3027
0.1	*FoM*	0.4053	0.4000	0.2005	0.1787	0.2807	0.2956	0.3948	0.3937	0.2014	0.1817
	ρ	0.5745	0.5769	0.3147	0.2796	0.4301	0.4621	0.5660	0.5687	0.3126	0.2811

These two types of conjunctive uninorms guarantee most of the good algebraic and morphological properties associated with the morphological operators obtained from them (see [10]). Here, the used idempotent uninorm is generated by the classical negation $N_C(x) = 1 - x$ and the representable one U_h by the additive generator $h(x) = \ln\left(\frac{x}{1-x}\right)$. Note that we use the continuous counterpart of the structuring elements B_1 and B_2 for the morphology based on nilpotent t-norms scaled by e for the case of uninorms, where e is the neutral element of the uninorm.

These different approaches have been applied to the ten images displayed in Fig. 2 corrupted with salt and pepper noise of parameter 0.02 to 0.1, with a step of 0.02. Thus 50 images with different amounts of noise have been considered. We have performed for each edge detector Algorithms 1 and 2 to transform the fuzzy edge image to the binary thin edge image. After that, the performance measures on

Table 3 Number of images for which a particular configuration of edge detector obtains the best marks according to some performance measure

Noise	Measure	T_{nM}		T_{LK}		U_h		U^N		Umbra	
		Alg. 1	Alg. 2	Alg. 1	Alg. 2	Alg. 1	Alg. 2	Alg. 1	Alg. 2	Alg. 1	Alg. 2
0.02	*FoM*	6	3	0	0	0	1	0	0	0	0
	ρ	2	6	0	0	0	1	0	1	0	0
0.04	*FoM*	6	2	0	0	0	1	0	1	0	0
	ρ	3	5	0	0	0	1	0	1	0	0
0.06	*FoM*	8	1	0	0	0	1	0	0	0	0
	ρ	3	4	0	0	0	1	2	0	0	0
0.08	*FoM*	8	1	0	0	0	0	0	1	0	0
	ρ	4	4	0	0	0	0	0	2	0	0
0.1	*FoM*	8	1	0	0	0	0	0	1	0	0
	ρ	4	5	0	0	0	0	0	1	0	0
Total	*FoM*	36	8	0	0	0	3	0	3	0	0
	ρ	16	24	0	0	0	3	2	5	0	0

edge detection have been computed and the overall results are presented in Table 2. In this table, the mean of the values given by a performance measure with respect to the binary thin edge images obtained by every edge detector is displayed. Note that we have computed the values depending on the amount of salt and pepper noise added to the original image. For example, for the ten images

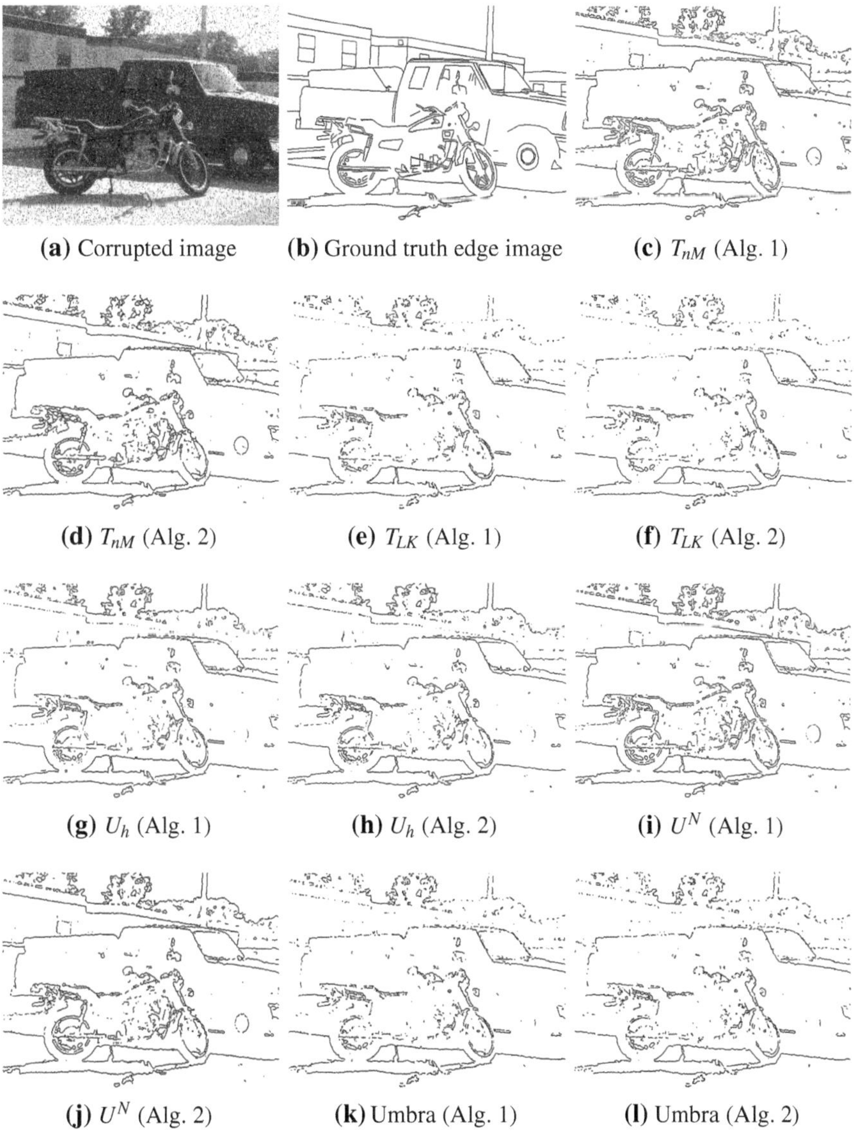

(a) Corrupted image **(b)** Ground truth edge image **(c)** T_{nM} (Alg. 1)

(d) T_{nM} (Alg. 2) **(e)** T_{LK} (Alg. 1) **(f)** T_{LK} (Alg. 2)

(g) U_h (Alg. 1) **(h)** U_h (Alg. 2) **(i)** U^N (Alg. 1)

(j) U^N (Alg. 2) **(k)** Umbra (Alg. 1) **(l)** Umbra (Alg. 2)

Fig. 6 Corrupted image with salt and pepper noise with parameter 0.1 and binary thin edge images obtained by the considered approaches corrupted with salt and pepper noise of parameter 0.02, T_{nM} with Algorithm 1 obtains *FoM* values with a mean value of 0.4057, while T_{nM} with Algorithm 2 obtains a mean value of 0.4063. In addition, in Table 3, we show the number of images for which a particular edge detector is the best one among the considered ones according to a specific performance measure. For example, T_{nM} with Algorithm 1 obtains the highest *FoM* value in 6 out of 10 images corrupted with salt and pepper noise of parameter 0.02.

Analysing these two tables, we can ensure that the edge detector based on T_{nM} outperforms the other approaches according to both performance measures. Only the edge detector based on the idempotent uninorm U^N obtains in some cases comparable results. After these approaches, the following one with respect to its performance is the edge detector based on the representable uninorm U_h, while worse results are obtained by the umbra approach and the Łukasiewicz t-norm. The visual observation of the results supports the previous statement. The edge images obtained with T_{nM} contain the main edges of the original images without being distorted by the presence of the noise in the initial images. Although the other methods remove the noise quite well, they do not obtain some main edges of the original images. This fact is clearly showed in Fig. 6, where the binary thin edge images obtained by the 10 considered edge detectors are displayed. Furthermore, in Fig. 7, note that the edge images obtained by the continuous Łukasiewicz t-norm are almost white, i.e., few edges are detected and specially, no part of the egg is recognisable.

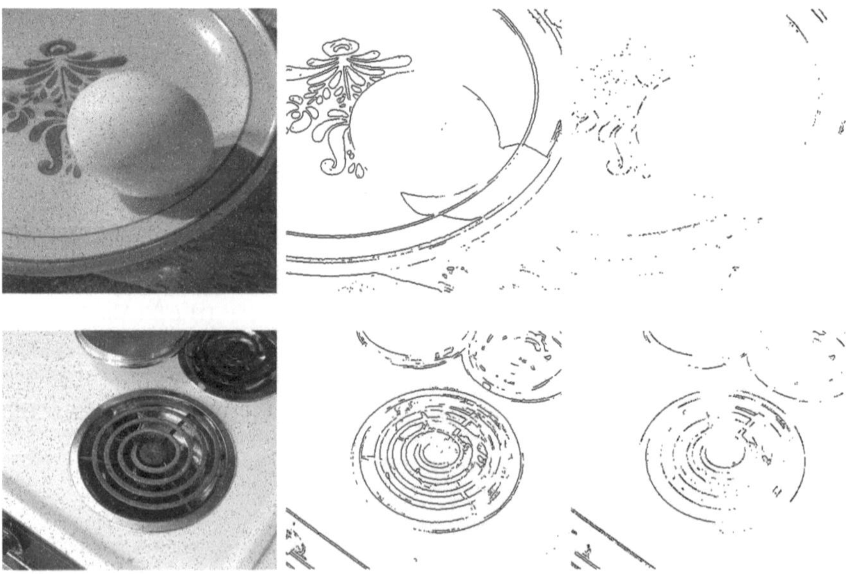

(a) Corrupted image **(b)** T_{nM} (Alg. 1) **(c)** T_{LK} (Alg. 1)

Fig. 7 Corrupted image with salt and pepper noise with parameter 0.02 and binary thin edge images obtained by T_{nM} and T_{LK} with Algorithm 1

Furthermore, the obtained numerical and visual results show that this classification of the edge detectors according to their performance does not depend on the amount of salt and pepper noise added to the original image. The superiority of the discrete approach remains although we increase the amount of noise. This fact is evident in Fig. 8 where the evolution of the measures obtained by the different approaches depending on the amount of noise is graphically displayed. Note that T_{nM} is the best edge detector according to both performance measures independently of the used method to transform the fuzzy edge image to the binary thin edge image. Recall that higher values of FoM and ρ are indicators of a better performance on edge detection.

However, although the discrete approach is pointed out by both performance measures as the best edge detector, they do not agree in which is the best method to binarize and perform the thinning operation to the fuzzy edge image. Taking into account the number of images for which an edge detector is the best configuration and the obtained mean value, T_{nM} with Algorithm 1 is the best configuration according to FoM, but Algorithm 2 has to be used to obtain better results

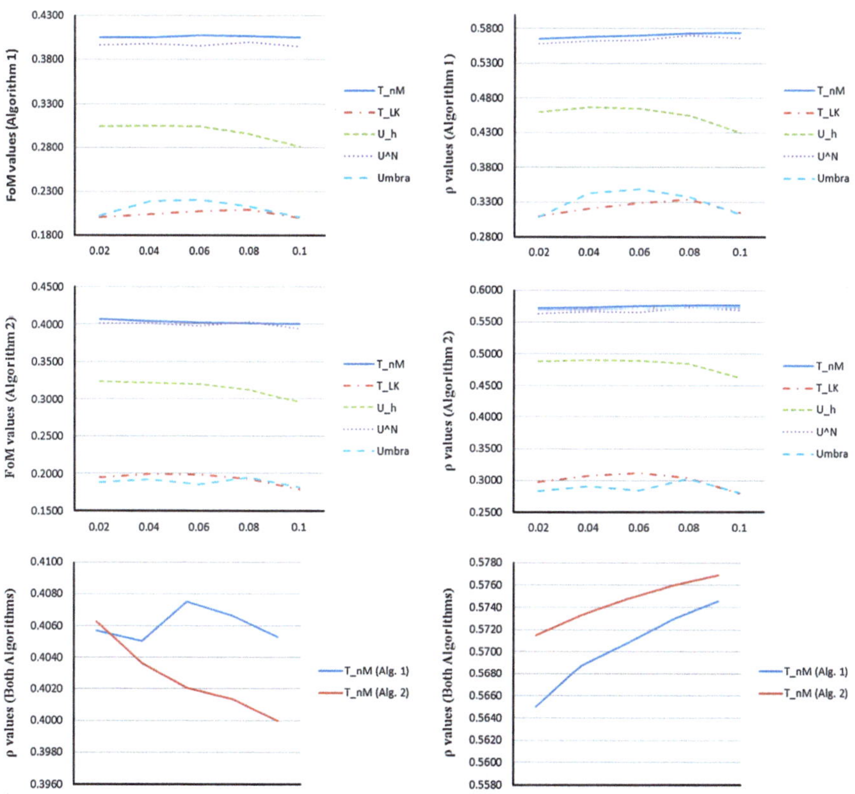

Fig. 8 Comparison of the mean values of the performance measures on edge detection depending on the amount of salt and pepper noise for the considered approaches

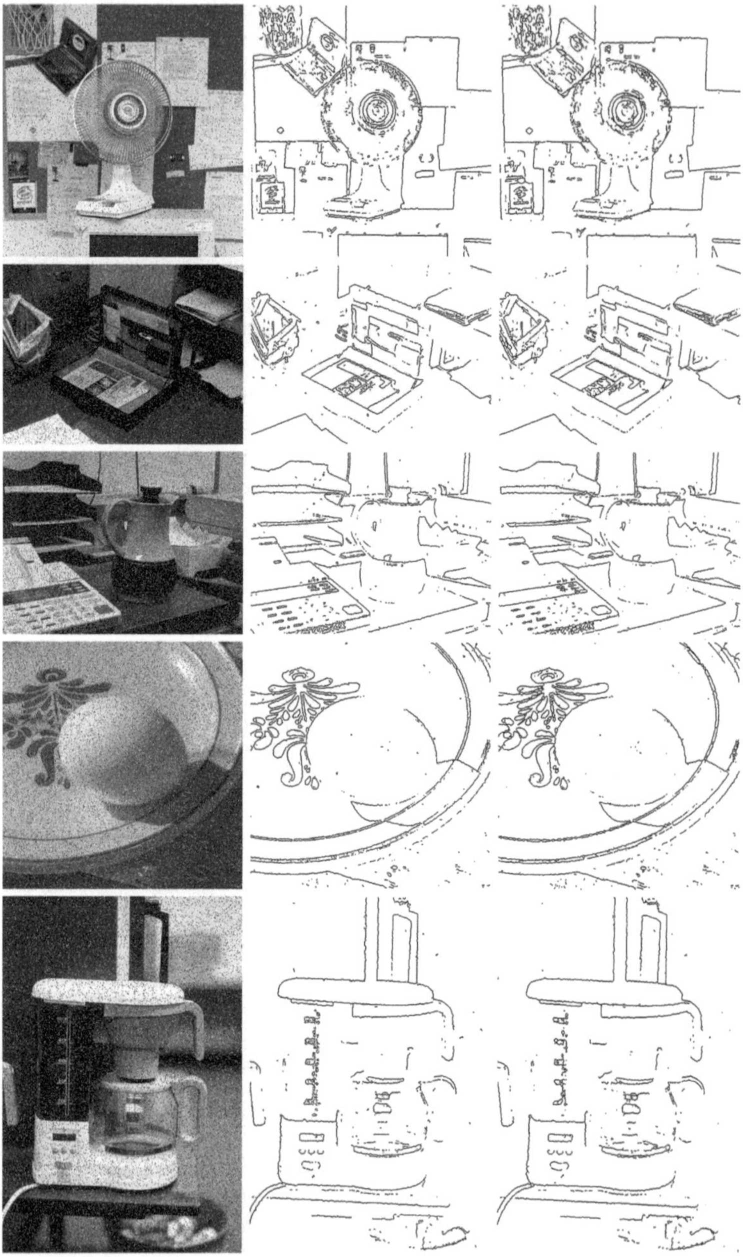

Fig. 9 From *left* to *right*, corrupted image with salt and pepper noise and binary thin edge images obtained by T_{nM} with Algorithms 1 and 2

according to ρ. If we turn our attention to the visual results, we will see that the binary thin edge images obtained by T_{nM} with Algorithm 1 maintain better the geometry of the original image again than the ones obtained by T_{nM} with Algorithm 2. In Fig. 9, this effect is present in the fan structure, the sheets in the portfolio and the omnifax word.

5 Conclusions and Future Work

In this work, an edge detection algorithm based on the fuzzy morphology using discrete t-norms, derived as a residual operator from the basic morphological operations, has been proposed. Such algorithm is able to detect edges and contours, and preserve them. To evaluate the performance of the algorithm, comparison experiments with other well known approaches have been carried out according to some performance measures. The results indicate that the proposed algorithm is robust against noisy images. Experimental results show that it outperforms other fuzzy morphological edge detection methods in detecting detailed edge features. Moreover, these edges can be preserved even though the image is corrupted by noise. Future work consists on one hand, in the study of the behaviour of the algorithm for other types of noise and, on the other hand in the selection of the size, shape and direction of the structuring element adapted to the edge features of the image and how we can improve performance.

Acknowledgments This paper has been partially supported by the Spanish Grant MTM2009-10320 with FEDER support.

References

1. Bloch I, Maître H (1995) Fuzzy mathematical morphologies: a comparative study. Pattern Recogn 28:1341–1387
2. Bowyer K, Kranenburg C, Dougherty S (1999) Edge detector evaluation using empirical ROC curves. Comput Vis Pattern Recogn 1:354–359
3. Bustince H, Barrenechea E, Pagola M, Fernandez J (2009) Interval-valued fuzzy sets constructed from matrices: application to edge detection. Fuzzy Sets Syst 160(13):1819–1840
4. Bustince H, Pagola M, Barrenechea E (2007) Construction of fuzzy indices from fuzzy DI-subsethood measures: application to the global comparison of images. Inform Sci 177:906–929
5. Canny J (1986) A computational approach to edge detection. IEEE Trans Pattern Anal Mach Intell 8(6):679–698
6. González-Hidalgo M, Massanet S (2011) Towards an objective edge detection algorithm based on discrete t-norms. In: Galichet S, Montero J, Mauris G (eds) Proceedings of the 7th conference of the european society for fuzzy logic and technology (EUSFLAT-2011) and LFA-2011, Advances in Intelligent Systems Research, pp 319–326
7. González-Hidalgo M, Massanet S, Torrens J (2010) Discrete t-norms in a fuzzy mathematical morphology: algebraic properties and experimental results. In: Proceedings of WCCI-FUZZ-IEEE, Barcelona, Spain, pp 1194–1201

8. González-Hidalgo M, Massanet S, Mir A (2011) Closing and opening based on discrete t-norms. Applications to natural image analysis. In: Galichet S, Montero J, Mauris G (eds) Proceedings of the 7th conference of the European society for fuzzy logic and technology (EUSFLAT-2011) and LFA-2011, Advances in intelligent systems research, pp 358–365
9. M. González-Hidalgo, A. Mir-Torres, and D. Ruiz-Aguilera. A robust edge detection algorithm based on a fuzzy mathematical morphology using uninorms (ϕ MM-U morphology). In J. M. R. Tavares and R. M. N. Jorge, editors, Computational Vision and Medical Image Processing: VIPIMAGE 2009, pages 630–635, Bristol, PA, USA, 2009. CRC Press, Taylor & Francis, Inc.
10. González-Hidalgo M, Mir-Torres A, Ruiz-Aguilera D, Torrens J (2009) Edge-images using a uninorm-based fuzzy mathematical morphology: Opening and closing. In: Tavares J, Jorge N (eds) Advances in computational vision and medical image processing, number 13 in computational methods in applied sciences, Chap. 8, Springer, Netherlands, pp 137–157
11. González-Hidalgo M, Mir-Torres A, Ruiz-Aguilera D, Torrens J (2009) Image analysis applications of morphological operators based on uninorms. In: Proceedings of the IFSA-EUSFLAT 2009 Conference, Lisbon, Portugal, pp 630–635
12. Grigorescu C, Petkov N, Westenberg MA (2003) Contour detection based on nonclassical receptive field inhibition. IEEE Trans Image Process 12(7):729–739
13. Jiang J-A, Chuang C-L, Lu Y-L, Fahn C-S (2007) Mathematical-morphology-based edge detectors for detection of thin edges in low-contrast regions. IET Image Process 1(3):269–277
14. Kovesi PD MATLAB and Octave functions for computer vision and image processing. Centre for exploration targeting, school of earth and environment, the university of western australia. http://www.csse.uwa.edu.au/~pk/research/matlabfns/
15. Mayor G, Torrens J (2005) Triangular norms in discrete settings. In: Klement E, Mesiar R (eds) Logical, Algebraic, Analytic, and Probabilistic aspects of triangular norms, Chap. 7, Elsevier, Amsterdam, pp 189–230
16. Nachtegael M, Kerre E (2000) Classical and fuzzy approaches towards mathematical morphology. In: Kerre EE, Nachtegael M (eds) Fuzzy techniques in image processing, number 52 in studies in fuzziness and soft computing, Chap. 1, Physica, New York, pp 3–57
17. Otsu N (1979) A threshold selection method from gray-level histograms. IEEE Trans Syst Man and Cybern 9:62–66
18. Pratt WK (2007) Digital image processing. 4 edn. Wiley-Interscience, New York
19. Serra J (1982,1988) Image analysis and mathematical morphology. vols. 1, 2. Academic Press, London
20. Wang Z, Bovik AC, Sheikh HR, Simoncelli EP (2004) Image quality assessment: From error visibility to structural similarity. IEEE Trans Image Process 13(4):600–612
21. Zhang TY, Suen CY (1984) A fast parallel algorithm for thinning digital patterns. Commun ACM 27:236–239

Colour Quantisation as a Preprocessing Step for Image Segmentation

Henryk Palus and Mariusz Frackiewicz

Abstract Colour quantisation is very often used as an auxiliary operation in colour image processing, e.g. this operation can reduce the complexity of image segmentation process. In this chapter the results of segmentation preceded by a colour quantisation have been compared with segmentation without such preprocessing step. The choice of tools for the experiment was, for obvious reasons, limited to some colour quantisation and image segmentation methods. The colour quantisation techniques based on clustering of pixels, i.e. the classic *k-means* technique (KM) and new *k-harmonic means* technique (KHM) were considered. For image segmentation the unseeded region growing (USRG) technique has been selected from a variety of known techniques. Evaluation of the results was based on empirically defined quality function used for segmentation results. Not every method of colour quantisation, carried out as preprocessing step in the process of segmentation, leads to improved segmentation result. Therefore, our approach needs a good quantisation technique, e.g. researched segmentation technique works better for KHM quantisation technique than KM technique. This study uses different images acquired from relatively simple scenes without significant highlights and shadows. An interesting open question is what kind of colour images needs to be quantised before the segmentation. Perhaps an estimation of image segmentation difficulty will help to answer this question. The further research should be focused on establishing the conditions and parameters of additional improvement in image segmentation preceded by a colour quantisation.

H. Palus (✉) · M. Frackiewicz
Silesian University of Technology, ul. Akademicka 16 44-100 Gliwice, Poland
e-mail: Henryk.Palus@polsl.pl

M. Frackiewicz
e-mail: Mariusz.Frackiewicz@polsl.pl

J. M. R. S. Tavares and R. M. Natal Jorge (eds.), *Topics in Medical Image Processing and Computational Vision*, Lecture Notes in Computational Vision and Biomechanics 8,
DOI: 10.1007/978-94-007-0726-9_7,

1 Introduction

In recent years the importance of colour in image processing cannot be understated: colour images are commonplace and grey-level images today are less common. Among many operations performed on colour images, the colour image segmentation plays an important role for practical applications (e.g., object recognition, image compression). The goal of colour image segmentation is to identify homogeneous regions in colour image that represent objects or meaningful parts of objects present in a scene. Sometimes is important to have a pre-processing stage in the chain of colour image processing. There are many different types of preprocessing before segmentation (e.g., colour space transformation, noise filtration, edge enhancement or colour quantisation). In this chapter our interests are limited to colour quantisation techniques before colour image segmentation. The application of such techniques may significantly improve segmentation results and therefore their influence on the segmentation results is studied.

Colour image quantisation is the process of transformation of a true colour image (typically eight bit onto each colour component) into an image consisting of a small number of specially selected colours (colour palette). New colours are selected by minimizing the colour difference between the original image and the quantised image. In other words, this is a special case of vector quantisation realized in three-dimensional colour space.

Colour quantisation is also very often used as an auxiliary operation in colour image processing. On example it can reduce the complexity of image segmentation process. In literature we can find examples that use the colour quantisation as pre-processing in image segmentation.

The chapter will be organized as follows. In Sect. 2, we will review former works that have been done to investigate a sense of colour quantisation in image segmentation. The idea of proposed experiment, used tools and final results will be described in Sects. 3 and 5. In Sect. 4, will be presented some autonomous problem of robustness of quantisation techniques to noise-corrupted images. Finally we will conclude the chapter in Sect. 6.

2 Related Works

Ten years ago the first important work about using colour quantisation in image segmentation process was published [5]. Deng and Manjunath proposed JSEG technique composed from two independent steps: colour quantisation by modified Generalized Lloyd Algorithm (GLA) and spatial segmentation based on quantised colours. This quantisation technique contained a special Peer Group Filtering (PGF), quantising in perceptual CIELUV colour space and merging close clusters with the use of a threshold value [6]. Authors emphasized the importance of good quality of quantisation technique and recommended the use of 10–20 colours in the images of natural scenes. Unfortunately, the colour quantisation technique is sensitive on selected value of parameter (a threshold of the quantisation). Improperly selected threshold badly affects the result of quantisation and leads to incorrect segmentation.

In last years the JSEG technique was many times modified. This also applies to colour quantisation technique. Good example is a JSEG version with variance-based quantisation method [3] that is faster than modified GLA. In other paper [23] a special attention has been paid to the need of searching better colour quantisation algorithms for JSEG technique. Another modified version of JSEG uses an adaptive mean-shift clustering technique (AMS) for non-parametric colour quantisation [22].

When the image segmentation is based on the clustering of pixels, the colour quantisation using the colour pixel statistics can be naturally used to determine the number of clusters and the initial location of their centres. An example of this approach is a sophisticated version of classical FCM algorithm, named Ant Colony-Fuzzy C-means Hybrid Algorithm (AFHA), that adaptively 'clusters' the image pixels viewed as three-dimensional points in the RGB colour space [25].

Sometimes attention is paid to decreasing the computational costs and reducing the sensitivity of segmentation to the noise data [7, 10]. The authors of both papers demonstrated that colour reduction by using a self-organizing map (SOM) simplifies further segmentation. Similarly some method of colour texture segmentation starts with a simple uniform colour quantisation [24].

Colour texture descriptors, e.g. histograms of various types, used in segmentation process are more easily extracted from quantised images [4]. Sometimes a specially selected quantisation technique is applied, which in this case is a cellular colour quantisation based on HSV colour space [15]. The choice of this colour space is a result of the relation with human visual system. Quantised image should have an adequate number of visually dominant colours. The quantisation process starts here with 21 (seven colours defined on H-S plane and three levels of V) specially selected from HSV space initial colours. Number of colours in the splitting stage of quantisation may be increased to 192 colours and next in colour merging stage is limited to a maximum 50 colours. The PSNR is used for terminating quantisation process. Other example of applying quantisation in colour texture segmentation is a method named by Authors *modal image segmentation* [11]. Also in this case the first step is the colour quantisation, which aim is extraction of coarse representation of image. The output colour quantisation is used for region growing based on proposed deformable model energy function. The idea of colour quantisation scheme proposed in this paper comes from JSEG framework. However, the node displacements of the deformable surface model, instead of each pixel's colour, are applied.

The colour quantisation is used for many years as preprocessing in segmentation of complex document images [27]. Additionally, recently developed quantisation techniques automatically estimate the final number of colours in segmented image [18]. Similar problems exist with text detection and separation of characters from colour signboard images captured by mobile devices [13]. These images have a large number of unique colours, which can be limit to three essential colours representing characters (foreground), background and noise. An adaptive approach proposed in this paper is based on colour quantisation and k-means clustering.

The colour quantisation is also a simplification step used in video segmentation [21]. A large number of unique colours in several frames of an image sequence is reduced to few quantised colours. All colours are clustered consistently for all frames. First frame of the sequence is quantised into 16 colours by utilizing the k-means technique working in the CIELAB colour space. In this way the colour quantisation simplify the first frame for subsequent processing. New colours appearing in the next frames are automatically identified and added to the colour palette.

3 Idea of Experiment and Used Tools

In an experiment the results of segmentation preceded by a colour quantisation have been compared with segmentation without such preprocessing step. Below we present tools for colour quantisation, image segmentation and evaluation of both quantisation and segmentation results, that were selected for this experiment.

3.1 Selected Techniques for Colour Quantisation

In this chapter were considered two colour quantisation techniques based on clustering of pixels: the classic *k-means* technique (KM) [16] and new *k-harmonic means* technique (KHM) proposed by Zhang [26]. The usefulness of both techniques for colour image quantisation has been shown by authors of this chapter in work [8].

Each colour image contains n pixels and is treated as clustering data set $X = \{x_1, \ldots, x_n\}$. After the initialization step the number of clusters k and values of starting cluster centres $C = \{c_1, \ldots, c_k\}$ are determined. The membership function $m(c_j|x_i)$ defines the degree of membership of x_i pixel in the cluster with the centre c_j. This function has following basic properties:

$$\begin{cases} m(c_j|x_i) \geq 0 \\ \sum_{j=1}^{k} m(c_j|x_i) = 1 \end{cases} \tag{1}$$

In contrast to KM, the KHM technique is based on "soft membership". The fuzzy membership (2) of pixel to cluster $m(c_j|x_i)$ was here applied and similarly was applied the dynamic weight function $w(x_i)$ (3), what means different influence an individual pixel x_i on calculating the new values c_j in each next iteration.

$$m(c_j|x_i) = \frac{\left\| x_i - c_j \right\|^{-p-2}}{\sum_{j=1}^{k} \left\| x_i - c_j \right\|^{-p-2}} \tag{2}$$

$$w(x_i) = \frac{\sum_{j=1}^{k} \left\| x_i - c_j \right\|^{-p-2}}{\left(\sum_{j=1}^{k} \left\| x_i - c_j \right\|^{-p} \right)^2} \tag{3}$$

The KHM technique requires defining an internal parameter p, which usually fulfils following condition: $p \geq 2$. We used here the value $p = 2.7$. KHM, basing on formulas (2) and (3), uses the following formula for calculating new cluster centres:

$$c_j = \frac{\sum_{i=1}^{n} m(c_j|x_i) w(x_i) x_i}{\sum_{i=1}^{n} m(c_j|x_i) w(x_i)} \tag{4}$$

The KHM technique minimizes following objective function:

$$KHM(X, C) = \sum_{i=1}^{n} \frac{k}{\sum_{j=1}^{k} \frac{1}{\left\| x_i - c_j \right\|^{p}}} \tag{5}$$

Both quantisation techniques are used here with the same deterministic initialization method marked as *SD*. This method uses a size of the pixel cloud of a colour image. First, the mean values and standard deviations (*SD*) for each RGB component of all image pixels are calculated. Then, around the point of mean colour a rectangular cuboid with side lengths equal to $2\sigma_R$, $2\sigma_G$ and $2\sigma_B$ is constructed. We assume that it lies within the RGB cube. Next, the main diagonal of cuboid is divided into k equal segments. The centres of these diagonal segments are used as initial cluster centres.

A disadvantage of KHM in relation to KM is a greater computational complexity, resulting in longer computation time. This time, however, can be reduced by the use of multithreaded programming (multicore processors, GPGPU etc.).

As a background for the quantisation techniques described above were applied two simpler splitting techniques. The splitting techniques divide the colour space into smaller subspaces and then a colour palette is built by choosing representative colours from subspaces. We used here a technique implemented in IrfanView ver.4.0 and designated as IV and more complicated Wu's algorithm implemented in Ximagic plug-in developed for IrfanView.

3.2 Tools for Evaluation of Quantisers

Objective image quality measures are very important in the evaluation process of different colour quantisers. Commonly used measures are Mean Squared Error (MSE) and average colour difference in CIELAB colour space (ΔE). The MSE for colour image is defined by:

$$MSE = \frac{1}{MN}\sum_{i=1}^{M}\sum_{j=1}^{N}\left[(R_{ij} - R^*{}_{ij})^2 + (G_{ij} - G^*{}_{ij})^2 + (B_{ij} - B^*{}_{ij})^2\right] \quad (6)$$

where M and N are the image dimensions in pixels, R_{ij}, G_{ij}, B_{ij} are colour components of the pixel of location (i,j) in original image and R^*_{ij}, G^*_{ij}, B^*_{ij} are colour components of this pixel in quantised image. The smaller the MSE value, the better is the quantised image. Unfortunately, this measure sometimes bad correlates with subjective visual quality of image. Other common error measure applied to evaluation of quantisation is Peak Signal-to-Noise Ratio (PSNR), related with MSE directly:

$$PSNR = 20\log_{10}\frac{255}{\sqrt{MSE}} \quad (7)$$

Next quality measure ΔE, which takes the colorimetric aspects into account, can be expressed as:

$$\Delta E = \frac{1}{MN}\sum_{i=1}^{M}\sum_{j=1}^{N}\sqrt{\left(L_{ij} - L^*{}_{ij}\right)^2 + \left(a_{ij} - a^*{}_{ij}\right)^2 + \left(b_{ij} - b^*{}_{ij}\right)^2} \quad (8)$$

where L_{ij}, a_{ij}, b_{ij} denote the CIELAB colour components of the pixel of location (i,j) in original image and L^*_{ij}, a^*_{ij}, b^*_{ij} are CIELAB colour components of this pixel in quantised image. The traditional Euclidean distance in perceptually uniform CIELAB colour space well expresses the colour differences between the pixels.

Additional third measure of quantisation error is based on the idea of colourfulness of the image. If we assume that the colourfulness of image calculated after colour quantisation should be equal to the colourfulness of original image, then we can use following difference of colourfulness as a tool for evaluation of quantisation [19]:

$$\Delta M = \left|M_{orig} - M_{quant}\right| \quad (9)$$

where M_{orig} is the colourfulness of original image and M_{quant} is the colourfulness of quantised image. According to [9] the colourfulness of image can be computed using following formula:

$$M = \sqrt{\sigma_{rg}^2 + \sigma_{yb}^2} + 0.3\sqrt{\mu_{rg}^2 + \mu_{yb}^2} \quad (10)$$

where σ_{rg}, σ_{yb} are the standard deviations and μ_{rg}, μ_{yb} are the mean values of opponent colour components of the image pixels. The opponent components are approximated by following simplified equations:

$$rg = R - G \tag{11}$$

$$yb = 0.5(R + G) - B \tag{12}$$

where *rg*—red-green opponency, *yb*—yellow-blue opponency. Formulas for computing of colourfulness are simple and good correlate with the perceptual colourfulness of the image, which was confirmed experimentally in [9].

3.3 Region-Based Image Segmentation

Image segmentation techniques are usually classified into following classes: pixel-based techniques, region-based techniques, edge-based techniques, physics-based techniques and hybrid techniques. Of the many techniques developed for image segmentation, the UnSeeded Region Growing (USRG) technique, described by Palus [20], has been selected. This is a typical bottom-up pixel aggregation technique. It is based on the concept of region growing without the need for seeds to start the segmentation process. At the beginning of the algorithm each pixel has its own label (single pixel regions). Neighbouring pixels are merged into regions, if their attributes, for example colours, are sufficiently similar. This similarity condition is often represented by a homogeneity criterion. If a pixel satisfied the homogeneity criterion, then the pixel can be included to the region. After such inclusion, the region's area and mean colour are updated. For this updating appropriate recurrent formulas are used.

Two simple raster scans of the colour image are applied in this technique: one pass from the left to the right and from the top to the bottom and second reverse pass over the image. The pixel aggregation process results in a set of regions characterized by their mean colours, their sizes and lists of pixels that belong to proper regions. The typical homogeneity criterion based on the Euclidean metric has following form:

$$\sqrt{(R - R^*)^2 + (G - G^*)^2 + (B - B^*)^2} \leq d \tag{13}$$

where: R, G, B are colour components of tested pixel, R^*, G^*, B^* are colour components of mean colour of creating region and d is the parameter, that is very important for segmentation results. If the value of parameter d increases, then the number of regions in the segmented image simultaneously decreases. Too low value of parameter d is leading to oversegmentation and too high value is a reason of undersegmentation.

The version of the algorithm described here, works in the RGB colour space. This algorithm can also work in other colour space when the homogeneity criterion will be formulated in this space. The following formula is an example of criterion defined in HSI colour space:

$$\sqrt{(I - I^*)^2 + S^2 + S^{*2} - 2SS^* \cos(H - H^*)} \leq d \tag{14}$$

where: H, S, I are hue, saturation and intensity components of tested pixel, H^*, S^*, I^* are HSI colour components of mean colour of creating region.

The segmentation of good quality images also results in a large number of small regions on the edges of objects. The USRG technique removes these regions from the segmented image by postprocessing. It is not difficult task, because after segmentation we have a list of regions that can be sorted according to their area. Postprocessing needs an additional pass from the top left corner of the image to the bottom right corner, whose goal is removing the regions which consist of a number of pixels smaller than a certain threshold. A threshold value of the area of small region A depends on the image. After merging of small region, the mean colour of new region is computed and a label of small region pixels is changed. In result of such postprocessing, the number of regions in the segmented image significantly decreases. Final goal of region merging is to receive the segmented image with homogeneous regions as large as possible.

This region-based segmentation technique is relatively fast and effective: a PC with a 3.2 GHz Intel processor segments a color image (512 × 512 pixels) in 0.1 s. Other properties of USRG technique have been described in detail in paper [20].

3.4 Tools for Evaluation of Image Segmentation

In the literature are few results in the field of evaluation of image segmentation. Often the evaluation is limited to tests on the small number of images. The reason is a lack of generally accepted criteria and uniform procedures for the evaluation. Among different methods we can find empirically defined function used for evaluation of segmentation results [2]:

$$Q(I) = \frac{1}{10000\,(M \cdot N)} \sqrt{R} \sum_{i=1}^{R} \left[\frac{e_i^2}{1 + \log A_i} + \left(\frac{R(A_i)}{A_i} \right)^2 \right] \tag{15}$$

where I is the segmented image, $M \cdot N$ is the size of the image, R is the number of regions in the segmented image, A_i is the area of the region i, $R(A_i)$ is the number of regions having an area equal to A_i and e_i is the colour error of region i. The colour error in RGB space is calculated as the sum of the Euclidean distances between colour components of pixels of region and components of average colour, which is an attribute of this region in the segmented image. The colour errors in different colour spaces are not comparable and therefore are transformed back to the RGB space. First term of Eq. (15) is a normalization factor, the second term penalizes results with too many regions (oversegmentation), and the third term penalizes results with non-homogeneous regions. Last term is scaled by the area factor because the colour error is higher for large regions. The main idea of using this kind of function can be formulated as follows: the lower the value of $Q(I)$, the better is the segmentation result.

4 Comparison of Robustness of Quantisation Techniques

Digital colour images are sometimes acquired in bad lighting conditions and transmitted by the channels of different transmission quality, which leads to a noticeable noise in these images. Below is presented the robustness to noise of KM and KHM quantisation techniques. The experiments were performed on the test image pairs with simple colour objects arranged on a uniform background.

4.1 Robustness to Natural Noise

Two pairs of images for the first test (Fig. 1) were acquired in good and worse lighting conditions. The noisy images from Fig. 1b, d .have larger numbers of unique colours and also have a different image colourfulness (Table 1). The higher value of PSNR for the second pair of images shows a lower level of noise in the image from Fig. 1d.

The following results were obtained from the KM and KHM quantisation of the first image in the pair and the second image in the pair (noisy) and the second image after denoising. The both techniques used $k = 10$, performed 15 iterations and applied the same, based on statistical parameters of pixel cloud in RGB space, *SD* method for initialization. In case of KHM technique the parameter $p = 2.7$ was adopted.

Two classical filters have been selected for impulsive noise filtering: VMF [1] and Kuwahara-Nagao filter [12, 17]. We have used most typical versions of filters working with 3×3 masks filter. We have limited the number of iterations for each filter to only one. The VMF filter is a popular filtration technique. It is an extension of the scalar median filter which orders the RGB colour vectors. Each pixel from the mask defines one RGB vector. For each vector the distances to all of vectors from the mask are calculated and the sum of distances is computed as a cumulative distance. Finally, the output of the VMF filter is the RGB colour vector with a minimal cumulative distance. The Euclidean metric can be used for distance calculations.

The 3×3 mask of Kuwahara-Nagao filter is splitted into four 2×2 slightly overlapping windows with the masks central pixel as a common part. In original monochromatic version of this filter the variance of grey levels is calculated for each window, and the new grey level of the central pixel is equal to the average of grey

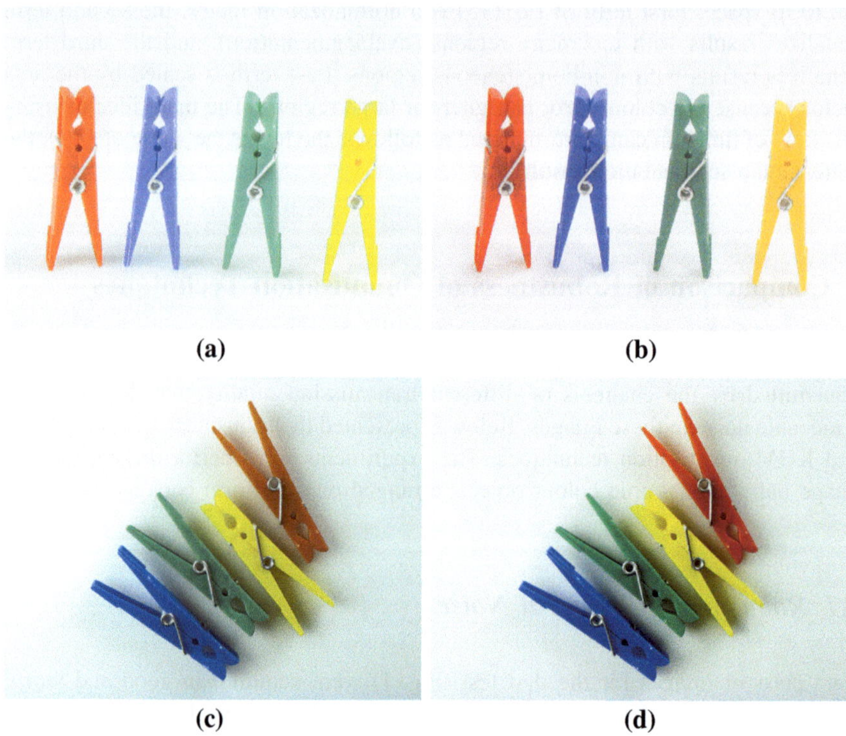

Fig. 1 Two pairs of test images: **a** good quality image, **b** noisy version of (**a**), **c** good quality image, **d** noisy version of (**c**)

Table 1 Properties of images from Fig. 1

Image	Unique colours	M	PSNR (dB)
Pair 1			
Image from Fig. 1a	47629	61.39	
Image from Fig. 1b (noisy)	73386	51.60	25.22
Pair 2			
Image from Fig. 1c	82160	58.44	
Image from Fig. 1d (noisy)	97913	63.07	27.96

levels in window with smallest variance. It is fairly straight-forward to extend this algorithm to the field of color images: for each window the covariance matrices with their Frobenius norms are calculated. The mean colour value of the window with minimal Frobenius norm is used as the output value of the central pixel.

Analysis of the data included in Tables 2 and 3 shows that the KHM technique gives better results, both for images with natural noise and their filtered versions. The information in Table 4 indicates that the quality indexes for KHM are more invariable than in the case of KM.

Table 2 Image quality indexes for the first pair of images

Image	PSNR (dB)	ΔE	ΔM
Image from Fig. 1a			
Image after KM	30.95	2.34	0.97
Image after KHM	31.61	2.17	0.76
Image from Fig. 1b (noisy)			
Image after KM	30.36	2.85	1.60
Image after KHM	31.39	2.68	1.08
Image from Fig. 1b (noisy) after VMF filtration			
Image after KM	31.06	2.34	1.35
Image after KHM	32.61	2.23	0.65
Image from Fig. 1b (noisy) after Kuwahara-Nagao filtration			
Image after KM	29.89	3.93	2.16
Image after KHM	32.10	2.09	0.76

Table 3 Image quality indexes for the second pair of images

Image	PSNR	ΔE	ΔM
Image from Fig. 1c			
Image after KM	25.55	6.85	5.81
Image after KHM	27.32	4.78	3.00
Image from Fig. 1d (noisy)			
Image after KM	23.46	8.82	8.80
Image after KHM	26.53	5.26	3.30
Image from Fig. 1d (noisy) after VMF filtration			
Image after KM	23.83	8.55	8.39
Image after KHM	26.88	4.94	3.11
Image from Fig. 1d (noisy) after Kuwahara-Nagao filtration			
Image after KM	24.53	7.81	7.22
Image after KHM	26.74	5.04	3.21

Table 4 Range of variability of image quality indexes

Quantisation technique	PSNR variability	ΔE variability	ΔM variability
Pair 1			
KM	1.17	1.59	1.19
KHM	1.22	0.59	0.43
Pair 2			
KM	2.09	1.97	2.99
KHM	0.79	0.48	0.30

4.2 Robustness to Noisy Pixels of Outlier Colours

For many data clustering techniques, which include KM and KHM techniques, a sensitivity to outlying points called *outliers*, is typical. In our case, the *outliers* are the outlier colours. The results of the clustering should not depend on these few points that are far away from the centres of clusters.

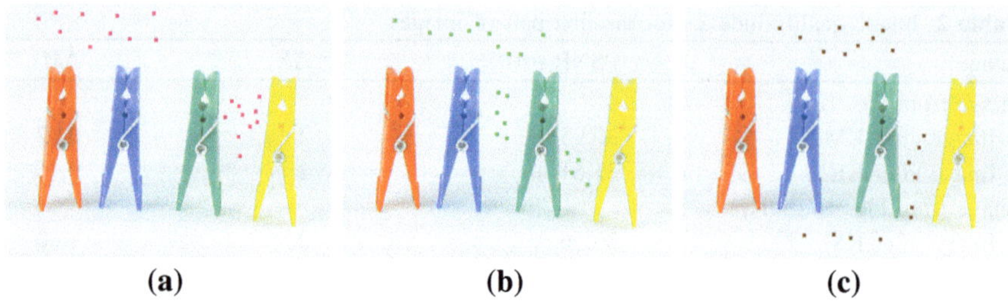

Fig. 2 Images corrupted by 2000 pixels of outlier colours: **a** (255, 0, 128); **b** (0, 255, 0); **c** (128, 64, 0)

Table 5 The values of the image quality indexes for images with pixels of outlier colours

Image	PSNR	ΔE	ΔM
Image 1(a) corrupted by 2000 pixels (255,0,128)			
Image after KM	29.69	2.64	1.60
Image after KHM	30.57	2.42	1.53
Image 1(a) corrupted by 2000 pixels (0,255,0)			
Image after KM	25.88	4.91	5.24
Image after KHM	30.82	2.41	0.95
Image 1(a) corrupted by 2000 pixels (128,64,0)			
Image after KM	29.24	3.90	2.16
Image after KHM	30.94	2.28	1.11

Table 6 Ranges of variability of image quality indexes for 3 images with pixels of outlier colours

	PSNR variability	ΔE variability	ΔM variability
KM	3.81	2.27	3.64
KHM	0.37	0.14	0.58

In order to check the robustness of both quantisation techniques to outlier colours were created images contaminated by noisy pixels with outlier colours. To the output image, i.e. the first image of the first image pair in the previous subsection, was introduced 2000 such pixels (Fig. 2). *Outliers* in one case were the purple pixels ($R = 255, G = 0, B = 128$), in the other case: the green pixels ($R = 0, G = 255, B = 0$) and in yet another case: the brown pixels ($R = 128, G = 64, B = 0$).

So corrupted images were subjected to the colour quantisation by both KM and KHM techniques. The results obtained for each of the corrupted images are shown in Table 5 and ranges of variability of image quality indexes for these images are contained in Table 6. The results of KM and KHM techniques for image Fig. 2b shows Fig. 3. Two extreme objects in Fig. 3a are the same colour (pixels in one cluster) different from the colours in original image. Therefore, it is possible to see the advantage of KHM, which is also confirmed by the values of quality indexes.

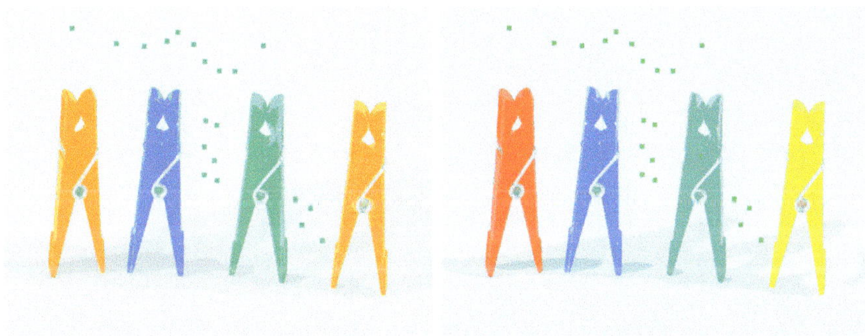

(a) (b)

Fig. 3 The quantisation results for image from Fig. 2b $k = 10$: **a** KM; **b** KHM

Analysis of the results contained in both the above tables shows that the KHM technique is much more robust to the presence of outlier colours in the images than the KM technique.

4.3 Robustness to Additional Impulsive Noise

Our test images were additionally contaminated by impulsive achromatic noise and colour noise. Result for the noise intensity $p = 6\,\%$ presents Fig. 4. These noisy images were quantised into 10 colours. Examples of the results for the noise intensity $p = 10\,\%$ are shown in Fig. 5.

The results of KHM technique are visually much better than the images after the KM technique. This is confirmed also in most cases by the values of image quality indexes. Table 7 contains the results for the image from Fig. 1a contaminated by achromatic "salt and pepper" noise, while Table 8 presents the results of the same image corrupted by impulsive colour noise. Table 9 presents the results for the image from Fig. 1c contaminated by achromatic "salt and pepper" noise, while Table 10 presents the results of the same image corrupted by impulsive colour noise.

Table 11 shows the values of image quality indexes for the image from Fig. 1a contaminated by impulsive colour noise, filtered by VMF filter and quantised by KM and KHM techniques. Table 12 presents the same data for the image from Fig. 1c. Again, the results for the KHM technique are clearly better than the results for KM technique.

The advantage of KHM technique over KM technique, expressed by the three indexes of image quality, is clearly visible if the images contain a natural noise or are corrupted by outlying pixels. If the images are corrupted by achromatic "salt and pepper" noise then KHM technique also gives better results than KM for both a visual evaluation and evaluation based on using quality indexes. In the case of

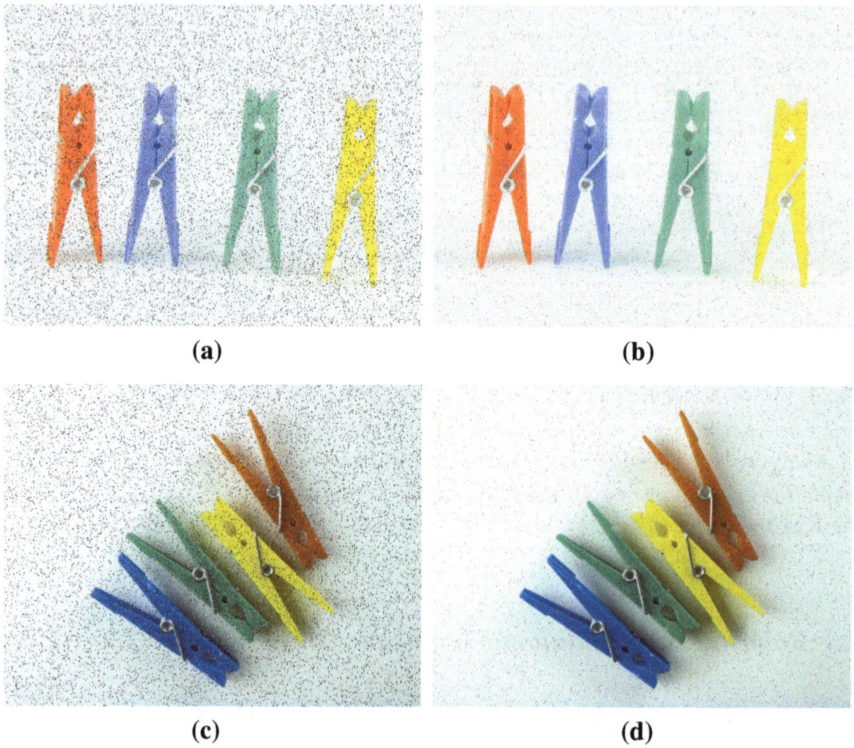

Fig. 4 Test images contaminated by impulsive noise, $p = 6\,\%$: **a**, **c** achromatic noise; **b**, **d** colour noise

colour impulsive noise, for ΔM index the situation is not entirely clear. However, after the VMF filtration the evaluation based on ΔM index is again better for the KHM technique. Other indexes give an advantage of KHM over KM technique.

5 Quantisation Before Image Segmentation

Preliminary tests were carried out on five images with relatively easy defined number of output colours. We assumed the number of clusters $k = 25$ for test image *Chart* (Fig. 6a), $k = 20$ for test image *DNA* (Fig. 6d) and $k = 10$ for other test images (Fig. 6b, c, e). In all cases the quantisation process used 15 iterations. The following parameter values were applied in the USRG segmentation technique: for image *Chart-d* $= 25$, $A = 1000$, for image *Objects-d* $= 25$, $A = 1000$, for image *Book-d* $= 25$, $A = 10$, for image *DNA-d* $= 10$, $A = 500$ and for image *Eye-d* $= 20$, $A = 100$.

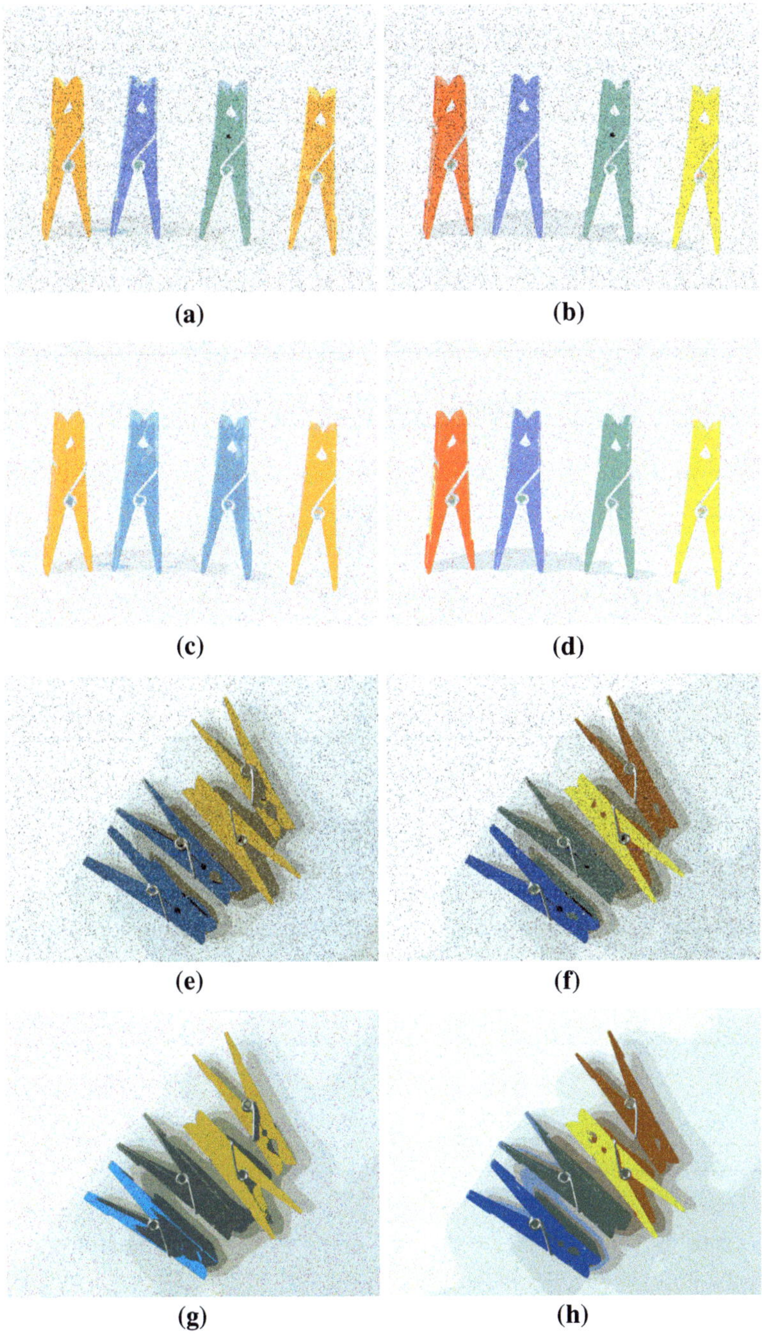

Fig. 5 The results of quantisation into 10 colours for images corrupted by noise $p = 10\,\%$: **a**, **e** KM, achromatic noise, **c**, **g** KM, colour noise, **b**, **f** KHM, achromatic noise, **d**, **h** KHM, colour noise

Table 7 Image quality indexes for the image from Fig. 1a in the presence of achromatic "salt and pepper" noise after KM and KHM quantisation

Noise (%)	PSNR		ΔE		ΔM	
	KM	KHM	KM	KHM	KM	KHM
$p = 2$	20.16	20.40	4.61	3.67	2.71	1.50
$p = 6$	15.55	15.87	7.48	5.48	6.05	3.08
$p = 10$	13.51	13.69	9.47	7.39	7.51	4.38
$p = 20$	10.64	10.69	12.90	12.82	7.45	7.49

Table 8 Image quality indexes for the image from Fig. 1a in the presence of impulsive colour noise after KM and KHM quantisation

Noise (%)	PSNR		ΔE		ΔM	
	KM	KHM	KM	KHM	KM	KHM
$p = 2$	23.41	26.28	5.47	3.14	0.79	0.98
$p = 6$	20.22	20.39	7.10	5.05	7.52	12.17
$p = 10$	17.91	18.45	10.08	6.72	15.51	19.20
$p = 20$	15.38	15.56	12.63	11.16	35.21	35.46

Table 9 Image quality indexes for the image from Fig. 1c in the presence of achromatic "salt and pepper" noise after KM and KHM quantisation

Noise (%)	PSNR		ΔE		ΔM	
	KM	KHM	KM	KHM	KM	KHM
$p = 2$	21.28	20.41	7.71	5.98	7.30	3.92
$p = 6$	15.82	16.14	10.21	7.90	7.90	4.91
$p = 10$	13.78	14.01	12.11	9.88	8.63	6.12
$p = 20$	10.98	11.09	16.19	14.88	11.20	8.96

Table 10 Image quality indexes for the image from Fig. 1c in the presence of impulsive colour noise after KM and KHM quantisation

Noise (%)	PSNR		ΔE		ΔM	
	KM	KHM	KM	KHM	KM	KHM
$p = 2$	23.54	24.17	7.07	5.40	3.15	1.51
$p = 6$	19.36	21.09	8.99	6.72	5.80	1.60
$p = 10$	17.74	20.04	11.24	7.87	12.46	3.82
$p = 20$	16.16	15.76	15.12	13.25	15.98	32.67

The data in Table 13 shows that not every method of colour quantisation, carried out as preprocessing step in the process of segmentation, leads to improved segmentation result. Good example is a case of IV technique: all $Q(I)$ values are higher than $Q(I)$ for segmentation without quantisation. A much better impact on the segmentation have the Wu's algorithm. The KHM technique reduces the values of $Q(I)$ index but the KM technique, on the contrary, can in some cases

Table 11 Image quality indexes for the image from Fig. 1a in the presence of impulsive colour noise after VMF filtration and KM and KHM quantisation

Noise (%)	PSNR		ΔE		ΔM	
	KM	KHM	KM	KHM	KM	KHM
$p = 2$	25.48	27.19	6.86	4.79	5.81	2.76
$p = 6$	25.38	27.05	6.89	4.82	5.90	2.93
$p = 10$	25.32	26.95	6.87	4.79	5.99	2.80
$p = 20$	24.56	25.88	6.98	4.96	6.17	3.40

Table 12 Image quality indexes for the image from Fig. 1c in the presence of impulsive colour noise after VMF filtration and KM and KHM quantisation

Noise (%)	PSNR		ΔE		ΔM	
	KM	KHM	KM	KHM	KM	KHM
$p = 2$	25.50	27.21	6.86	4.80	5.80	2.82
$p = 6$	25.48	27.19	6.86	4.79	5.80	2.74
$p = 10$	25.45	27.14	6.85	4.81	5.68	2.82
$p = 20$	25.38	27.05	6.89	4.83	5.71	2.91

increase it significantly. All this means that poorly quantised images badly affect the final result of segmentation.

It is easy to see that the usefulness of colour quantisation in segmentation process depends on the value of parameter k (number of clusters). Tables 14 and 15 show for two test images how, in the case of KHM, the number of clusters k affects the value of $Q(I)$. From these tables, one can see that for each of the tested images, there is a range of values of k which improves the image segmentation by initial colour quantisation.

6 Conclusions

We proposed and preliminary tested an idea to use initial colour quantisation as preprocessing step for colour image segmentation. The performance of segmentation can be limited by the quality of colour quantisation. Poorly quantised image badly affects the final result of image segmentation. Therefore, our approach needs a good quantisation technique, e.g. researched segmentation technique works better for KHM quantisation technique than KM technique, e.g. It is also important to properly select the size of the palette to the quantised image. Better quantisation techniques such as human-based colour quantisation or techniques that do not need a priori the number of final colours may further improve the usefulness of quantisation before segmentation.

It has long been known that the significant reduction of the number of image colours before segmentation simplifies and accelerates the execution of this

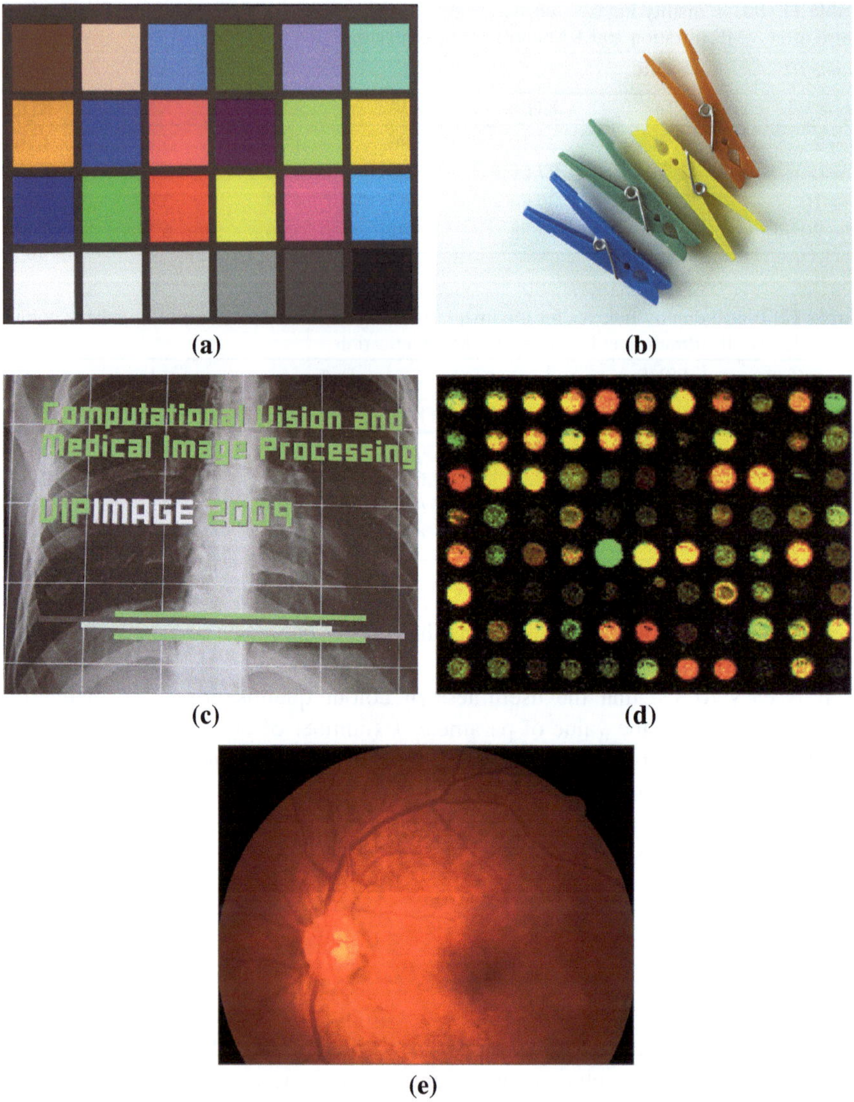

Fig. 6 Test images used in the experiment: **a** *Chart*, **b** *Objects*, **c** *Book*, **d** *DNA*, **e** *Eye*

Table 13 $Q(I)$ indexes for tested images

Image	*USRG*	*IV + USRG*	*Wu + USRG*	*KM + USRG*	*KHM + USRG*
Chart	617	823	759	959	**478**
Objects	998	8139	1204	650	**409**
Book	387	477	415	463	**348**
DNA	4647	8592	**881**	944	2628
Eye	613	1325	397	386	**287**

Table 14 Dependence of $Q(I)$ on assumed number of clusters

Chart, k =	10	15	20	25	30	35	40	45
USRG	617							
KHM + USRG	2312	839	**467**	**478**	**445**	682	756	725

Table 15 Dependence of $Q(I)$ on assumed number of clusters

Objects, k =	5	8	10	15	20	25	30	35
USRG	998							
KHM + USRG	2142	**637**	**409**	1506	1608	1504	721	1183

difficult operation. In this chapter we searched for the conditions of additional improvement in image segmentation preceded by a colour quantisation. The further research will be focused on establishing the conditions and parameters of the tested approach.

Our study uses different images acquired from relatively simple scenes without significant highlights and shadows. For more complex images the results will not be so good. Therefore, an interesting question is what kind of colour images need to be quantised before the segmentation. Perhaps the estimation of image segmentation difficulty will help answer this question [14].

Acknowledgments This work was supported by Polish Ministry for Science and Higher Education under internal grant BK-/RAu1/2012 for Institute of Automatic Control, Silesian University of Technology, Gliwice, Poland.

References

1. Astola J, Haavisto P, Neuvo Y (1990) Vector median filters. Proc IEEE 78(4):678–689
2. Borsotti M, Campadelli P, Schettini R (1998) Quantitative evaluation of color image segmentation results. Pattern Recognit Lett 19(8):741–747
3. Celebi ME, Aslandogan YA, Bergstresser PR (2005) Unsupervised border detection of skin lesion images. In: international conference on information technology, vol 2. pp 123–128
4. Chen KM, Chen SY (2002) Color texture segmentation using feature distributions. Pattern Recognit Lett 23(7):755–771
5. Deng Y, Manjunath B (2001) Unsupervised segmentation of color-texture regions in images and video. IEEE Trans Pattern Anal Mach Intell 23(8):800–810
6. Deng Y, Kenney C, Moore MS, Manjunath BS (1999) Peer group filtering and perceptual color image quantization. In: Proceeding IEEE international symposium on circuits and systems ISCAS '99, vol 4, pp 21–24
7. Dong G, Xie M (2005) Color clustering and learning for image segmentation based on neural networks. IEEE Trans Neural Netw 16:925–936
8. Frackiewicz M, Palus H (2011) KM and KHM clustering techniques for colour image quantisation. In: Tavares JMRS, Jorge RMN (eds) Computational vision and Medical image processing. Springer, Netherlands, pp 161–174

9. Hasler D, Suesstrunk S (2003) Measuring colourfulness for natural images. In: Proceedings of SPIE electronic imaging 2003: human vision and electronic imaging VIII, vol 5007, pp 87–95
10. Ilea DE, Whelan PF (2008) Ctex—an adaptive unsupervised segmentation algorithm based on color-texture coherence. IEEE Trans Image Process 17(10):1926–1939
11. Krinidis M, Pitas I (2009) Color texture segmentation based on the modal energy of deformable surfaces. IEEE Trans Image Process 18(7):1613–1622
12. Kuwahara M, Hachimura K, Eiho S, Kinoshita M (1976) Digital processing of biomedical images, chap. In: Processing of ri-angiocardiographic images, Plenum Press, pp 187–202
13. Lai AN, Park K, Kumar M, Lee G (2009) Korean text extraction by local color quantization and k-means clustering in natural scene. In: Proceedings of the 2009 First Asian conference on intelligent information and database systems. IEEE Computer Society, Washington, DC, USA, pp 138–143
14. Liu D, Xiong Y, Pulli K, Shapiro L (2011) Estimating image segmentation difficulty. In: Proceedings of 7th international conference on machine learning and data mining, MLDM'11. Springer-Verlag, Berlin, Heidelberg, pp 484–495
15. Lo C, Chen S (1999) Image classification using cellular color decomposition. In: Proceedings of IPPR conference on computer vision, graphics, and image processing, vol 2. Taipei, Taiwan, pp 681–688
16. MacQueen JB (1967) Some methods for classification and analysis of multivariate observations. In: Cam LML, Neyman J (eds) Proceedings of the fifth Berkeley symposium on mathematical statistics and probability, vol 1. University of California Press, University Berkeley and Los Angeles, CA, USA, pp 281–297
17. Nagao M, Matsuyama T (1979) Edge preserving smoothing. Comput Graph Image Process 9(4):394–407
18. Nikolaou N, Papamarkos N (2009) Color reduction for complex document images. Int J Imaging Syst Technol 19(1):14–26
19. Palus H (2004) On color image quantization by the k-means algorithm. In: Droege D, Paulus D (eds) Proceedings of 10 workshop Farbbildverarbeitung. Germany, pp 58–65
20. Palus H (2006) Color image segmentation: selected techniques. In: Lukac R, Plataniotis K (eds) Color image processing: methods and applications. CRC Press, Boca Raton, pp 103–108
21. Smith M (2008) Unsupervised object-based video segmentation using color, texture and motion. Ph.D. thesis, Southern Methodist University, Dallas, TX, USA
22. Wang Y, Yang J, Peng N (2006) Unsupervised color-texture segmentation based on soft criterion with adaptive mean-shift clustering. Pattern Recognit Lett 27(5):386–392
23. Wang YG, Yang J, Chang YC (2006) Color-texture image segmentation by integrating directional operators into JSEG method. Pattern Recognit Lett 27(16):1983–1990
24. Weng SK, Kuo CM, Kang WC (2005) Unsupervised texture segmentation using color quantization and color feature distributions. In: Proceedings IEEE International Conference Image Processing ICIP 2005, vol 3. Genoa, Italy, pp 1136–1139
25. Yu Z, Au OC, Zou R, Yu W, Tian J (2010) An adaptive unsupervised approach toward pixel clustering and color image segmentation. Pattern Recognit 43:1889–1906
26. Zhang B (2000) Generalized k-harmonic means—boosting in unsupervised learning. Technical Report, TR HPL-2000-137, Hewlett Packard Labs, Palo Alto, CA, USA
27. Zhong Y, Karu K, Jain AK (1995) Locating text in complex color images. Pattern Recognit 28(10):1523–1535

Medical Imaging and Computational Flow Models in Deformable Ducts

Marc Thiriet

1 Introduction

Fluids, especially physiological fluids, either incompressible such as blood or compressible such as air, can flow through strongly deformed vessels in certain circumstances. In particular, veins and intrathoracic segments of the respiratory tract can collapse when they experience strong external pressure. In addition, the digestive tract launches an active peristaltism, i.e., unidirectional waves of radially symmetrical contraction and relaxation of mural smooth muscles, to propel nutrients to destination. However, the present chapter focuses on passive deformations due to changes in transmural pressure, i.e., the difference between the external and internal pressure ($p = p_{\rm i} - p_{\rm e}$). Usually, the distribution of the external pressure is supposed to be uniform, whereas the non-linear distribution of the internal pressure is given by the flow in an entrance segment of the deformed pipe.

Medical imaging techniques are used to build computational meshes or to non-invasively yield in vivo validation of measurements. The present chapter thus briefly introduce the major medical imaging techniques and various methods of three-dimensional reconstruction and meshing before giving 2 examples devoted on flows in collapsible tubes. The first example illustrates image-based flow simulations; the second provides non-invasive estimation of flow quantities for comparison with numerical and experimental data in simple and representative flow models.

M. Thiriet (✉)
INRIA Rocquencourt-BP 105, 78153 Le Chesnay Cedex, France
e-mail: marc.thiriet@inria.fr

J. M. R. S. Tavares and R. M. Natal Jorge (eds.), *Topics in Medical Image Processing and Computational Vision*, Lecture Notes in Computational Vision and Biomechanics 8,
DOI: 10.1007/978-94-007-0726-9_8,

1.1 Medical Imaging Techniques

Computerized medical imaging provides subject-dependent 3D geometry of any body organ. Medical images of the human body mainly display the body in three main planes: (1) coronal planes which divide the body into front and back regions; (2) sagittal planes which separate the body into left and right parts; and (3) transverse planes, perpendicular to the body axis, which split the body into upper and lower domains.

Since the end of the last century, numerical simulations are carried out in computational domains based on imaging data after 3D reconstruction. Input data for the surface reconstruction of the target body's compartment come from X-ray computed tomography (CT) [1–3], nuclear magnetic resonance imaging [4–7], or 3D ultrasonography [8].

Computed tomography (CT) scans regions of interest of the human body. To enhance vascular anatomy, an intravenous injection of a radio-opaque solution can be made prior to or during the scan (computed angiography [CA]). In spiral CT (SCT), or helical CT (HCT), data acquisition is combined with a continuous motion of the acquisition system. This procedure image entire anatomical regions in a 20- to 30-s apnea, hence reducing motion artifacts. Body's organs are then reconstructed to get external surface displays as well as virtual endoscopies of hollow organs and anatomical ducts. Multi-slice spiral CT (MSSCT) acquires many slices in a single rotation. Sixteen-slice MSSCT has high spatial resolution and reduces examination time. On the other hand, electron beam CT (EBCT) that does not use motion of the X-ray source allows very quick scanning in 50–100 ms [9]. Features of these main CTs are summarized in Tables 1, 2, and 3.

Nuclear magnetic resonance imaging (MRI) uses magnetic fields and radio-frequency waves to stimulate hydrogen nuclei in selected regions of the body that emit radio waves. The emerging signals have frequency, amplitude, and phase components that are processed to construct images of the human body. Magnetic field gradients are introduced to determine the spatial location of re-emitted microwaves. Frequency and timing characteristics of excitation pulses are modified to image particular types of molecules and motions. Magnetic resonance angiography (MRA) focuses on blood vessels without necessarily using any contrast material [10]. Functional MRI (FMR) explores the function of strongly moving and deformable organs such as the myocardium [11]. High-performance

Table 1 Main features [(size (mm) and time] of computed tomography

	SCT	MSSCT	EBCT
Slice thickness	10	$1.5 \rightarrow 0.6$	8
Between-slice thickness		30–50 % Overlapping	Pair gap of 4, contiguous dual slicing
Scanning acquisition time (s)	≥ 160	20	8–12
Slice acquisition time (ms)			100

Table 2 Spatial resolution of X-ray scanners

CT	$\Delta x, \Delta y$ (mm)	Δz (mm)	Matrix	Slice number
MSSCT function mode	0.5	0.6	512 × 512	4
MSSCT volume mode	0.5	0.6	512 × 512	$\mathcal{O}(100)$
SS-EBCT	0.7	1.5–3	512 × 512	$\sim$100
MS-EBCT	1	8	360 × 360	2–8

Table 3 Temporal resolution of X-ray scanners

CT	Slice scan time (ms)	Temporal image number
MSSCT function mode	300	60
MSSCT volume mode	300	4
SS-EBCT	50	1
MS-EBCT	30	6–40

magnetic resonance imaging allows high resolution and quick image acquisition, which adequately delineate organs and thin-walled vessels. Phase-locking MRI can then be used to record the vasculature deformation at different phases of the cardiac cycle. Magnetic resonance tagging assesses soft tissue dynamics [12–16]. Diffusion tensor MRI (DTMRI) estimate the myofiber orientation in the cardiac wall [17]. Magnetic particle imaging (MPI) is another technique [18].

Ultrasound imaging (USI) involves US propagation through biological tissues where US are partially reflected at each acoustical interface on its path. The echoing waves are then interpreted to create anatomical images. The quality of echographic images depends on the: (1) axial (in the US propagation direction) and transverse resolution, (2) ultrasonic attenuation, and (3) echo dynamics. Because resulting images are associated with the interaction between US waves and tissues, the collected information can reveal the mechanical properties of the tissues through which US travel (compressibility and density). Ultrasound attenuation by diffusion and absorption can also yield additional data on tissue heterogeneity level at the wavelength scale and between-cell cohesion, respectively. Three-dimensional transthoracic and transesophageal echocardiographies are used for cardiac valve explorations. Intravascular ultrasound imaging (IVUS) is a catheter-based technique that provides real-time high resolution images of both the lumen and arterial wall of a vascular segment (axial and transverse resolutions are 80–100 and 200–250 μm, respectively; 30 images/s). Tissue-Doppler US is applied for tissue motion estimation using appropriate signal processing. Intravascular ultrasound palpography assesses the mechanical properties of the vessel wall using the deformation caused by intraluminal pressure [19]. Ultrasound ECG-triggered elastography can provide real-time strain data [20].

Nuclear medicine imaging (NMI) relies on radioactive tracers with short life time. Tagging molecules seek specific sites. The distribution within the body of the radioactive isotope provides information on irrigation and functions of the explored organ. This technique yields images with low resolution and a high amount of noise, due to necessary low-radiation doses. The two most common types of NMI are single photon emission computed tomography (SPECT) and positron emission tomography (PET). The former uses photon-emitting radiotracers, the latter radiotracers that produce positron-electron pairs. Data fusion with CT or MRI images couples physiologic activity to the underlying anatomy.

1.2 3D Reconstruction

Imaging devices provide non-invasively accurate and very large datasets of discrete information on explored organs. However, output data are usually not suitable for archiving and data processing, as well as for representing 3D geometry; polygonal models are largely preferred. This requirement for piecewise approximations of the domain boundaries is reinforced by numerical applications. Most of the current reconstruction algorithms convert the initial sampled data into surface triangulations. Surface simplification algorithms are aimed at finding a compromise between the minimal number of triangles and the preservation of the geometric accuracy of the surface model.

Mesh creation from imaging data relies on image segmentation and facetization. Automatic mesh generator must be able to cope with surfaces that are frequently full of gaps, overlaps, and other imperfections. Three main classes of 3D reconstruction algorithms can be defined. Slice connection algorithms work for a series of planar parallel sections of target organs. At first, a closed contour is extracted in each slice, then contours are connected to each other between each pair of adjacent slices [21, 22]. Marching-cube approaches extract an implicit surface from a 3D range image based on a "voxelhood" analysis. Delaunay tetrahedralization algorithms first generate 3D triangulations over a point cloud and then extract a bounded surface triangulation from this set of tetrahedra using suitable topological and geometrical criteria [23].

In some circumstances, the surface is reconstructed from a point set, which defines planar parallel contours of vessels. A triangulated surface is drawn between each pair of consecutive sections, ensuring that each point in a contour is connected to its closest point in the next contour. To fit up a surface on a set of contours amounts to constructing a volume enclosed by these contours. The global volume is considered as the union of independent pieces resulting from pair treatment. Consider a set of input points that define the vessel contours obtained by the level set method. After a cubic-spline fit of each contour associated with smoothing, a new node set can be defined by equally spaced points along the vessel contour. Then two successive slices are projected orthogonally to the local axis in a same plane and a 2D constrained Delaunay triangulation is built. The surface triangles are finally extracted by elevation of the two planes. The projection direction based on the set of intrinsic vessel axes gives a better slice-pair treatment than using a projection direction normal to the slice planes.

The marching cube algorithm is used in volume rendering to reconstruct an isosurface from a 3D field of values [24]. The space is subdivided into a series of cubes, or cells. Their matrices is defined by the set of voxel barycenters. Mean intensity values of voxels are assigned to the corresponding barycenters. The algorithm instructs to "march" through each of the cubes, testing the corner points and replacing the cube with an appropriate set of polygons, most often triangles. This step is done by inserting vertices at the cell edges using linear interpolation. The result formed by joining the vertices with facets is a piecewise surface that approximates the isosurface. The isosurface can be defined by the set of intersection points between the voxel mesh and a 3D implicit function, the value of which is given from image thresholding.

Level set methods track the evolution of fronts [25]. They exploit the link between moving fronts and equations from computational fluid equations [26]. This technique handles problems in which separating fronts develop, the existence of sharp corners and cusps, and topology changes, as well as simultaneously forward and backward moving fronts according to different sites.

Contour shape can be a priori known, as closed contour with a regular surface of a given region of the image. It can then be considered as an elastic contour in equilibrium under a set of forces. An average template mesh for the organ of interest undergoes elastic deformations to fit the image data [27].

Any tube can be placed in a cube that is subdivided into octants of length scale determined by the mesh size to suit the possible caliber changes of the explored vascular segment [28]. The octants containing the vessel walls are trimmed to match the wall surface with a given tolerance level. Smoothing can then be performed. The octants within the vessel are subdivided into tetrahedra.

Smooth implicit functions for 3D reconstruction have been associated with spectral/hp high order elements for blood flow computations [29]. The vessel edges are first detected, segmented, and smoothed using B-spline interpolation in each image of the slice set. The resulting contours are fitted by an implicit function defined as a linear combination of radial basis functions associated with the contour nodes and a set of interior constraint points along the normal direction to the spline at the corresponding nodes. An isosurface extraction leads to vessel surface triangulation using an implicit surface polygonizer. The vessel surface is then smoothed using a boundary representation of its edges and surfaces by spline curves and surfaces, preserving the main curvatures. Bicubic spline patches, which are interactively defined and projected onto the implicit surface, serve as the initial element for meshing [30]. Mesh size and shape optimization is determined by the eigenvalues of the Hessian matrix of the implicit function.

Snakes, or active closed contours defined within an image domain, can be used for image segmentation [31]. Snakes move under the influence of internal forces coming from the curve and external forces computed from image data. The functional to be minimized is analog to the deformation energy of an elastic material subjected to a loading. The properties of deformable snakes are specified by a potential associated with a contraction–expansion term by analogy to a mechanical thin heterogeneous membrane [32]. The internal and external forces are defined so that the snake will conform to an object boundary (image intensity gradient) within an image. The initial contour can be a small circle centered on a selected point. The iterative deformation of the initial curve in the force field can be done by convoluing gradient images to Gaussian-type functions and modeling the deformable curve by splines. The coefficient number of these splines rises during the iterations to progressively decrease the curve energy. An additional force has been proposed to deform the snakes avoiding to track spurious isolated edge points [32]. External force, like gradient vector flow, can be computed as a diffusion of the gradient vectors of a gray-level or binary edge map derived from the image [33]. A simplicial grid can be superimposed to the image domain and used to iteratively reparameterize the deforming snakes model. This procedure is able to adapt to complex shapes with significant protrusions or branches, and dynamically change topology [34].

Bioconduit modeling can be based on vessel-axis determination. Once the set of axes is known, a "response function" is computed for each vessel slice from a vector rotating around the axis point and the intensity gradient. The voxel positions for which the response function is maximum give the vessel contour in the investigated slices when the axis is correctly determined. Precisely approximated contours a posteriori confirm that the vessel axis was reasonably well estimated. Several techniques may be used for axis determination. The vessel contours can be detected by derivative operators. The eigenvalues of the Hessian matrix of the intensity can be computed; the eigenvalue that is the nearest to zero estimates the axis location [35]. Reconstruction of complex vessel trees can use a marking procedure to detect all the connected components of the lumen of the vessel network and set up a mark for each of them serving as a starting subset for high-order reconstruction. A suitable morphological filter is then needed. A morphological filter based on selective marking and depth constrained connection cost labels the vessel by binarization of the difference between original image and connection cost image [36]. An energy-based aggregation model is applied to the marking set with respect to voxel values. The marking set progressively grows by state change of boundary voxels, according to local minimization of an energy functional (Markov process-like method). The energy functional is composed of 3 propagation potentials, a potential associated with the pipe topography, another based on similar density for all ducts, and a limiting growth potential for bounded growth within lumen limits [36]. The state is determined with respect to the states of 26-connected adjoining voxels and their gray levels. The smoothing is adaptive according to vessel caliber based on adaptation of Gaussian kernel to size of labeled vessels. Vessel axis computation is based on geodesic front propagation with respect to a source point, the axis being defined by the set of centroids of successive fronts. The determination of the axis tree uses a geodesic front propagation combined to 3D distance map associated with vessel wall geometry, which allows space partitioning. This method provides robust branching point detection with axis hierarchy preservation [37].

Despite being efficient and robust, 3D reconstruction generally suffers several drawbacks. Discrete data may be very noisy, i.e., points do not belong to the surface. The dataset density that is not necessarily related to the local geometric complexity yields very large polygonal models. Reconstruction algorithms often introduce artefacts in the polygonal approximation, such as "staircase" effects. The element shape quality do not always fit requirements of numerical simulations. To overcome these problems, a 2-step integrated approach consists of first generating a simplified geometric surface mesh, possibly preceded by a surface smoothing stage, and then constructing a computational surface mesh by taking into account shape and size requirements for the mesh elements.

1.3 Meshing

Two main issues in mesh studies applied to numerical analysis are the surface mesh quality that must not significantly affect the problem solution, and algorithms associated with volumic meshes that are automatically generated [38–40]. The second work class focuses on mesh adaptation and adaptativity, including mesh refinement and coarsening, edge refinement and swapping, and node displacement, based either on metrics and error estimations independently of equation types [41, 42] or minimization of the hierarchical estimator norm [43–46].

Surface meshes must match strong requirements related to the accuracy of the surface approximation (geometry) and boundary conditioning as well as the computational element shape and size quality. Patches, such as B-splines and non-uniform rational basis spline (NURBS), that fit the facetization can be meshed. However, facetization can be directly processed. Determined corners and ridges define patches that are triangulated by an advancing front technique [1].

In any case, the first stage consists of simplifying the initial dense surface mesh to produce a geometric surface mesh. First, the initial reference mesh must be simplified to remove redundant elements while preserving the accuracy of the geometric approximation of the underlying surface. A simplification procedure based on the Hausdorff distance can thus be used. This algorithm involves vertex deletion, edge flipping, and node smoothing local mesh modifications. Often, especially for surface triangulations supplied by marching-cube algorithms, a smoothing stage based on a bi-Laplacian operator is required to remove the "staircase" artifacts [47]. This stage yields a geometric surface mesh that is a good approximation of the surface geometry and contains far fewer nodes than the initial reference mesh [48].

Surface discretization obtained from the 3D reconstruction needs further treatment to be suitable for numerical simulations. Boundary conditions must be set sufficiently far from the exploration volume, otherwise they affect the flow within the fluid domain. Moreover, any duct geometry change (curvature, branching, lumen narrowing or enlargement, wall cavity, taper, etc.) induces flow disturbances over a given length both upstream and downstream from it [49]. Consequently, short straight ducts in the direction of the local axis is connected to every vessel end. Furthermore, entry and exit sections must correspond to cross sections to assume an uniform pressure distribution in these sections.

Computational cell shapes and sizes must be controlled as they usually impact the accuracy of the numerical results. An anisotropic geometric metric map based on the local principal directions and radii of curvatures is constructed in tangent planes related to mesh vertices. This metric map prescribes element sizes proportional to the local curvature of the surface [50]. The metric map can also be combined with a computational metric map, e.g., supplied by an a posteriori error estimate, and eventually modified to account for a desired mesh gradation. Then, a surface mesh generation algorithm is governed by the metric map and based on local topological and geometrical mesh modifications. This approach can be easily extended to mesh adaptation as it already involves mixing geometric and computational metrics to govern the mesh generation stage.

1.4 Collapsible Tubes

Under positive transmural pressures, the tube cross-section is circular; the pressure force are balanced by tangential stresses. The deformed cross-section remains circular. The tube in its reference configuration is supposed to be stress free, in particular $p = 0$. Physiological vessels and their polymeric models more often have non-circular cross section. The unstressed (subscript 0) cross-sectional shape is commonly assumed to be elliptical (the tube ellipticity k_0 is the ratio between the major semi axis a_0 and the minor semi axis of the neutral wall mid-line in the unstressed tube configuration).

Once they are subjected to negative transmural pressures, deformable tubes collapse, i.e., experience changes in both cross-sectional area and shape, although locally the transmural pressure is uniformly distributed in the entire cross-section. The thinner the vessel wall, the easier the collapse. The set of conservation equations that govern fluid flow in deformable duct is closed by the relationships between the transmural pressure and the cross-sectional area A_i (state law). The fluid dynamics are indeed strongly coupled to the mechanics of the flexible vessel wall via the non-linear tube law $p(A_i)$ [51, 52]. The constitutive laws of involved materials depend on the microstructure.

The tube law depends strongly on both tube geometry (length, shape of the unstressed cross-section—circular or elliptical—, and in the latter case, tube ellipticity [k_0] [53], and wall thickness [h_0] [54]) and rheology in the unstressed state. When the unstressed cross-section is circular and the transmural pressure is slightly negative, the flexible duct keeps its circular cross-section down to the buckling pressure p_b. In other words, the compliant tube buckles under a slightly negative transmural pressure.

Three characteristic transmural pressures are of interest during the tube collapse: (1) the ovalisation pressure p_p, for which the wall cross curvature radius becomes locally infinite (i.e., at the material point $(0, b_0/k_0)$ thus causing an oval-shaped cross-section with parallel opposite edges; (2) the point-contact pressure

p_c, at which the opposite sides touch for the first time; (3) the line-contact pressure p_ℓ, the radius of curvature at the contact point being infinite.

Three modes of collapse are then distinguished. Mode 1 that corresponds to the collapse before wall contact ($p_c < p \leq 0$) is characterized by a high tube compliance, i.e., large variations in cross sectional area under small variations of transmural pressures. Mode 2 is defined by a contact set at the tube axis, when the opposite edges of the wetted perimeter touch ($p_\ell < p \leq p_c$); the curvature at the contact point decreases from a finite value down to zero with increasing loading. Mode 3 is defined by a contact on a line segment ($p \leq p_\ell$); the contact segment lengthens (the flat region of contact spreads laterally), whereas the transmural pressure continue to decrease. The lumen of any straight deformable vessel of unstressed elliptical cross-section is reduced to 2 parallel narrow tear-drop channels separated by the wall contact region.

Huge changes in tube transverse configuration for slightly negative transmural pressure occur in any compliant pipe, whether the unstressed cross-section is elliptical [53] or circular [55], whether the deformable vessel has a uniform homogeneous wall or is a composite material of non-uniform geometry [56], in vitro as well as in vivo [9], especially when its wall is thin and in the absence of stiff surrounding biological tissues.

The contact reactions induce discontinuities in the first $\partial A_i/\partial p\big|_{p_c}$ and second derivative $\partial^2 A_i/\partial p^2\big|_{p_\ell}$ [52, 57]. Such discontinuities affect probably the mechanical behavior of the fluid–tube couple. The discontinuity in the first derivative at p_c is exhibited by a break in the slope of the tube law [53]. Ultrasound imaging can be used to measure the cross-sectional area in experimental setup. A careful positioning of the probes is then required.

When the unstressed cross-section is circular, different modes of collapse can occur according to the number N of lobes (i.e., opened regions of the collapsed tube lumen, which are associated with symmetry axes; bifurcation problem). The buckling pressure is proportional to $N^2 - 1$ in computational shell models of deformation of tube of infinite length and purely elastic wall [58, 59]. The lobe number N depends on the tube geometry and rheology in its unstressed and deformed states. The cross-section shape usually displays 3 or 4 lobes either in tubes subjected to longitudinal bending effects [60] or in short and thin-walled pipes [55].

The tube collapse has been theoretically investigated in infinitely long straight tube with a thin homogeneous isotropic and purely elastic wall and with uniform geometry and rheology [53, 54, 58, 61]. The transmural pressure is supposed to be uniformly distributed in every tube section and bending effects are assumed to be predominant. The floppy duct is subjected to a uniform transmural pressure. The wall thickness, small relative to the wall mid-line curvature, is assumed to remain constant during the collapse. The neutral mid-surface is deformed without circumferential extension as checked experimentally [62]. The tube collapses then according to a bilobal collapsing mode, even in the presence of a very slight ellipticity (Fig. 1).

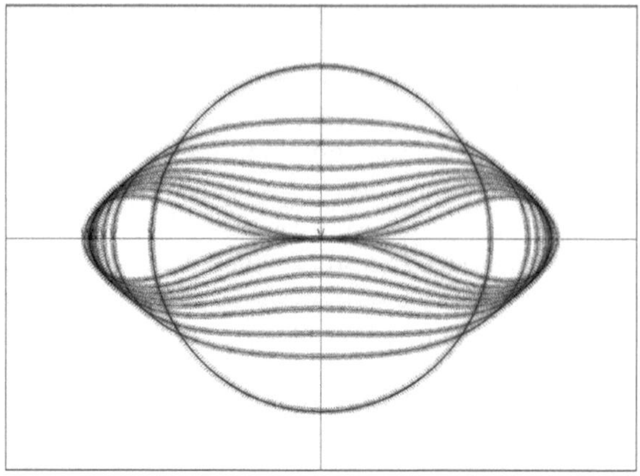

Fig. 1 Computational wall displacement during the collapse of a tube ($k_0 = 1.005, h_0 = 0$) with the following set of dimensionless quantities ($\tilde{p}, \tilde{A}_i$): (0, 1), (−1.60, 0.89), (−1.70, 0.79), (−1.85, 0.67), (−2.00, 0.57), (−2.15, 0.48), (−2.35, 0.38), ($p_c = -2.64$, 0.27), ($p_\ell = -5.20$, 0.21)

The tube deformation, from rest to the line-contact pressure p_ℓ, is illustrated in Fig. 2, using the dimensionless quantities $\tilde{p} = p/\mathtt{K}$ and $\tilde{A}_i = A_i/A_{i_0}$. The bending stiffness K, used as the pressure scale, depends on the tube geometry and is proportional to the flexural rigidity $\mathtt{D} = Eh_0^3/(12(1 - \nu_P^2))$: $\mathtt{K} = 2\mathtt{D}/a_0^3$, where E and ν_P are the Young modulus and the Poisson coefficient, respectively. The tube law is affected by the unstressed ellipticity (Fig. 2).

The speed (c) of the elasto-hydrodynamics coupling wave is computed from the tube law.[1] The speed of propagation of small pressure wave in a long straight collapsible tube containing an incompressible fluid of mass density ρ is assumed to be given by the Moens-Korteweg equation:

$$c^2 = (A_i/\rho)(\partial p/\partial A_i) \tag{1}$$

The pressure wave of small amplitude, which propagates with the speed c, depends thus on the fluid inertia and the wall compliance (transverse propagation mode). This simple relationship is valid under the following additional assumptions: (1) purely elastic thin wall and constant geometry along the whole tube length of the reference configuration and negligible wall inertia; and (2) one-dimensional motion of the fluid.

Experimental observations have shown that the wave speed reaches its minimum when a contact between the opposite walls occurs [52]. In the slightly negative range of transmural pressures, both the tube cross-sectional area and the high compliance entail a low wave speed associated to a high fluid velocity. Critical conditions (superscript ★) are reached when the local cross-sectional average fluid velocity ($U_q(\mathbf{x})$ becomes equal to the wave speed (Mach number Ma = 1).

[1] The speed scale $(\mathrm{K}/\rho)^{1/2}$ is used to calculate the dimensionless quantity $\tilde{c}$.

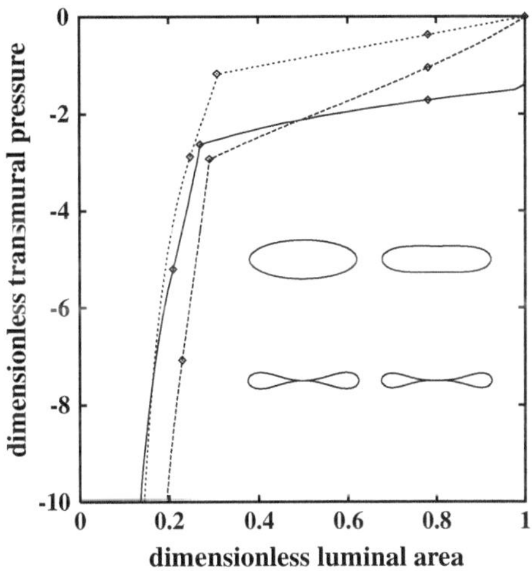

Fig. 2 Numerical $\tilde{p}(\tilde{A}_i)$ laws for three ellipticities in the unstressed state: $k_0 = 1,005$ (*continuous line*), 2.8 (*dashed line*), and 10 (*dotted line*), with the characteristic values ($\diamond$) corresponding to the displayed characteristic shapes in the bottom right region (unstressed elliptical, oval-shaped, and point- and line-contact cross-section from *left* to *right* and *top* to *bottom*)

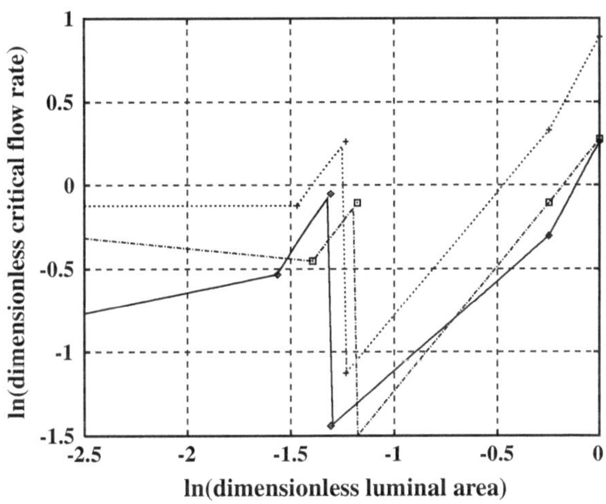

Fig. 3 Relationships between the cross-sectional area ($\ln(\tilde{A}_i)$) and the critical flow rate ($\ln(\tilde{q}^\star)$) for different tube ellipticities $k_0 = 1.005$ (*continuous line*), 2.8 (*dotted line*), and 10 (*dashed line*), with the following characteristic values ($\tilde{A}_{i0}$, $\tilde{A}_{ip}$, $\tilde{A}_{ic}$, $\tilde{A}_{i\ell}$). When $p \leq p_\ell$, both the value and the sign of the slope of the relationship are affected by the tube ellipticity

At each cross section can be associated a critical flow rate $q^\star$ that is related to the luminal area by $q^\star = A_i c$. Due to the discontinuity induced by the wall contact, the critical conditions are different on the right ($q^\star_{c+}$) and on the left ($q^\star_{c-}$) side of the discontinuity (Fig. 3).

2 Computational Exploration of a Three-Dimensional Steady Flow in a Strongly Collapsed Tube

A first example illustrate the use of imaging to build a computational mesh from experimental observations and, in particular, to assess the three-dimensional velocity field. When the transmural pressure is negative, the vessel collapses;

opposite walls can come into contact. As an illustration, the laminar, 3D, steady flow is computed in a rigid pipe, the configuration of which corresponds to a highly collapsed tube (frozen state) with wall contact (critical flow; Reynolds number calculated from the diameter and the cross-sectional average velocity in the inlet rigid tube of 1210).[2] The Navier-Stokes equations, associated to the classical boundary conditions, were solved using a finite element method.

2.1 Tube Configuration

A collapsible tube is attached on circular rigid tubes at both ends inside of a transparent box filled with water [63, 64]. The downstream part of the tube is connected to a constant-level reservoir via a rigid tube. Water supply is ensured by gravity forces from a constant-head tank. Thin-walled elastic tubes of elliptical unstressed cross-sections, have a density close to the water one.

The tube shape, in both axial and transverse planes, was designed from ultrasound echographic measurements in steady conditions on an actual Starling resistor. The thin-walled collapsible tube ($a_0 = 7.5$ mm, $k_0 = 1.2$, $h_0 = 0.3$ mm, $h_0/a_0 = 0.04$), attached to rigid pipes (internal diameter of 13.5 mm) was subjected to an initial lengthening of 1.5 %. The wall material was supposed to be incompressible (Poisson ratio 0.5). The elastic modulus was calculated with an indirect method [65]. The measured point-contact pressure $p_c = 90$ Pa and the theoretical normalized point-contact pressure for the geometrically defined compliant tube $\tilde{p}_c = -2.9$; therefore $K = 31$ Pa and $E = 2.2\,10^6$ N.m^{-2}.

The imaged stations that serve as input cross sections of known size of the geometrical domain were located at the following axial positions: $z = 210$, 300, 320, 340, 350, 356, 363, 370, and 377 mm. The digitized cross-sectional contours are compared to equivalent cross-section geometry derived from a theoretical model of an infinitely long flexible tube submitted to a negative transmural pressure [54]. The coordinates of points of the wetted perimeter are computed from the coordinates of the mid line and the corresponding angle between the local horizontal and tangent, knowing the wall thickness.

The entire tube (length 604.3 mm) is decomposed into 3 main segments (Fig. 4): (1) a set of 2 uniform circular entrance pipe in series (length 83.7 and 23.5 mm, radius 8.54 and 6.75 mm, respectively), the second short pipe representing the rigid attachment; (2) the collapsed tube (length 383 mm) that terminates on (3) a set of 2 uniform cylindrical pipes (length 30.4 and 83.7 mm, radius 6.75 and 8.54 mm, respectively), the first short pipe being the exit attachment.

[2] The critical state is defined by a localized throat near the tube outlet with a local speed equal to 20 times the entrance cross-sectional average velocity.

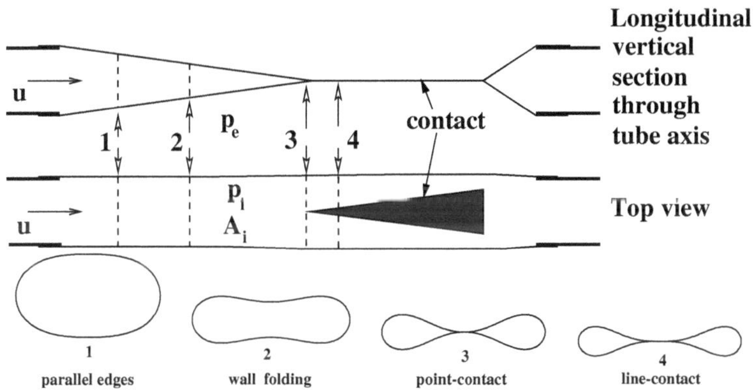

Fig. 4 Stationary collapse of a horizontal straight flexible tube attached at both ends to rigid circular ducts. The thin-walled tube has an unstressed elliptical cross section. The cross-sectional area and shape depend on the transmural pressure distribution, i.e. from the flow-dependent internal pressure field when the external pressure is uniform. A contact occurs between opposite walls; the tube lumen is then composed of 2 lobes in the present example. *Top* pipe axial configuration in the vertical centerplane. *Mid* upper tube face with the contact region (*dark area*). *Bottom* cross-sectional shape, before and after contact, are given for some labeled stations (1–4)

The collapsed tube is also subdivided in the streamwise direction into 3 successive segments: (1) a tapered segment (length 364.5 mm); (2) a contact zone (axial distance between the point-contact and the line-contact input cross sections of $\sim$7 mm (i.e., 1.16 % of the entire tube length or 1.83 % of the collapsed tube length); and (3) the downstream reopened segment (length 11.5 mm) attached to a circular uniform exit duct.

The contact zone is equivalent to a set of 2 symmetrical outward channels; the edge x coordinate increases and the lumen height decreases, whereas the central contact segment rises in length. The reopened segment is only partially divergent: whereas the top and bottom walls diverge, its edges are convergent.

Fourteen segments are defined in the test section: (1) 2 in the set of entry rigid pipes (T1 and T2); (2) 10 in the collapsed tube, T3 to T9 in the tapered segment, T10 the contact zone, T11 and T12 the reopened segment; and (3) 2 in the set of exit rigid conduits (T13 and T14). Each segment is bounded in the streamwise direction z by 2 input cross sections; the generatrices running axially along the tube wall are linearly interpolated lines between corresponding points of the cross-section walls.

2.2 Tube Mesh

Each input cross section quarter is meshed. The quarter of the wall is defined by the minimal number of nodes (15) to fit the original data (100 points). The segment regions in the planes $x = 0$ (plane normal to the centerplane at the tube axis) and

$y = 0$ (centerplane) and the segment wall are meshed using corresponding cross-section nodes. The 5 surfaces are then assembled to give the segment of interest. The 14 segments are merged to provide the whole quarter of the test section surface, the three-dimensional domain of which is then meshed using the software ghs3d [39]. The entire pipe is obtained by symmetry. The numbers of vertices and tetrahedra are equal to 15538 and 76484, respectively.

2.3 Computational Flow Model

The flow in the collapsed rigid straight tube is governed by the classical equations of fluid dynamics, i.e., mass and momentum conservation in a Cartesian reference frame. The body forces can be neglected. The fluid is homogeneous, incompressible, and Newtonian, with the water physical properties. The flow is supposed to be steady.

The variational formulation of the set of governing equations, associated with classical boundary conditions, were solved by a finite element method designed for unsteady flow. Hence, the time was used as an iterative parameter of the solution.

A variational formulation of the Navier-Stokes equations is used:

$$\frac{d}{dt}(\mathbf{u}, \mathbf{v}) + B(\mathbf{u}, \mathbf{v}) + T(\mathbf{u}; \mathbf{u}, \mathbf{v}) + B'(\mathbf{v}, p) = \langle l, \mathbf{v}, \rangle, \ \forall \mathbf{v} \in V \subset H^1(\Omega)^3 \quad (2)$$

$$B'(\mathbf{u}, q) = 0, \ \forall q \in Q \subset L^2(\Omega) \quad (3)$$

where $(\mathbf{u}, \mathbf{v})$ is the scalar product associated to the space $L^2(\Omega)$, B et B' are bilinear forms $(B(\mathbf{u}, \mathbf{v}) = \frac{1}{Re}\left[(\nabla \times \mathbf{u}, \nabla \times \mathbf{v})_{L^2(\Omega)} + (\nabla \cdot \mathbf{u}, \nabla \cdot \mathbf{v})_{L^2(\Omega)}\right]$ for the set of boundary conditions given in [66], $B' = -(\nabla \cdot \mathbf{v}, p))$, T is a trilinear form $(T(\mathbf{u}; \mathbf{u}, \mathbf{v}) = [(\mathbf{u} \cdot \nabla)\mathbf{u}] \cdot \mathbf{v})$, and $\langle l, \mathbf{v} \rangle$ the dual product. The functional space V is defined by:

$$V : \{\mathbf{v} \in H^1(\Omega)^3, \ \mathbf{v}|_{\Gamma_1} = 0, \mathbf{v}|_{\Gamma_2} = v_{z_{in}}, \ (\mathbf{v} \times \hat{\mathbf{n}})|_{\Gamma_3} = 0, \ p(\Gamma_3) = p|_{\Gamma_3}\},$$

$\{\Gamma_i\}_1^3$ being a partition of the boundary Γ of the fluid domain $\Omega : \Gamma_1$ is the wall on which the classical no-slip condition is applied, Γ_2 and Γ_3 are the flow inlet and outlet sections. The inlet boundary condition is a uniform injection velocity. The pressure is set equal to zero at the tube exit ($p|_{\Gamma_3} = 0$).

The pressure p is defined at the 4 vertices of the tetrahedron (P_1 element) and the velocity $\mathbf{u}$ at both the vertices and the barycenter (P_1 bubble element). The order of the method is $\mathcal{O}(\xi^2)$ for $\mathbf{u}$ and $\mathcal{O}(\xi)$ for p in the L^2 norm, ξ being the mesh step [67]. The convective term is approximated by the method of characteristics [68].

The computation is initialized as a potential flow. The solution is obtained via a generalized Uzawa-preconditioned-conjugate gradient method [69].

The convergence was supposed to be reached when the L^2 norm of the residuals of the flow quantities are divided at least by a factor 10^{-5}. It is usually obtained at a time lower than the duration of a characteristic path of 4 tube length, with the suitable time step.

2.4 Results

Usual modes of the velocity field representation are used: (1) velocity vector maps in selected planes; (2) isovelocity contours with a entire scale from zero speed to the maximal velocity ($1.4\ m \cdot s^{-1}$) for an entrance uniform velocity of $0.07\ m \cdot s^{-1}$ in the explored planes; and (3) streamlines either in the planes of interest or in the three-dimensional fluid domain. The flow velocity has thus been increased 20 times (critical situation). The investigated planes are (1) input and interpolated cross sections (planes $z = cst$, cross view); (2) planes $x = cst$ (side view) and $y = cst$ (top view) in the cartesian reference frame, from the symmetry plane to the wall.

Scans of the velocity field in a set of cross sections, from the middle part of the collapsed tube to the outlet rigid duct are given in Fig. 5. The flow is convectively accelerated in its proximal collapsed segment and decelerated in the reopened segment. In the reopened segment, 4 jets exiting from the side lobes of the contact zone, head for the top (bottom) wall and for the vertical symmetry plane $x = 0$, due to both the divergence of the opposite tube walls and convergence of the tube edges. In the reopened segment, secondary flows are totally different from those observed in symmetrical junctions, characterized by a rapid merge in side jets. In each quarter of cross section, twinned vortices appear. The outer swirl widen from the top (bottom) wall to the lateral wall from station $\tilde{z} = 0.811$ to $\tilde{z} = 0.822$, whereas the transverse near-axis vortex center gets a back-and-forth motion from the symmetry planes.

Scans of the velocity field in a set of planes normal to the centerplane $x = cst$ from the symmetry plane to the tube edge are given in Fig. 6 (isovelocity contours) and Fig. 7 (streamlines). The greater part of the side jet is observed in plane close to the tube edge. A saddle point takes place at the single point of contact upstream from the reopening of the flexible tube lumen. The flow separation region along the top (bottom) wall of the distal segment of the reopened segment cross the vertical symmetry plane and becomes larger near the tube edges. Upstream from it, another flow separation region develops both sides of the vertical mid plane in the proximal segment of the reopened segment. Eddies are located both sides of the centerplane and near the top and bottom walls in the entrance region of the rigid outlet duct near the vertical mid plane.

Scans of the velocity field in a set of planes parallel to the centerplane $y = cst$ from the symmetry plane to the tube edge are given in Fig. 8 (isovelocity contours)

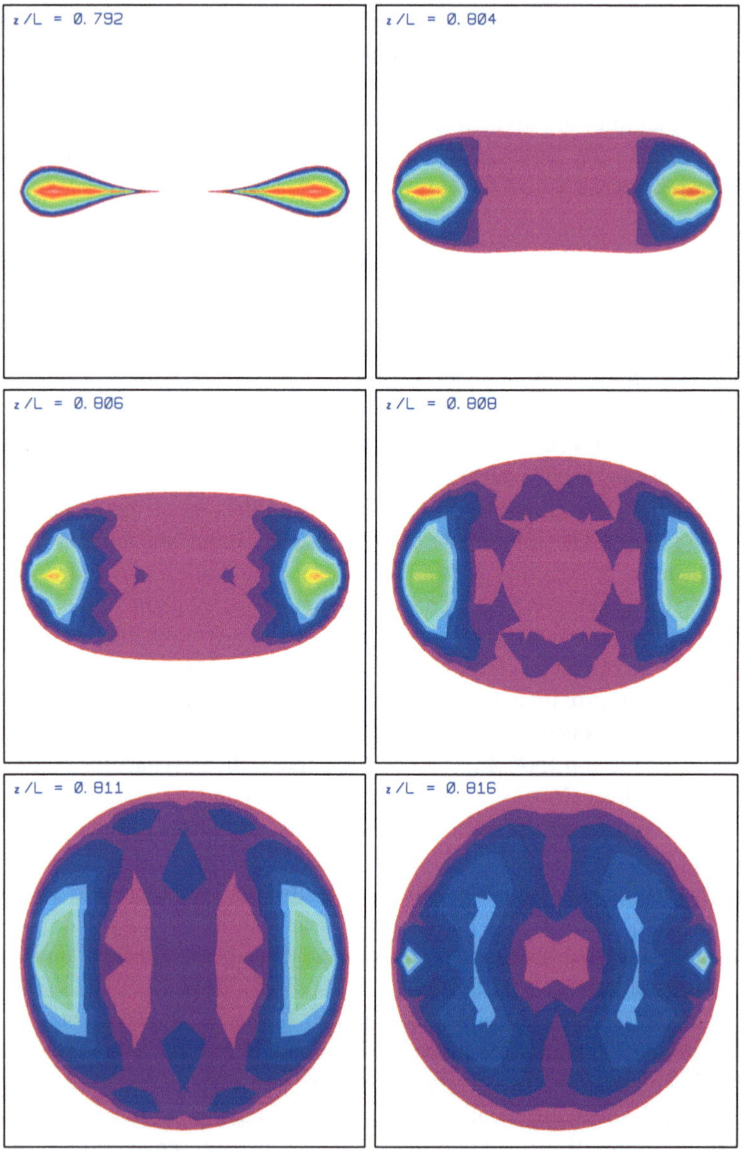

Fig. 5 Isovelocity contours of the transverse component in a set of cross sections downstream from the contact-point station (the dimensionless axial position is given in the figure and corresponds to S9, S10, the first and the second intermediate mesh section of T12, S11 and the first intermediate mesh section of T13, respectively)

and Fig. 9 (streamlines). The side jets are associated to flow separation regions at the edges of the rigid outlet duct, which becomes closer to the compliant tube exit in plane near the top and bottom walls than near the centerplane. In each top

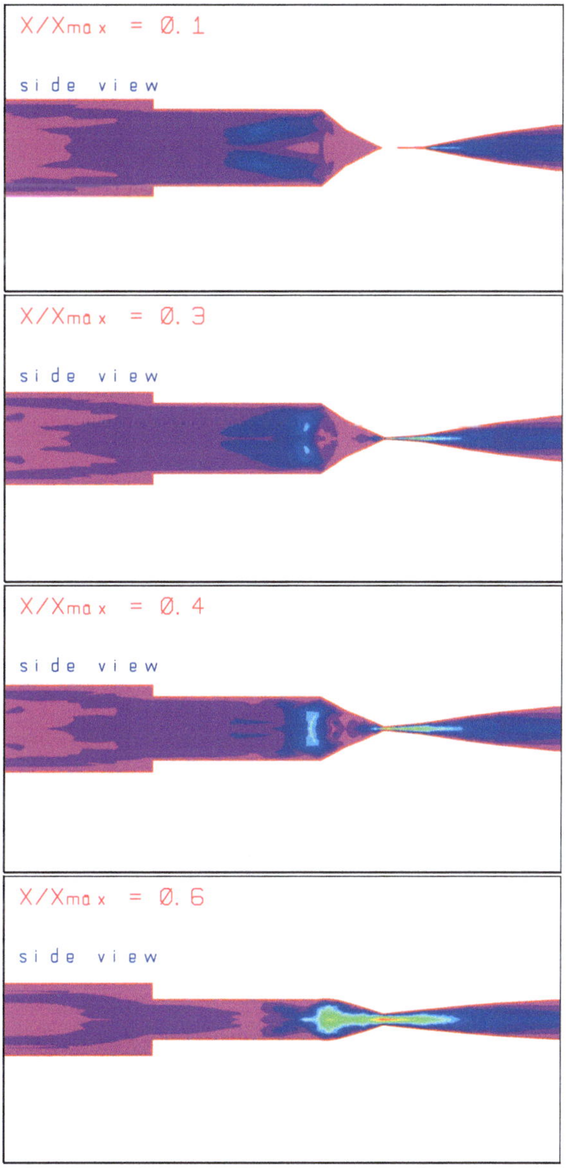

Fig. 6 Isovelocity contours in the set of sections normal to the centerplane of the collapsed tube and of the exit rigid ducts, downstream from the contact region (duct exit on the *left* side)

(bottom) half of the collapsed tube, 2 swirls occur behind the contact zone, the center of which is located in the entrance section of the rigid outlet duct.

Steady flow at very low Reynolds number was studied in a collapsing elastic tube = [70]. More or less collapse was observed according to the flow rate and external pressure values, without opposite wall contact. The streamlines of the cross flow in the collapsed segment upstream from the throat are similar to those in our model.

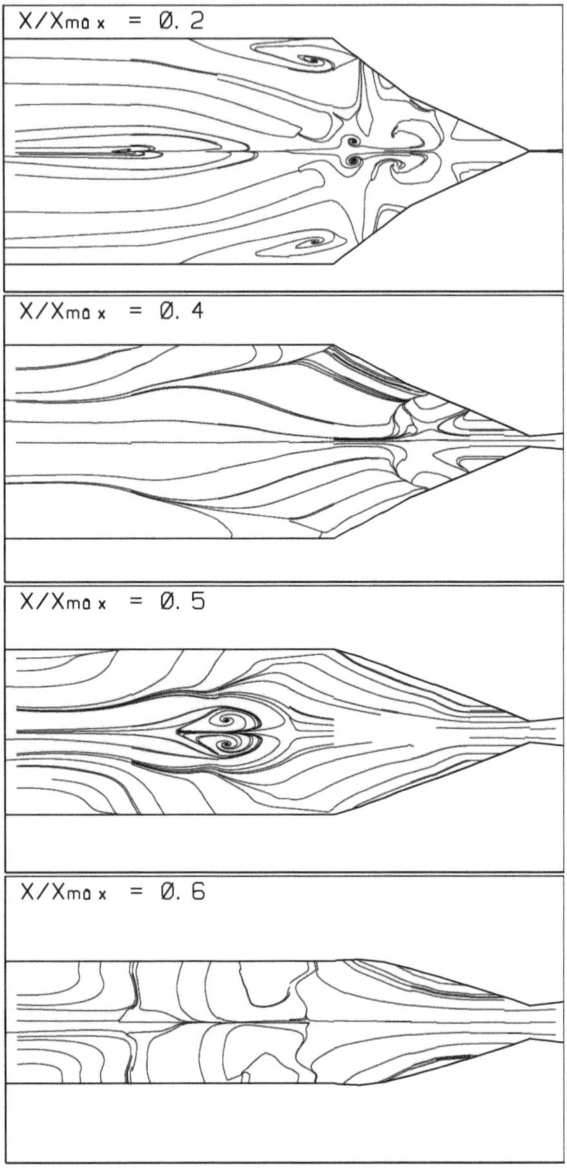

Fig. 7 *Streamlines* in 4 selected sections normal to the centerplane of the collapsed tube and of the exit rigid ducts, downstream from the contact region (duct exit on the *bottom*)

3 Image-Based Deformation of the Tracheobronchial Tree During Forced Expiration

A second example is given by an usual maneuver of lung function testing: forced expiration. This maneuver is characterized by a flow limitation that appears early. The strategy was typical of those currently adopted in physics. Simple and

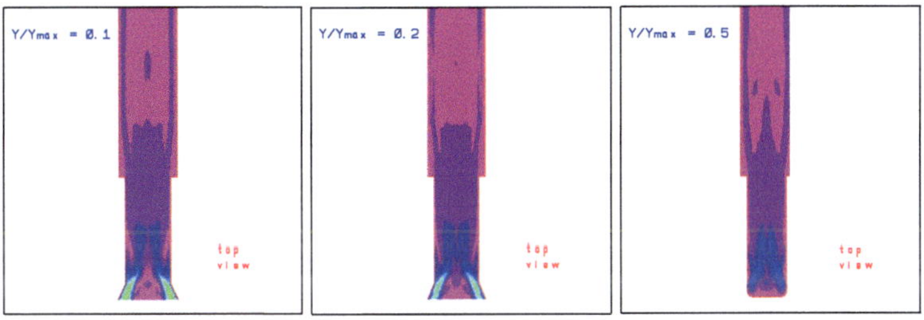

Fig. 8 Isovelocity contours in the set of sections parallel to the centerplane of the collapsed tube and of the exit rigid ducts, downstream from the contact region (upward streamwise direction)

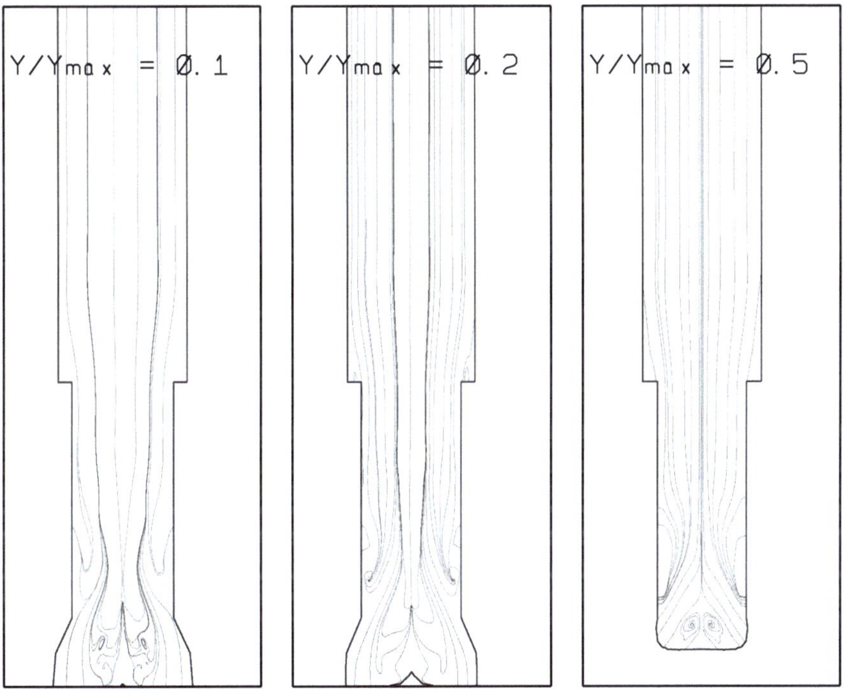

Fig. 9 *Streamlines* in 3 selected sections parallel to the centerplane of the collapsed tube and of the exit rigid ducts, downstream from the contact region

representative models of the complex reality are designed to understand underlying processes. Simplification is erroneous, but remains necessary to understand observation facts. In the present work, the three-dimensional feature of the flow caused by successive bends and airway branchings is neglected, whereas the airway deformability is emphasized to demonstrate the physical mechanisms responsible of the forced expiratory flow limitation. Measurements and numerical results in deformable mono- and bialveolar lung models made from tubes and

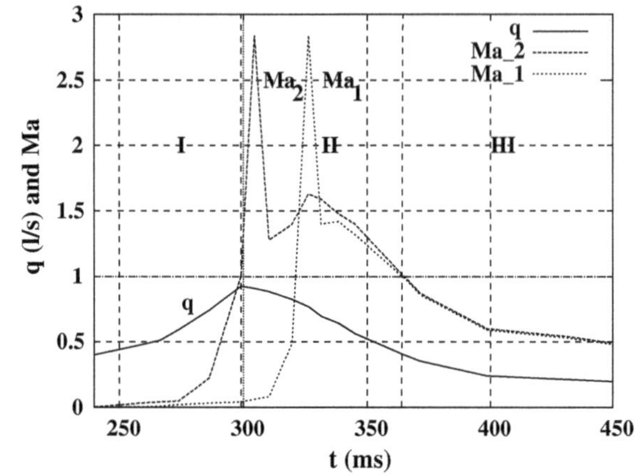

Fig. 10 Time variations of the volume flow rate q and of the Mach number computed at measuring stations of the upstream (index 1) and downstream (index 2) transmural pressure p in a monoalveolar compliant model. Three phases are defined: phase I of flow acceleration, II of wave-speed flow limitation, and III of viscous flow limitation in a strongly collapsed tube

balloons in series in unsteady conditions[3] demonstrate the occurrence of a transient trans- and supercritical flow simultaneously with the peak flow and at the beginning of the decelerating phase [71, 72]. A flow-limiting section (Mach number 1) appears near the exit of the tube from the pressurized chamber (Fig. 10).[4] The flow-limiting site then travel upstream with the airway collapse. Here, this example is given to show the non-invasive support given by medical imaging to validate numerical and experimental results obtained in a simple and representative model.

Spirometry is a procedure aimed at quantifying both air volumes and flow rates at given times during normal and deep breathing. Forced expiration corresponds to the quickest possible exhalation starting from the maximal lung volume (total lung capacity) down to the minimal lung volume (residual capacity). It is mainly used to separate obstructive lung diseases (decreased flow rates in a higher amount than reduced volumes) from restrictive pulmonary pathologies (same lowering rate of volumes and flow rates).

During a forced expiration, the trachea conveys a highly unsteady flow generated by the respiratory pump. Both in normal subjects and in patients with lung disease, the expiratory flow becomes limited. An early peak flow is reached (50–200 ms after the test onset) [9]. The flow limitation takes place although the

[3] Unsteadiness in collapsible tube flow can arise from occurrence of self-excited oscillations, although the flow is steady. This section is, however, devoted to unsteady flow in collapsible tubes subjected to pressure ramps. Another medical application is given by venous flow under muscle contraction such as flow in inferior limb veins during walking.

[4] The air compressibility is much lower than the tube distensibility and can be neglected. The first and second factor are associated with typical small-amplitude pressure wave speed of $\mathcal{O}$[100 m/s] and $\mathcal{O}$[10 m/s], respectively. Trans- and supercritical flows can then be more easily obtained in compliant ducts than in rigid pipes with a nozzle (a neck between a convergent and divergent segment) conveying a gas.

pressure exerted by the respiratory pump continues to rise. Associated with flow limitation, large intrathoracic airways collapse.

Mechanisms of flow limitation are tightly coupled to airway collapse. A large decrease in area of the central airway and an increase in volumetric flow rate induce rise in flow velocity. Simultaneously, airway collapse locally reduces the value of the wave speed ($c^2 = A/(\rho\partial A/\partial p$; $(1/A)\partial A/\partial p$ being the local airway compliance. Consequently, a catastrophic decrease in area associated with a transient increase in airway compliance can be associated with a rise in the propagation wave speed.

The thoracic trachea and the proximal portion of the major bronchi were imaged in normal volunteers during a forced expiration maneuver using a cine CT system. Sixteen images of 2 contiguous slices were obtained in less than 1 s while expiratory flow was recorded at the mouth. The area of the thoracic trachea decreased rapidly as flow rate rose to its maximum and the wave of collapse propagated distally (Fig. 11). The compressive narrowing of both the pars membranacea and the ventrolateral wall was asymmetric. A contact area appeared between the posterior and the left lateral walls. The measured maximum air

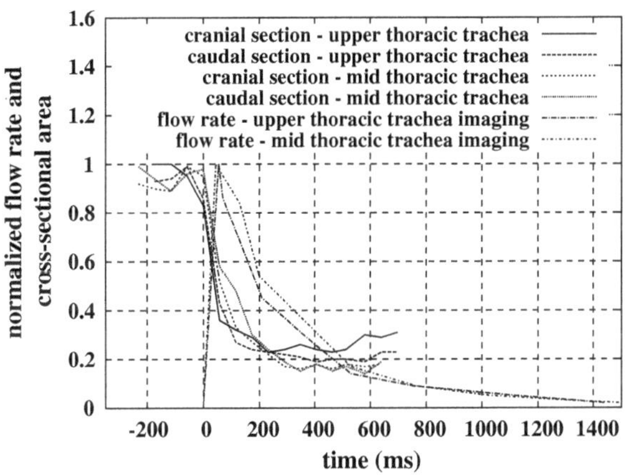

Fig. 11 Temporal variations of normalized flow rate (q/q_{max}) and area of (A/A_{max}) imaged tracheal sections in a normal human male volunteer (A_{max} and q_{max} are the maximal values measured before and during forced expiration, respectively). Two contiguous tracheal slices perpendicular to the craniocaudal axis of the body are simultaneously imaged: a cranial and caudal slice (slice thickness 8 mm; tracheal segment thickness 16 mm; between-image interval 58 ms). *Upper* and *mid* segments of the intrathoracic trachea are imaged successively, i.e., during 2 reproducible forced expiration maneuvers (q_{max} = 15.5 and 14.4 l/s, respectively). The *upper* boundary of the cranial slice of the *mid* thoracic trachea corresponded to the lower boundary of the caudal slice of the upper tracheal segment. The surface areas of the tracheal lumens in the cranial and caudal slices equal 37 and 40 % of their initial values 17 ms after the peak expiratory flow, respectively. During the rapid collapse, the cranial slice is always narrower than the caudal slice. After the peak flow the tracheal area continues to decay. It reaches its minimum 190 ms after the peak flow. The same degree of collapse is observed in both the cranial and caudal slices (minimal relative area $\sim$0.20)

velocity was greater than the estimated local wave velocity. In one subject, the trachea was imaged during the entire maneuver with a lower scan frequency. By 725 ms after the beginning of the forced expiration, the area had first decreased to 15 % of its initial value and then reincreased to 46 % of its initial value. It stayed constant for the remainder of the maneuver.

The time variations of the lumen surface area of imaged sections of the intrathoracic trachea are similar to those observed in pressurized elastomeric tubes. The instantaneous air velocity in a given tracheal section was computed using the mouth flow. A velocity equal to 170 m/s is computed at peak flow (Fig. 12). The corresponding relative area A/A_{max} equals 0.37. This study clearly shows that the area of the thoracic trachea experiences a catastrophic decrease very early during forced expiration. When the peak flow occurs, the outlet of the thoracic trachea is already very collapsed. The compressive narrowing of a given segment increases during the early phase of the maneuver as the peritracheal pressure continues to rise. Simultaneously the wave of collapse travels rapidly upstream. The tracheal collapse is asymmetrical and more marked on the left side than on the right side due to an observed bending of the trachea during forced expiration. In the upper thoracic trachea the air velocity reaches its maximum simultaneously with the peak flow. A transcritical flow may then occur in the trachea. The segment of the trachea that limits the flow may travel toward the carina as the airway collapse moves upstream.

Three major features of the time changes in the surface area of the tracheal lumen are: (1) all of the surface areas of tracheal slices decrease very early during the maneuver; (2) the intrathoracic trachea collapses very rapidly; and (3) all surface areas are greatly reduced.

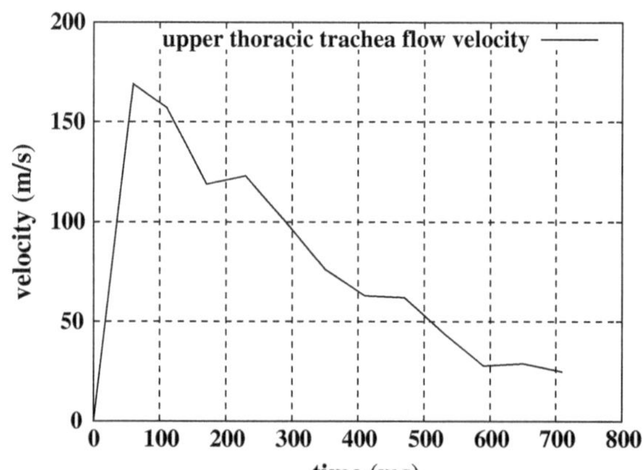

Fig. 12 Variations as a function of time of estimated air velocity during forced expiration. The flow rate is measured during imaging of the upper segment of the intrathoracic trachea (Fig. 11). With respect to sound speed in compressible air at ambient temperature, the flow remains subsonic ($\mathrm{Ma}_{\text{air compressibility}} = 0.5$). With respect to the propagation speed of pressure waves in deformable duct, the flow may become trans- and supercritical ($\mathrm{Ma}_{\text{wall compliance}} \geq 1$).

4 Concluding Remarks

Biofluids (air, blood, lymph, urine,...) are conveyed in vessels that can undergo strong deformations. Medical image acquisition and processing usually used to get configurations of anatomical pipes in normal and pathological conditions. Three-dimensional reconstruction also allows to derive meshes to solve equation set of continuum mechanics to yield further informations to clinicians. Furthermore, medical imaging can non-invasively provides functional data, especially MRI with associated MR velocimetry using hyperpolarized^{3}He gas, form which local velocity maps can be obtained [73]. Last, but not least, dynamical medical imaging associated with flow rate measurements using a pneumotachograph at the mouth allow assess flow quantities to validate models and numerical tests.

References

1. Cebral JR, Löhner R (2001) From medical images to anatomically accurate finite element grids. Int J Numer Methods Eng 51:985–1008
2. Thiriet M, Brugières P, Bittoun J, Gaston A (2001) Computational flow models in cerebral congenital aneurisms I: Steady flow. Revue Mécanique et Ind 2:107–118
3. Salmon S, Thiriet M, Gerbeau J-F (2003) Medical image-based computational model of pulsatile flow in saccular aneurisms. Math Model Numer Anal 37:663–679
4. Milner JS, Moore JA, Rutt BK, Steinman DA (1998) Hemodynamics of human carotid artery bifurcations: computational studies with models reconstructed from magnetic resonance imaging of normal subjects. J Vasc Surg 1998:143–156
5. Moore JA, Rutt BK, Karlik SJ, Yin K, Ethier CR (1999) Computational blood flow modeling based on in vivo measurements. Ann Biomed Eng 27:627–640
6. Ladak HM, Milner JS, Steinman DA (2000) Rapid 3D segmentation of the carotid bifurcation from serial MR images. J Biomech Eng 122:96–99
7. Papaharilaou Y, Doorly DJ, Sherwin SJ, Peiró J, Griffith C, Chesire N, Zervas V, Anderson J, Sanghera B, Watkins N, Caro CG (2002) Combined MRI and computational fluid dynamics detailed investigation of flow in idealised and realistic arterial bypass graft models. Biorheology 39:525–532
8. Gill JD, Ladak HM, Steinman DA, Fenster A (2000) Accuracy and variability assessment of a semiautomatic technique for segmentation of the carotid arteries from 3D ultrasound images. Med Phys 27:1333–1342
9. Thiriet M, Maarek JM, Chartrand DA, Delpuech C, Davis L, Hatzfeld C, Chang HK (1989) Transverse images of the human thoracic trachea during forced expiration. J Appl Physiol 67:1032–1040
10. Singer JR (1959) Blood flow rates by nuclear magnetic resonance measurements. Science 130:1652–1653
11. McCready VR, Leach M, Ell PJ (1987) Functional studies using NMR. Springer, New York
12. Zerhouni EA, Parish DM, Rogers WJ, Yang A, Shapiro EP (1988) Human heart: tagging with MR imaging—a method for noninvasive assessment of myocardial motion. Radiology 169:59–63
13. Axel L, Dougherty L (1989) Heart wall motion: improved method of spatial modulation of magnetization for MR imaging. Radiology 172:349–350
14. Mosher TJ, Smith MB (1990) A DANTE tagging sequence for the evaluation of translational sample motion. Magn Reson Med 15:334–339

15. Fischer SE, McKinnon GC, Maier SE, Boesiger P (1993) Improved myocardial tagging contrast. Magn Reson Med 30:191–200
16. McVeigh ER (1996) MRI of myocardial function: motion tracking techniques. Magn Reson Imaging 14:137–150
17. Basser PJ, Mattiello J, LeBihan D (1994) MR diffusion tensor spectroscopy and imaging. Biophys J 66:259–267
18. Gleich B, Weizenecker J (2005) Tomographic imaging using the nonlinear response of magnetic particles. Nature 435:1214–1217
19. Schaar JA, de Korte CL, Mastik F, Baldewsing R, Regar E, de Feyter P, Slager CJ, van der Steen AF, Serruys PW (2003) Intravascular palpography for high-risk vulnerable plaque assessment. Herz 28:488–495
20. Kanai H, Hasegawa H, Chubachi N, Koiwa Y, Tanaka M (1997) Noninvasive evaluation of local myocardial thickening and its color-coded imaging. IEEE Trans Ultrason Ferroelectr Freq Control 44:752–768
21. Boissonnat J-D (1988) Shape reconstruction from planar cross-sections. Comput Vis Graph Image Process 44:1–29
22. Boissonnat J-D, Chaine R, Frey P, Malandain G, Salmon S, Saltel E, Thiriet M (2005) From arteriographies to computational flow in saccular aneurisms: the INRIA experience. Med Image Anal 9:133–143
23. Boissonnat J-D, Cazals F (2002) Smooth surface reconstruction via natural neighbour interpolation of distance functions. Comput Geom 22:185–203
24. Lorensen WE, Cline HE (1987) Marching cubes: a high resolution 3D surface construction algorithm. Comput Graph 21:163–169
25. Osher S, Sethian JA (1988) Fronts propagating with curvature-dependent speed: algorithms based on Hamilton-Jacobi formulations. J Comput Phys 79:12–49
26. Sethian JA (1996) Level set methods: evolving interfaces in geometry, fluid mechanics, computer vision, and materials science. Cambridge University Press, Cambridge
27. Delingette H, Hébert M, Ikeuchi K (1992) Shape representation and image segmentation using deformable surfaces. Image Vis Comput 10:132–144
28. Taylor CA, Hughes TJR, Zarins CK (1998) Finite element modeling of blood flow in arteries. Comput Methods Appl Mech Eng 158:155–196
29. Peiró J, Giordana S, Griffith C, Sherwin SJ (2002) High-order algorithms for vascular flow modelling. Int J Numer Methods Fluids 40:137–151
30. Sherwin SJ, Peiró J (2002) Mesh generation in curvilinear domains using high-order elements. Int J Numer Methods Eng 53:207–223
31. Giachetti A, Tuveri M, Zanetti G (2003) Reconstruction and web distribution of measurable arterial models. Med Image Anal 7:79–93
32. Cohen LD (1991) On active contour models and balloons. Comput Vis Graph Image Process 53:211–218
33. Xu C, Prince JL (1998) Snakes, shapes and gradient vector flow. IEEE Trans Image Process 7:359–369
34. McInerney T, Terzopoulos D (1995) Topologically adaptable snakes. In: Proceedings of the fifth international conference on computer vision (ICCV'95), Cambridge, MA, pp 840–845
35. Krissian K, Malandain G, Ayache N (1998) Model based multiscale detection and reconstruction of 3D vessels. INRIA research report RR-3442
36. Fetita C, Prêteux F, Beigelman-Aubry C, Grenier P (2004) Pulmonary airways: 3D reconstruction from multi-slice CT and clinical investigation. IEEE Trans Med Imaging 23:1353–1364
37. Perchet D, Fetita CI, Vial L, Prêteux F, Sbiêrlea-Apiou G, Thiriet M (2004) Virtual investigation of pulmonary airways in volumetric computed tomography. Comput Animat Virtual Worlds 15:361–376
38. George PL, Hecht H, Saltel E (1990) Fully automatic mesh generator for 3D domains of any shape. Impact Comput Sci Eng 2:187–218

39. George PL, Borouchaki H (1997) Triangulation de Delaunay et maillage [Delaunay triangulation and mesh]. Hermès, Paris
40. Frey PJ, George PL (1999) Maillages [Meshes]. Hermès, Paris
41. George PL, Hecht F (1999) Nonisotropic grid. In: Thompson JF, Soni BK, Weatherill NP (eds) Handbook of grid generation. CRC Press, Boca Raton
42. Mohammadi B, George PL, Hecht F, Saltel E (2000) 3D Mesh adaptation by metric control for CFD. Revue européenne des éléments finis 9:439–449
43. Habashi WG, Dompierre J, Bourgault Y, Fortin M (1998) Vallet MG (1998) Certifiable computational fluid mechanics through mesh optimization. AIAA J 36:703–711
44. Fortin M (2000) Anisotropic mesh adaptation through hierarchical error estimators. In: Minev P, Yanping L (eds) Scientific computing and applications. Nova Science Publishers, Commack
45. Dompierre J, Vallet MG, Bourgault Y, Fortin M, Habashi WG (2002) Anisotropic mesh adaptation: towards user-independent, mesh-independent and solver-independent CFD III: unstructured meshes. Int J Numer Methods Fluids 39:675–702
46. Fortin A, Bertrand F, Fortin M, Boulanger-Nadeau PE, El Maliki A, Najeh N (2004) Adaptive remeshing strategy for shear-thinning fluid flow simulations. Comput Chem Eng 28:2363–2375
47. Taubin G (1995) Curve and surface smoothing without shrinkage. In: Proceedings of the fifth international conference on computer vision, IEEE, pp 852–857
48. Frey PJ, Borouchaki H (1998) Geometric surface mesh optimization. Comput Vis Sci 1:113–121
49. Thiriet M, Graham JMR, Issa RI (1992) A pulsatile developing flow in a bend. J de Phys III 2:995–1013
50. Frey PJ, Borouchaki H (2003) Surface meshing using a geometric error estimate. Int J Numer Methods Eng 58:227–245
51. Shapiro AH (1977) Steady flow in collapsible tubes. J Biomech Eng 99:126–147
52. Bonis M, Ribreau C (1981) Wave speed in non circular collapsible ducts. J Biomech Eng 103:27–31
53. Bonis M, Ribreau C, Verchery G (1981) Etude théorique et expérimentale de l'aplatissement d'un tube élastique en dépression. J de Mécanique Appliquée 5:123–144
54. Ribreau C, Naili S, Bonis M, Langlet A (1993) Collapse of thin-walled elliptical tubes for high values of major-to-minor axis ratio. J Biomech Eng 115:432–440
55. Dion B, Naili S, Renaudeaux JP, Ribreau C (1995) Buckling of elastic tubes: study of highly compliant device. Med Biol Eng Comput 33:196–201
56. Begis D, Delpuech C, Le Tallec P, Loth L, Thiriet M, Vidrascu M (1988) A finite element model of tracheal collapse. J Appl Physiol 64:1359–1368
57. Kresch E (1979) Compliance of flexible tubes. J Biomech 12:825–839
58. Flaherty JE, Keller JB, Rubinow SI (1972) Post buckling behavior of elastic tubes and rings with opposite sides in contact. SIAM J Appl Math 23:446–455
59. Tadjbakhsh I, Odeh F (1967) Equilibrium states of elastic rings. J Math Anal Appl 18:59–74
60. Palermo T, Flaud P (1987) Etude de l'effondrement à deux et trois lobes de tubes élastiques. J de Biophysique et de Biomécanique 11:105–111
61. Kresch E, Noordegraaf A (1972) Cross-sectional shape of collapsible tubes. Biophys J 12:274–294
62. Nahmias J (1980) Pertes de charge dans les tuyaux collabab採les. Thèse, Université Pierre and Marie Curie
63. Thiriet M, Ribreau C (2000) Computational flow in a collapsed tube with wall contact. Revue Mécanique et Ind 1:349–364
64. Naili S, Thiriet M, Ribreau C (2005) Wall shear stress in a laminar flow through a collapsed tube with wall contact. Eur Phys J Appl Phys 31:195–209
65. Ribreau C, Merle D, Bonis M (1986) Détermination expérimentale du module d'Young transversal d'une conduite élastique en dépression lors de son aplatissement. Conditions d'application aux veines. J de Biophysique et de Biomécanique 10:57–62

66. Conca C, Pares C, Pironneau O, Thiriet M (1995) A computational model of Navier-Stokes equations with imposed pressure and velocity fluxes. Int J Numerl Methods Fluids 20:267–287
67. Arnold DN, Brezzi F, Fortin M (1984) A stable finite element for the Stokes equation. Calcolo 21:337–344
68. Pironneau O (1982) On the transport-diffusion algorithm and its application to the Navier-Stokes equations. Numerische Mathematik 38:309–332
69. Glowinski R (1984) Numerical methods for nonlinear variational problems. Springer, New York
70. Heil M (1997) Stokes flow in collapsible tubes: computation and experiment. J Fluid Mech 353:285–312
71. Thiriet M, Bonis M (1983) Experiments on flow limitation during forced expiration in a monoalveolar lung model. Med Biol Eng Comput 21:681–687
72. Thiriet M, Bonis M, Adedjouma AS, Hatzfeld C, Yvon JP (1987) Experimental and theoretical models of flow during forced expiration: pressure and pressure history dependence of flow rate. Med Biol Eng Comput 25:551–559
73. de Rochefort L, Vial L, Fodil R, Maître X, Louis B, Isabey D, Caillibotte G, Thiriet M, Bittoun J, Durand E, Sbirlea-Apiou G (2007) In vitro validation of computational fluid dynamic simulation in human proximal airways with hyperpolarized 3He magnetic resonance phase-contrast velocimetry. J Appl Physiol 102:2012–2023

Tracking Red Blood Cells in Microchannels: A Comparative Study Between an Automatic and a Manual Method

D. Pinho, R. Lima, A. I. Pereira and F. Gayubo

Abstract Image analysis is extremely important to obtain crucial information about the blood phenomena in microcirculation. The current study proposes an automatic method for segmentation and tracking red blood cells (RBCs) flowing through a 100 μm glass capillary. The original images were obtained by means of a confocal system and then processed in MatLab using the Image Processing Toolbox. The automatic measurements with the proposed automatic method are compared with a manual tracking method performed by ImageJ. The comparison of the two methods is performed using a statistical Bland–Altman analysis. The numerical results have shown a good agreement between the two methods. Additionally, no significant difference was found between the two methods and as a result the proposed automatic method is demonstrated to be a rapid and accurate way to track RBCs in microchannels.

D. Pinho · R. Lima (✉) · A. I. Pereira
ESTiG, IPB, C. Sta. Apolonia, Braganca 5301-857, Portugal
e-mail: ruimec@ipb.pt

D. Pinho
FEUP, R. Dr. Roberto Frias, Porto 4200-465, Portugal

R. Lima
CEFT, FEUP, R. Dr. Roberto Frias, Porto 4200-465, Portugal

A. I. Pereira
ALGORITMI, Campus de Azurém, Minho University, Guimarães 4800-058, Portugal

F. Gayubo
Fundación CARTIF, División de Robótica y Visión Artificial, Parque Tecnológico de Boecillo, Parc 205, BOECILLO, Valladolid 47151, Spain

J. M. R. S. Tavares and R. M. Natal Jorge (eds.), *Topics in Medical Image Processing and Computational Vision*, Lecture Notes in Computational Vision and Biomechanics 8,
DOI: 10.1007/978-94-007-0726-9_9,

1 Introduction

Over the years, several experimental techniques were performed in both environments, *in vivo* [1–3] and *in vitro*, in an attempt to understand the flow behavior of blood and microcirculation. Several of these studies on the blood flow in glass capillaries [4–9] and in microvessels produced significant results with respect to rheological properties of blood. One way to study blood flow behavior in detail is by measuring velocity fields with Eulerian methods such as the conventional micro-Particle Image Velocimetry (PIV) [10–15] or the confocal micro-PIV [7, 16–18]. By using these Eulerian methods the most common methodology to determine velocity profiles is by using a cross-correlation technique. For high concentration of particles, the micro-PIV technique is the most suitable methodology to study blood flow phenomena in microcirculation. However, most of *in vivo* measurements contain physiological fluids with high concentrations of blood cells and as a result the amount of tracer particles captured within the fluid is often very low [17]. If the number of particles or cells within the interrogation area is small, it is recommended to measure the displacements by tracking each particle or cell in a Lagrangian way [16]. This kind of PIV mode (low-image-density PIV) is often referred as Particle Tracking Velocimetry (PTV) [14, 15]. Although this method is becoming indispensable in microcirculation [7, 14–26] most of these studies were performed with manual tracking methods. For *in vitro* blood flow in microchannels, manual tracking methods have been extensively used to track individual RBCs flowing through glass capillaries [7, 16, 23, 24], straight polydimethylsiloxane (PDMS) microchannels [26], stenosis [4], hyperbolic contractions [27, 28], bifurcations [29, 30].

In microcirculation and, in particular, the study of the red blood cells (RBCs) flowing in microvessels and microchannels, it is very important to provide a better understanding on the blood rheological properties and disorders in microvessels in a fast and accurate way. In this kind of study, the image analysis plays an essential part to obtain crucial information about the blood rheology. However, manual tracking methods are extremely time consuming and may introduce operator errors. Hence, it is crucial to develop versatile and automatic tracking methods able to compute automatically multiple cell trajectories and remove errors from the user evaluation.

Image analysis processing is a huge area which provides a large number of viable applications. Segmentation is one of the most important elements in automated image analysis, mainly because at this step the objects or other entities of interest are extracted from the original image for subsequent processing, such as description and recognition [31].

Image segmentation is the process of partitioning an image into meaningful parts and is perhaps the most studied topic in image analysis. This can be attributed to the importance of segmentation in image analysis and the fact that a universal method that can segment all kinds of images does not exist [32]. A method is usually developed taking into consideration the properties of a particular class of images, of the image quality and the general image artifacts, such as noise. Some segmentation methods may require image preprocessing prior to the segmentation algorithm [32, 33]. On the other hand, some other methods apply postprocessing to overcome the problems arising from oversegmentation. Segmentation methods can be grouped into thresholding, boundary detection, and region growing.

Thresholding methods assign pixels with intensities below a certain threshold value into one class and the remaining pixels into another class and form regions by connecting adjacent pixels of the same class, i.e., in the thresholding process each pixel in a grayscale is recognized as either an object or background. More advanced method creates histograms, oriented to the intensity of grayscale or color, showing the frequency of occurrence of certain intensities in an image so that the regions and objects are recognized from these data [33–35]. Thresholding methods work well on simple images where the objects and background have distinctively different intensity distributions. Boundary extraction methods use information about intensity differences between adjacent regions to separate the regions from each other. If the intensities within a region vary gradually but the difference of intensities between adjacent regions remains large, boundary detection methods can successfully delineate the regions [32–35]. Region growing methods form regions by combining pixels of similar properties [32].

In this study we have used mainly thresholding method available in MatLab, combined with filtering, segmentation and feature extraction functions. The main purpose of this work is to develop an image analysis approach able to track the RBCs automatically and examine its accuracy and efficiency comparing with a manual tracking method.

2 Materials and Methods

2.1 Physiological Fluid, RBC Labeling and Microchannel

The working fluid was dextran 40 (Dx-40; Otsuka Medicine, Tokyo, Japan) containing 12 % of human RBCs, i. e., hematocrit (Hct) of 12 %. The blood used was collected from a healthy adult, heparin was added to prevent coagulation, and it was stored hermetical at 4 °C until the experiment was performed at room temperature (25 ± 2 °C). The RBCs were fluorescently labeled with a lipophilic carbocyanime derivative dye, chloromethylbenzamido (CM-Dil, C-7000, Molecular Probes) using a procedure previously described elsewhere [7, 17]. Briefly the RBCs where separated from the bulk blood by centrifugation and aspiration of the plasma and buffy coat and then washed twice with physiological saline. The washed RBCs were then incubated in the dye solution and the fluorescently labeled RBCs were washed to remove any excess dye and suspended with Dx40 to make up the required RBCs concentration by volume. This dye was well retained by the RBCs and had a strong light intensity able to track labeled RBCs flowing in concentrated suspensions of cells.

The microchannel used in this study was a 100 μm circular borosilicate glass capillary fabricated by Vitrocom (Mountain Lakes, NJ, USA). The capillary was mounted on a slide glass with a thickness of 170 ± 20 μm and was immersed in glycerol in order to minimize the refraction from the walls. Schematic illustration of the microdevice used in this study can be found elsewhere [36].

2.2 Experimental Set-Up

The confocal micro-PIV system consists of an inverted microscope (IX71; Olympus) combined with a confocal scanning unit (CSU22; Yokogawa), a diode-pumped solid-state (DPSS) laser (Laser Quantum) with an excitation wavelength of 532 nm and a high-speed camera (Phantom v7.1; Vision Research) (Fig. 1). The microdevice was placed on the microscope stage and by means of a syringe pump (KD Scientific) a pressure-driven flow was kept constant (Re $\sim$ 0.008). More detailed information about this confocal system can be found elsewhere [7, 17, 24, 25].

2.3 Image Analysis

The laser beam was illuminated from below the microscope stage through a dry 40× objective lens with a numerical aperture (NA) equal to 0.9. The confocal images were captured in middle of the capillary with a resolution of 640 × 480 pixel at a rate of 100 frames/s with an exposure time of 9.4 ms.

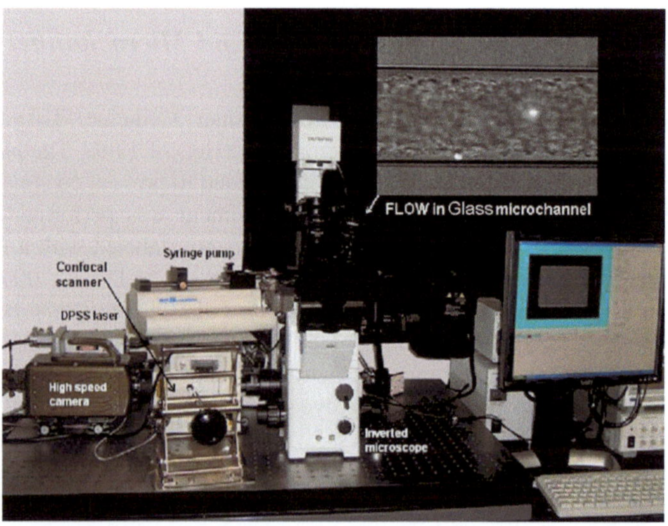

Fig. 1 Experimental set-up, confocal micro-PIV system

The recorded images were transferred to the computer and then two image analyses methods were used in this study: manual method (MM) and automatic method (AM).

2.3.1 Manual Method

In manual method, individual RBCs flowing through the microchannel were tracked manually by examining images sequences. For this purpose, a manual tracking plugin (MTrackJ) [37] of an image analysis software (Image J, NIH) [38] was used (Fig. 2).

With this plug-in, the bright centroid of the selected RBC was automatically computed and its position was defined by x and y coordinate. By following the identical RBC in the successive images, it is possible to record its trajectory with the set of these (x, y) positions. Setting the time interval of 10 ms, it is also possible to calculate the velocity of the travelling cells.

2.3.2 Automatic Method

The analysis of microscopical images requires essentially two parts, the image processing where preprocessing filter is applied and segmentation where the objects of interest (red blood cells) are isolated. In this study, the digital image processing procedure was performed with a processing software package, the Image Processing Toolbox from MatLab [39].

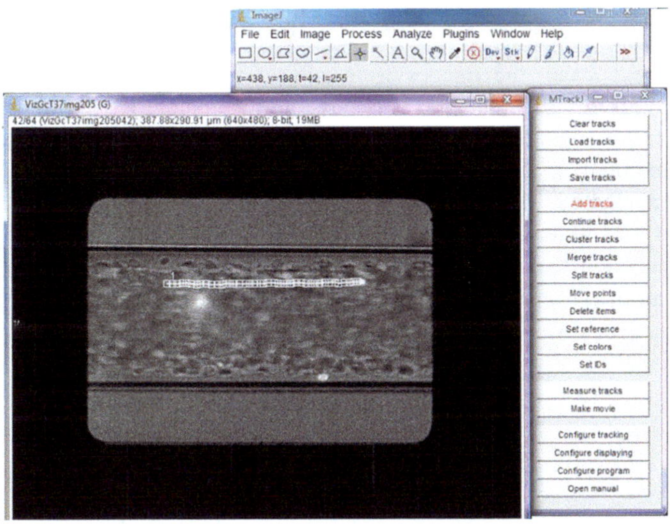

Fig. 2 Manual tracking by using the manual method from image J, plugin MtrackJ

Algorithm
The application must detect and track in time interval all objects that are present in a video sequence. The follow-up of objects that remain visible throughout the sequence is a relatively simple task; however, when certain situations arise (ex. high Hcts) where objects are temporarily not visible in the area of focus camera, the tracking task becomes much more complex. The algorithm used in the present tries to cover the entire situation to avoid losing the trajectory of the following objects. The algorithm is based on the steps as follows:

- A preprocessing is performed in order to correct the sequence of images defects (such as noise and brightness), and to enhance specific features of the image for increasing the robustness of the tracking procedure;
- Segmentation is applied, in which it is possible to divide the image into different parts or objects. The result of this step is a binary image with a clear division between background and objects of interest. The segmentation requires a thresholding method;
- Extraction procedure is done, to obtain the objects characteristics, necessary for the study.

Firstly, all the extracted images were loaded to MatLab. Then the region of interest was cropped from the original images with the function *imcrop* [39]. With this operation, we can work only with the region which needs to be analyzed (the region between the microchannel walls), that makes it easier to handle the images for the next steps.

The next operation is the elimination of the noise 'salt and pepper' which represents randomly occurring white and black pixels due to electrical interface interruption during acquisition or transmission [40]. By appling the median filter, *medfilt2*, with one mask 5×5 pixel, the images were enhanced with the objects to follow preserving the edges. In Fig. 3 the result of these processes described so far are presented.

In the next stage, the images were subject to a segmentation filter, Sobel [34, 35]. With this segmentation it is possible to separate RBCs from the background, i.e. differentiate the area of interest (the RBCs) from the not-interest area (background image). This is possible using a threshold method, where a definition of one or more values of separation is enough to divide the image into one or more regions (Fig. 4). Mathematically, the operation thresholding can be described as an image processing technique in which an input image $f(x, y)$ of N gray levels produces an image $g(x, y)$, called thresholded image, where the number of gray levels is less than N. Typically, $g(x, y)$ is described as follows:

$$g(x,y) = \left\{ \begin{matrix} 1 \text{ if } & T_1 \leq f(x,y) \leq T_2 \\ 0 & Otherwise \end{matrix} \right\}$$

where pixels labeled with 1 correspond to the objects and the pixels labeled 0 correspond to the background (background) and T_1, T_2 is different level value, for different objects [34, 35].

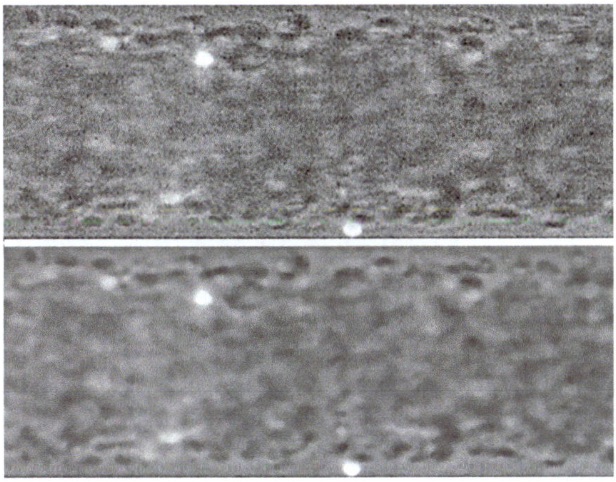

Fig. 3 The region of interest (*above*) and the image filtered by using the median function *medfilt2*

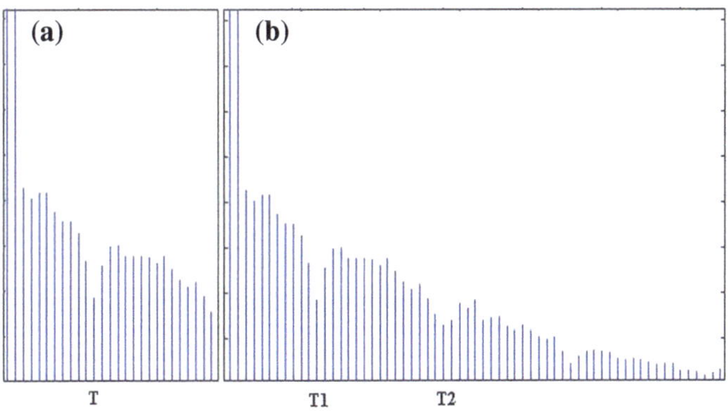

Fig. 4 Examples of threshold levels, **a** background and object, **b** background and two objects

Fig. 5 Result of the iterative threshold method and the filter Sobel

After thresholding, the objects were defined with the Sobel filter (see Fig. 5), which shows only the edge of the objects. The Sobel computes an approximation of the gradient of the image intensity. At each pixel point in the image, the result

Fig. 6 RBCs tracking and data extraction

of the Sobel operator is either the corresponding gradient vector or the norm of this vector [33].

After the segmentation processing, the RBCs were tracked and sets of data (x and y positions) were obtained with the MatLab function stored in the image processing toolbox, *regionprops* [39] (see Fig. 6). This function measures a set of properties (area, centroid, etc.) for each connected component (RBC) in the binary image.

Another approach for this type of application is underway, that is the optical flow. Optical flow is a technique used in computer vision algorithms to measure the speed of the pixels based on comparisons of frames, creating a field that describes the displacement that occurred between two consecutive frames of a video sequence. In other words, the optical flow consists in a dense field of speed where each pixel in the image plane is associated with a single velocity vector [41]. There is a great potential in this technique to follow moving objects, such as the RBCs flowing through a glass capillary, however due to the complexity of the method and the need for multiple variables which have to be standard for all video, this approach is still under study.

3 Results and Discussion

The captured videos were analyzed according to the system "confocal micro-PTV" in the center of the glass microchannel with 100 μm in diameter, at a temperature of 37 °C and a hematocrit of around 12 %. Numerical data were extracted from twenty five cells, from the analyzed videos. The Fig. 7 shows the trajectories of individual labeled RBCs, flowing in center plane of the micro-channel, determined by the manual tracking (MM) and the proposed automatic tracking method (AM).

For the twenty five cells we calculated the dispersion coefficient [28] of RBCs over the microchannel. The radial dispersion coefficient is given by:

$$D_{yy}(t) = \frac{1}{N}\sum_{i=1}^{N}\frac{\left(R_{i,y}(t) - R_{i,y}(0)\right)^2}{2t}$$

Fig. 7 Trajectories of individual labeled RBCs determined by manual and automatic method

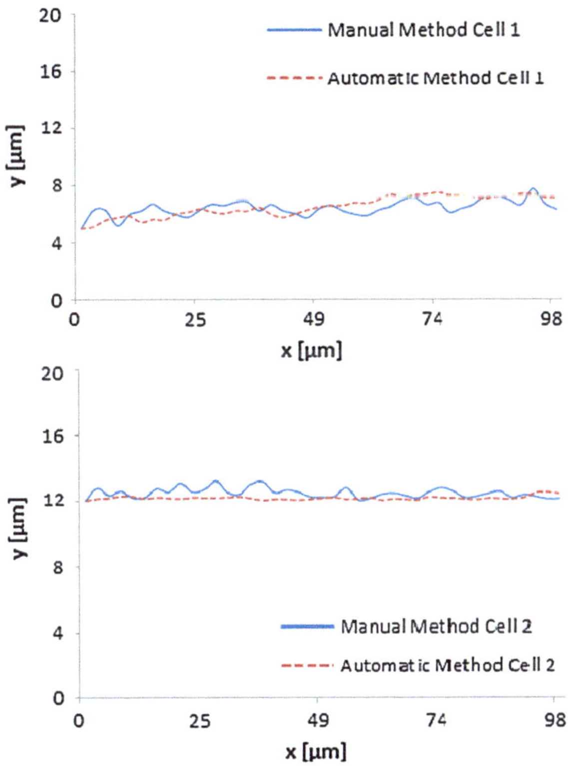

where $R_{i,y}$ is the radial displacements, and $R_{i,y}(t) - R_{i,y}(0)$ is the radial distance of each RBC in the position y, during the time interval t.

The time interval considered was [0.01, 0.2], where for each RBC 20 measurement were considered. The D_{yy} over time tends to stabilize to a constant. Figure 8 presents two RBCs with the radial dispersion of the both methods, for the considered time interval.

For a better visualization and comparison, the average of the radial dispersion and the respective standard deviation are presented in the next figure, to make a comparison between the two methods. The standard deviation was calculated by using the equation:

$$\sigma m = \frac{\sigma * t}{\sqrt{N}}$$

where N > 20, t = 1.64 with 95% of confidence level.

Analyzing the graph of Fig. 9 we can conclude that the both manual and automatic methods, although initially they have a slight discrepancy, tend to have a constant value with increasing time interval. In the Table 1 it is presented the results at $t = 0.20$ s and the respective standard deviation.

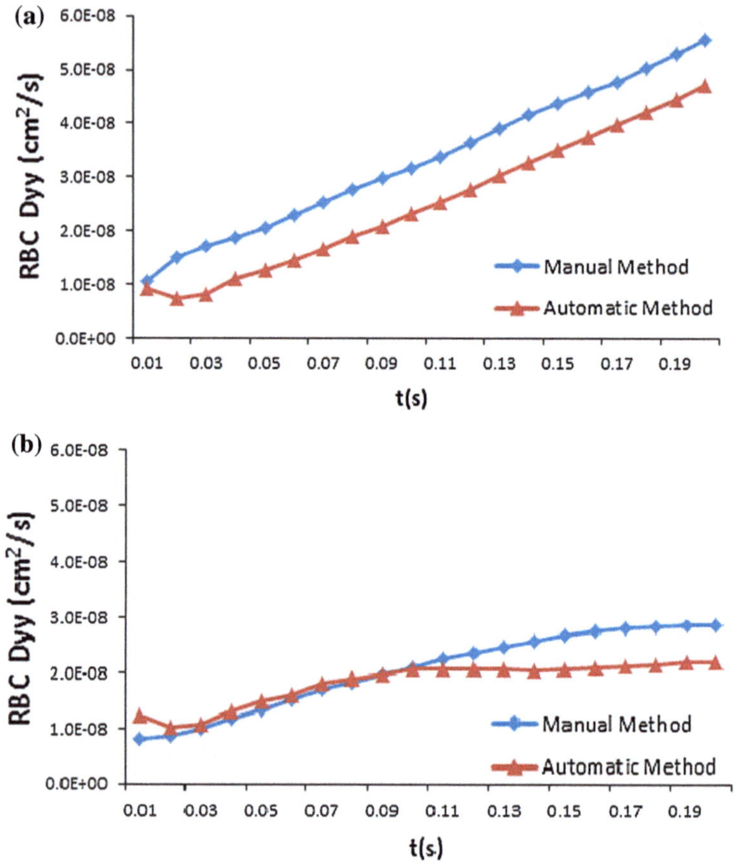

Fig. 8 Radial dispersion off two RBCs, (**a**) and (**b**), for the both method

To examine the accuracy of the proposed automatic method, the Bland–Altman analysis was performed. The Bland–Altman analysis provides a more extensive analysis of the agreement between two different methods of measurements. Furthermore, this method is a graphical method, which is suitable for comparing two measurements techniques. In this method the differences between the manual and automatic methods are plotted against the average of these two methods. If the difference obtained from the two techniques is not large enough and fell within the acceptable limit with a 95 % confidence, then the automatic method is considered to be similar to the manual method. For this analysis it was considered the manual measurement as the reference. To performed the Bland–Altman analysis it was use the commercial statistical software package, MedCalc Software [42, 43].

Figure 10 presents the Bland–Altman results of manual and automatic methods for the average of the radial dispersion coefficient of RBC with a 95 % confidence level. The Bland–Altman plot presents the mean difference and agreement limits,

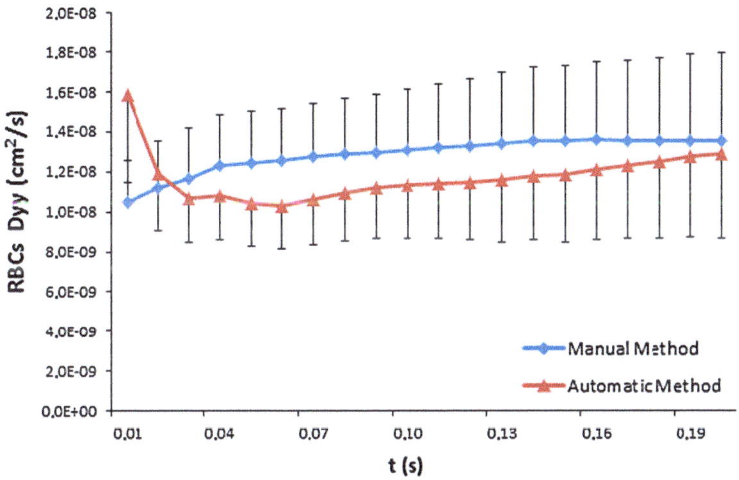

Fig. 9 Average radial dispersion coefficient of RBC with a 95 % confidence level

Table 1 Radial dispersion and standard deviation for $t = 0.20s$

	Manual method	Automatic method
Dyy [cm^2/s]	1.351E-08	1.288E-08
Standard deviation	4.438E-09	4.189E-09

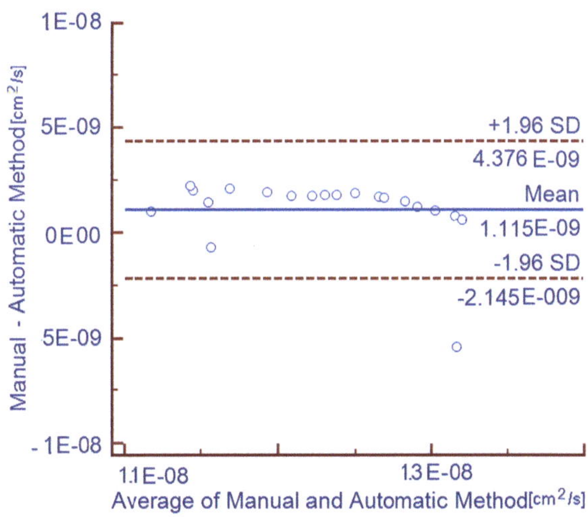

Fig. 10 Bland–Altman analyses for comparison of manual and automatic measurements in the average radial dispersion coefficient of RBC with a 95 % confidence level

which are defined as the mean difference plus and minus 1.96 times the standard deviation of the differences. In the Fig. 11 it is presented a Bland–Altman analysis for the two RBCs presented in the Fig. 8.

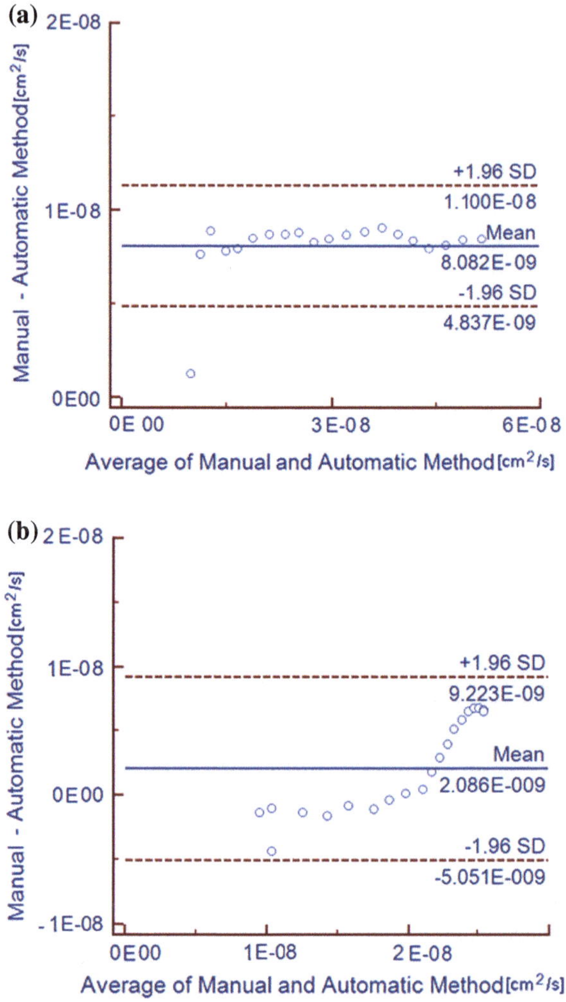

Fig. 11 Statistical compartion of the manual and automatic method, Bland–Altman analysis for two RBCs

From these results, it is possible to conclude that no significant difference between the two methods was found. Therefore, these results indicate a good agreement between the measurements obtained by the manual and automatic methods.

Regarding to the second study, the dispersion in a radial microchannel of 100 μm to different Hcts (Fig. 12), we conclude that the radial dispersion coefficient tends to increase with increasing Hct and Hcts for the values of 24 and 35 %, the magnitude is much higher than that of a 2 % Hct.

The results of Fig. 12 shows that high Hcts lead to a radial displacement of the RBC more irregular than in more dilute concentrations, because at high concentrations results in a higher number of collisions since different RBC concentrations were diluted and there is a very small number of RBC. Please note that the average

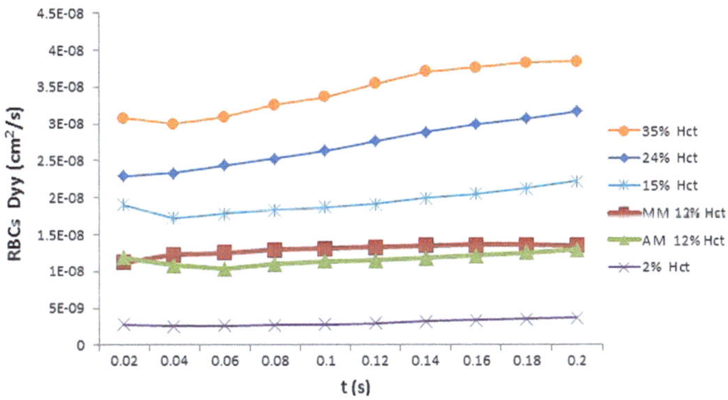

Fig. 12 Dispersion coefficient at different Hcts to a glass capillary of 100 μm

values of D_{yy} for the automatic and manual method, both with Hct 12 %, are within the range expected, because as shown in Fig. 12, they are among the Hct 15 and 2 %. These studies are consistent with existing literature [7, 24].

4 Limitations and Future Directions

The continuity of this work aims at an implementation of the image analysis application able to track in real time the flowing RBCs and consequently extract various features of the RBCs that can be used in other applications for further studies such as measuring the size of the cell-free layer or deformation of RBCs.

Another method, the optical flow, was also tested, which is still under study, in particular the Kalman Filter and Lucas Kanade Pyramidal, which can be used in the future for data collection. However the use of complex filters makes their applicability to this type of applications very difficult, due to the need of multiple variables and difficulty of standardization for the vast quantity and quality of images obtained experimentally.

The dimensions of work depend of the aims of the study and there is no unique and versatile technique for image processing. Our next study will focus on exploring more techniques to obtain quantitative measurements of the RBCs trajectories.

5 Conclusions

The present study compares two different methods, a manual method and an automatic method, to track the RBCs flowing through a 100 μm glass capillary. The automatic method is based on a threshold algorithm, with the aim to provide a convenient, accurate and automated process to track and measure the RBCs flowing in microchannels.

The comparison of the data obtained with the two methods showed good agreements. Furthermore, a statistical analysis reinforced the fact that there is no significant difference between the two results. As a result, the proposed automatic method is a promising image analysis technique for tracking blood cells in a fast and accurate way and can be successfully integrated with a confocal system for fast blood flow measurements and analysis.

Acknowledgments The authors acknowledge the financial support provided by: Student Mobility Placements with the program Lifelong Learning (Erasmus Program), PTDC/SAU-BEB/108728/2008, PTDC/SAU-BEB/105650/2008, PTDC/EME-MFE/099109/2008 and PTDC/SAU-ENB/116929/2010 from FCT (Science and Technology Foundation), COMPETE, QREN and European Union (FEDER).

References

1. Maeda N (1996) Erythrocyte rheology in microcirculation. Jpn J Physiol 46:1–14
2. Pries A, Secomb T (1994) Resistance to blood flow in microvessels in vivo. Circ Res 75:904–915
3. Suzuki Y, Tateishi N, Soutani M, Maeda N (1996) Deformation of erythrocytes in microvessels and glass capillaries: effects of erythrocyte deformability. Microcirculation 3:49–57
4. Fujiwara H, Ishikawa T et al (2009) Red blood cell motions in high-hematocrit blood flowing through a stenosed microchannel. J Biomech 42:838–843
5. Goldsmith H, Turitto V (1986) Rheological aspects of thrombosis and haemostasis: basic principles and applications. ICTH-Report-Subcommittee on Rheology of the International Committee on thrombosis and haemostasis. Thromb Haemost 55:415–435
6. Lima R, Wada S et al (2006) Confocal micro-PIV measurements of three dimensional profiles of cell suspension flow in a square microchannel. Meas Sci Tech 17:797–808
7. Lima R, Ishikawa T et al (2009) Measurement of individual red blood cell motions under high hematocrit conditions using a confocal micro-PTV system. Ann Biomed Eng 37:1546–1559
8. Lima R, Ishikawa T et al (2010) Blood flow behavior in microchannels: advances and future trends. In: Single and two-phase flows on chemical and biomedical engineering. Bentham
9. Pinho D, Pereira A, Lima R (2010) Measurement of the red blood cell (RBC) dispersion in microchannels: the effect of the temperature. In: Proceedings of the 6th World congress of biomechanics, p 471
10. Nakano A, Sugii Y, Minamiyama M, Niimi H (2003) Measurement of red cell velocity in microvessels using particle image velocimetry (PIV). Clin Hemorheol Micro 29:445–455
11. Sugii Y, Okuda R, Okamoto K, Madarame H (2005) Velocity measurement of both red blood cells and plasma of in vitro blood flow using high-speed micro PIV technique. Meas Sci Technol 16:1126–1130
12. Vennemann P, Kiger K, Lindken R, Groenendijk B, Stekelenburg-de Vos S, Hagen T, Ursem N, Rpoelmann R, Westerweel J, Hierk B (2006) In vivo micro particle image velocimetry measurements of blood-plasma in the embryonic avian heart. J Biomech 39:1191–1200
13. Wereley ST, Meinhart CD (2010) Recent advances in micro-particle image velocimetry. Annu Rev Fluid Mech 42:557–576
14. Adrian R (1991) Particle-imaging techniques for experimental fluid mechanics. Annu Rev Fluid Mech 23:261–304

15. Sbalzarini IF, Koumoutsakos P (2005) Feature point tracking and trajectory analysis for video imaging in cell biology. J Struct Biol 151(2):182–195
16. Lima R, Ishikawa T, Imai Y, Yamaguchi T (2012) Confocal micro-PIV/PTV measurements of the blood flow in micro-channels. In: Collins MW, Koenig CS (eds) Nano and micro flow systems for bioanalysis. Springer
17. Lima R (2007) Analysis of the blood flow behavior through microchannels by a confocal micro-PIV/PTV system. PhD (Eng), Bioengineering and robotics Department, Tohoku University, Sendai
18. Lima R, Ishikawa T, Imai Y, Yamaguchi T (2012) Blood flow behavior in microchannels: advances and future trends, In: Dias et al (eds) Single and two-phase flows on chemical and biomedical engineering, Bentham Science Publishers
19. Pinho D, Pereira A, Lima R (2010) Red blood cells motion in a glass microchannel. Numer Anal Appl Math 1281:963–966
20. Machin M, Santomaso A, Mazzucato M, Cozzi MR, Battiston M, Marco L, Canu P (2006) Single particle tracking across sequences of microscopical images: application to platelet adhesion under flow. Ann Biomed Eng 34(5) 833–846. doi:10.1007/s10439-006-9086-8
21. Acton ST, Wethmar K, Ley K (2002) Brief communication: automatic tracking of rolling leukocytes *in Vivo*. Microvasc Res 63:139–148. doi:10.1006/mvre.2001.2373
22. Lima R, Wada S, Tsubota K, Yamaguchi T (2006) Confocal micro-PIV measurements of three dimensional profiles of cell suspension flow in a square microchannel. Meas Sci Technol 17:797–808
23. Lima R, Wada S, Takeda M, Tsubota K, Yamaguchi T (2007) In vitro confocal micro-PIV measurements of blood flow in a square microchannel: the effect of the haematocrit on instantaneous velocity profiles. J Biomech 40:2752–2757
24. Lima R, Ishikawa T, Imai Y, Takeda M, Wada S, Yamaguchi T (2008) Radial dispersion of red blood cells in blood flowing through glass capillaries: role of heamatocrit and geometry. J Biomech 44:2188–2196
25. Lima R, Wada S, Tanaka S, Takeda M, Ishikawa T, Tsubota K, Imai Y, Yamaguchi T (2008) In vitro blood flow in a rectangular PDMS microchannel: experimental observations using a confocal micro-PIV system. Biomed Microdevices 10(2):153–167
26. Lima R, Oliveira MSN, Ishikawa T, Kaji H, Tanaka S, Nishizawa M, Yamaguchi T (2009) Axisymmetric PDMS microchannels for in vitro haemodynamics studies. Biofabrication 1(3):035005
27. Yaginuma T, Oliveira MSN, Lima R, Ishikawa T, Yamaguchi T (2011) Red blood cell deformation in flows through a PDMS hyperbolic microchannel. In: Proceedings of techconnect world 2011—microtech conference and expo, vol 2. Boston, p 505
28. Yaginuma T, Oliveira MSN, Lima R, Dias R, Ishikawa T, Imai Y, Yamaguchi T (2012) Flow visualization of trace particles and red blood cells in a microchannel with a diverging and converging bifurcation. In: Proceedings of the ECCOMAS thematic conference on computational vision and medical image processing, pp 209–211
29. Leble V, Lima R, Dias R, Fernandes C, Ishikawa T, Imai Y, Yamaguchi T (2011) Asymmetry of red blood cell motions in a microchannel with a diverging and converging bifurcation. Biomicrofluidics 5:044120
30. Lima R, Fernandes C, Dias R, Ishikawa T, Imai Y, Yamaguchi T (2011) Microscale flow dynamics of red blood cells in microchannels: an experimental and numerical analysis. In: Tavares, Jorge (eds) Computational vision and medical image processing: recent trends, vol 19. Springer, pp 297–309
31. Acharya T, Ray AK (2005) Image processing principles and applications. John Wiley & Sons, Inc, Hoboken
32. Goshtasby AA (2005) 2-D and 3-D image registration. John Wiley & Sons, Inc, Hoboken
33. Eddins SL, Gonzalez RC, Woods RE (2002) Digital image processing using Matlab. Prentice-Hall, Upper Saddle River
34. Al Bovik (2009) The essential Guide to Image Processing. Elsevier

35. Pinho D (2011) Determination and characterization of red blood cells trajectories: a semi-automatic method, master in biomedical technology. Polytechnic Institute of Bragança, Portugal (in portuguese)
36. Pinho D, Lima R, Pereira AI, Gayubo F (2012) Automatic tracking of labeled red blood cells in microchannels. International Journal for Numerical Methods in Biomedical Engineering. doi:10.1002/cnm.2526
37. Meijering E, Smal I, Danuser G (2006) Tracking in molecular bioimaging. IEEE Signal Process Mag 23:46–53
38. Abramoff M, Magelhaes P, Ram S (2004) Image processing with image. J Biophotonics Int 11:36–42
39. MatLab (2010) The MathWorks Inc, version 7.11. Image processing toolbox version 7.1 user's guide
40. Chan RH, Ho CW, Nikolova M (2005) Salt-pepper noise removal by median-type noise detectors and detail-preserving regularization. IEEE Trans Image Process 14:1479–1485
41. Horn BKP, Schunck BG (1981) Determining optical flow. Artif Intell 17:185–203
42. MedCalc Software, Version 12.1.4 Broekstraat 52, 9030 Mariakerke, Belgium
43. Bland JM, Altman DG (1986) Statistical methods for assessing agreement between two methods of clinical measurement. Lancet i:307–310

A Survey for the Automatic Classification of Bone Tissue Images

J. E. Gil, J. P. Aranda, E. Mérida-Casermeiro and M. Ujaldón

Abstract In this chapter, a computer-assisted system aimed to assess the degree of regeneration of bone tissue from stem cells is built. We deal with phenotype and color analysis to describe a wide variety of microscopic biomedical images. Then we investigate several trained and non-parametric classifiers based on neural networks, decision trees, bayesian classifiers and association rules, whose effectiveness is analyzed to distinguish between bone and cartilage versus other existing types of tissue existing in our input biomedical images. The features selection includes texture, shape and color descriptors, among which we consider color histograms, Zernike moments and Fourier coefficients. Our study evaluates different selections for the feature vectors to compare accuracy and computational time as well as different stainings for revealing tissue properties. Overall, picrosirius reveals as the best staining and multilayer perceptron as the most effective classifier to distinguish between bone and cartilage tissue.

1 Introduction

The computer technology has made a tremendous impact on medical imaging technology, for instance, in development of new imaging modalities such as computed tomography and magnetic resonance imaging, as well as developing computer aided diagnosis systems which assists medical experts in their decision making process.

J. E. Gil · J. P. Aranda · E. Mérida-Casermeiro
Applied Mathematics Department, University of Malaga, Málaga, Spain

E. Mérida-Casermeiro · M. Ujaldón (✉)
Computer Architecture Department, University of Malaga, Málaga, Spain
e-mail: ujaldon@uma.es

J. M. R. S. Tavares and R. M. Natal Jorge (eds.), *Topics in Medical Image Processing and Computational Vision*, Lecture Notes in Computational Vision and Biomechanics 8,
DOI: 10.1007/978-94-007-0726-9_10,

We are developing a computer-assisted system to assess the degree of regeneration of bone tissue to minimize the human role in this process. Our contribution aims to (1) stability (to reduce intra- and inter-reader variability of visual inspection), (2) speed (introducing Multilayer Perceptron—MLP—and Radial Basis Functions—RBF—to tune the classification process), (3) accuracy (using a wide range of features to compose the input vectors to classifiers). The computation of those features requires sophisticated algorithms for different types of automated decision making procedures such as determining the phenotype or the morphological characteristics of the analyzed tissue.

Classification success may require the selection of a different set of parameters to constitute a solid discriminant on every case. For our target application of cartilage and bone regeneration from pluripotent mesenchymal stem cells [2], approximately 500 slices of tissue sample are obtained, each being a microscopic 2560 × 1920 RGB color image in TIFF format. Image analysis is quite sensitive to the staining used for revealing image features during the acquisition phase. In this respect, we enrich our analysis considering three typical cases: picrosirius, alcian blue and safranin blue (see Fig. 1). For example, using picrosirius, bone tissue is revealed by the presence of type I collagen in solid red, whereas using alcian blue, cartilage tissue is identified by the presence of type II collagen (see Fig. 1).

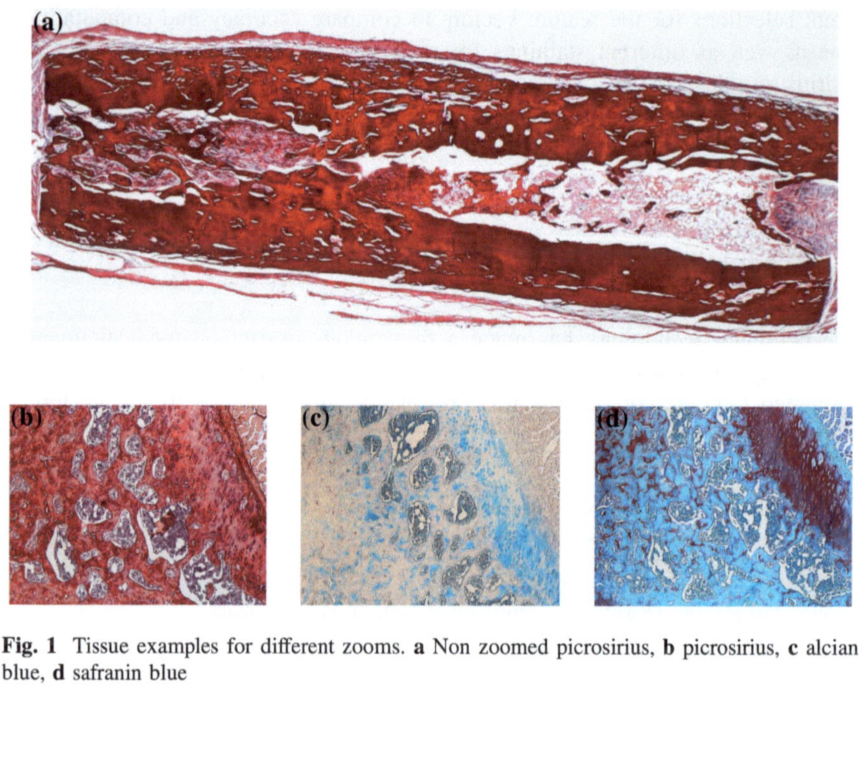

Fig. 1 Tissue examples for different zooms. **a** Non zoomed picrosirius, **b** picrosirius, **c** alcian blue, **d** safranin blue

2 Our System for Biomedical Image Analysis

The primary goal of our work is to segment bone tissue images into five different regions: bone, cartilage, fibrous, muscle and spinal. Different techniques for segmentation have been proposed depending on input images [15], but despite all these efforts, image segmentation still remains as a challenge for many types of input images and biomedical applications. In our particular case, we have built a tool where the clinical expert selects samples for each tissue type through a list of tissue tiles or windows, indicating the percentage of each tissue type contained within each window.

The window size may vary from 16×16 to 128×128 pixels according to the input images size. For each window, a vector of parameters is built as input to the classifier. After a preliminary analysis, we consider a vector composed of 25 features, basically using histograms built from red, green and blue channels as color descriptors and central moments, Zernike moments and Fourier components as phenotype descriptors. More precisely, we have:

- Color histograms for the red, green and blue channels (H_R, H_G, H_B).
- Normalized color histograms (H_R^N, H_G^N, H_B^N).
- Histogram deciles by color (D_R, D_G, D_B).
- Normalized histograms deciles by color (D_R^N, D_G^N, D_B^N).
- Zernike moment of order 4 (Z_4). In a previous work [11], we demonstrate the lower computational complexity and higher significance of low order moments on biomedical images. The fact that lowest moments capture similar information than the histograms and the typical deviation, leads us to choose the moment of order 4 as the more convenient to be part of our set of parameters.
- Zernike moment of order 4 by color and normalized $(Z_{4R}^N, Z_{4G}^N, Z_{4B}^N)$.
- Typical deviation by color and normalized $(\sigma_R, \sigma_G, \sigma_B)$.
- Central moment $(\mu_{1,1,1})$.
- Components of the Fourier Transform by color and normalized $(C_1, C_2, C_3, C_4, C_5)$.

Histograms are represented through bins which measure the number of image pixels containing the same color intensity. When these intensities are discretized in just ten intervals (histogram resolution), we say we use *deciles*. Zernike moments and the normalization process require further explanations is subsequent sections.

2.1 Zernike Moments

Zernike moments contribute with a mathematical concept to characterize cell phenotype [1], showing great performance about information redundancy [10]. These moments are defined using orthogonal basis, which simplifies the reconstruction of the original function from those generated by moments.

Zernike moments compose a set of complex functions defined within a unit circle, which, applied to digital imaging represent the length of the orthogonal projection from the base functions to the image. They are based on Zernike polynomials defined in 1, with $p - |q|$ being an even number and $|q| \leq p$; being q a positive integer, p a positive integer and (p, θ) the polar coordinates of $(x, y) \in R^2$, we have:

$$R_{pq}(\rho) = \sum_{s=0}^{(p-|q|/2)} \frac{(-1)^s (p-s)!}{s!\left(\frac{p+|q|}{2} - s\right)!\left(\frac{p-|q|}{2} - s\right)!} \rho^{p-2s} \tag{1}$$

Base functions are calculated by the following expression:

$$V(x, y) = V_{pq}(\rho cos\theta, \rho sin\theta) = R_{pq}(\rho) exp(iq\theta) \tag{2}$$

And using previous values, Zernike moments of an order p are defined as:

$$Z_{pq} = \frac{p+1}{\pi} \sum_{x^2+y^2 \leq 1} \sum Vpq^* f(x, y) \tag{3}$$

where V_{pq}^* represent the conjugate of V_{pq}.

As Zernike moments are defined over the circle $x^2 + y^2 \leq 1$, it is required to transform the image to polar coordinates prior to compute moments:

$$\rho = \sqrt{x^2 + y^2} \tag{4}$$

$$\theta = tan^{-1}\left(\frac{x}{y}\right) \tag{5}$$

where ρ represent the radius for the (x, y) point and θ represents the angle between the horizontal axis and ρ. To fulfill that those moments are invariant to translation and scaling, it is required to move the center of masses (Z_{00}) to the center of circular unit. Also, all images must be normalized to a radius of the same number of pixels. When these requirements are met, and knowing that rotation invariant is achieved by using only moments magnitudes (a rotation of the original image only produces a phase change), we can calculate Zernike moments invariant to rotation, translation and scaling:

$$Npq = \frac{Z_{pq}}{Z_{00}} \tag{6}$$

Finally, those Zernike moment values extracted from an image via the expression (3) are normalized in (6) and used as index to the image. In this way, each moment highlights a particular shape when such shape matches the intrinsic function of that moment. For example, first order moments recognize elliptical shapes, fourth order moments recognize spherical shapes, and in general, each moment corresponds to a different shape (see Fig. 2).

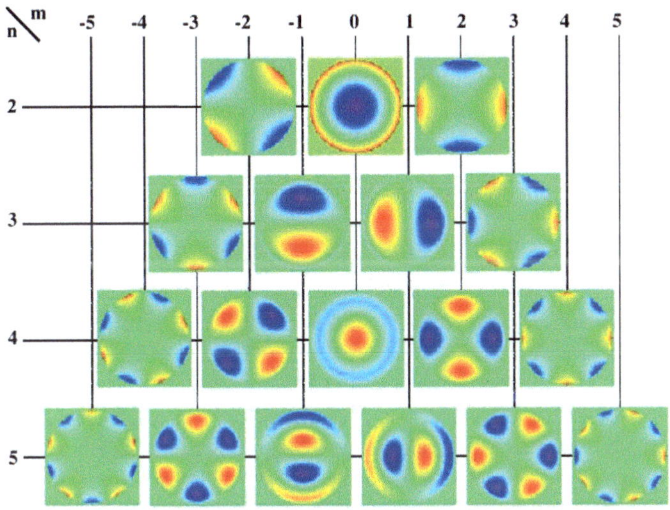

Fig. 2 Example of shapes and textures detected by Zernike moments of order n, repetition m

2.2 The Normalization Process

The normalization process is performed by applying the following procedure: Given a set X of elements, and an element $x \in X$, be $M = \max(X)$ and $m = \min(X)$. Let it be $A = M - m$, $M_a = M + 0.2 \times A$ an estimation for the maximum and $M_i = m - 0.2 \times A$ an estimation for the minimum. The normalization function is then defined as follows:

$$f(x) = \frac{x - M_i}{M_a - M_i} \tag{7}$$

And the central moment $\mu_{1,1,1}$ is defined by the following expression:

$$\mu_{1,1,1} = \sum_{i=0}^{N-1} \frac{(r_i - \overline{r}) \times (g_i - \overline{g}) \times (b_i - \overline{b})}{N} \tag{8}$$

With all the 25 parameters listed above, we have created 7 different running tests, each with a different features vector, such as illustrated in Table 1.

3 Principal Component Analysis

Once the vector of features is set, we apply Principal Component Analysis (PCA) to increase performance prior to the classifier analysis. PCA [6] is a technique widely used in data mining to reduce the number of components of a data set [7]. This technique identifies the reasons of the variability for a features space, and

Table 1 Parameters used for each running test performed by our tissue classifiers

	T1	T2	T3	T4	T5	T6	T7
H_R, H_G, H_B	•						
D_R, D_G, D_B	•						
H_R^N, H_G^N, H_B^N		•	•	•	•	•	•
D_R^N, D_G^N, D_B^N		•	•	•	•	•	•
Z_4	•						
$Z_{4R}^N, Z_{4G}^N, Z_{4B}^N$		•	•	•	•	•	•
$\sigma_R, \sigma_G, \sigma_B$			•	•	•	•	•
$\mu_{1,1,1}$			•	•	•	•	•
C_1				•			•
C_2, C_3				•	•	•	•
C_4, C_5						•	•

sorts them from higher to lower relevance. The goal is to transform a data set, X, of a given dimension $n \times m$, into another data set, Y, of lower dimension, so that the loss of information be minimal.

PCA involves the computation of eigenvalues decomposition for a covariance matrix, usually after centering data on the average of each attribute. The departure point is a set of n samples, each of them containing m variables which describe them. This way, covariance matrix is calculated as follows:

$$cov(X) = \frac{X^T X}{n-1} \tag{9}$$

Once covariance matrix is defined, we compute its eigenvalues (λ_a) and eigenvectors (p_a), and they are normalized to have a unit module. The absolute value for each autovector λ_a informs about the total variability gathered by the associated autovector from the sample. To reduce the sample to l components, they are selected from those l autovectors corresponding to those l autovalues of greater absolute value, and a matrix V is built with them arranged by columns:

$$V = [p_1 p_2 \cdots p_l] \tag{10}$$

Finally, the new data set, of dimension $n \times l$ is obtained by multiplying the data set X by the matrix V, that is:

$$Y = V^T X^T \tag{11}$$

4 Classifiers

4.1 Multilayer Perceptron

The core of our research has been conducted with the Multi-Layer Perceptron (MLP) neural network. This network contains a single layer of hidden neurons and

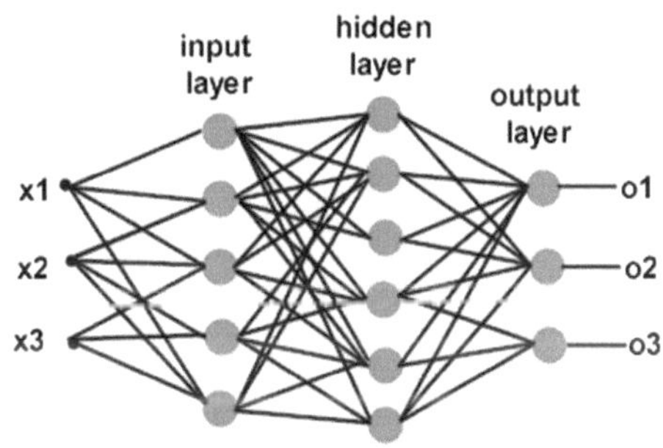

Fig. 3 A typical topology for a Multi-Layer Perceptron (MLP) neural network

is capable of making an approximation to whichever continuous function given a sufficient number of hidden neurons [5] (Fig. 3).

$$g(x, w) = \sum_{j=0}^{N_s} w_{k,j} f\left(\sum_{i=0}^{N_e} w_{j,i} x_i\right) \tag{12}$$

Using MLP, we can partition the features space via simple linear borders. We may also use complex linear borders at the expense of either adding layers to the network or neurons to the hidden layer.

Among those parameters to be defined when designing a MLP, we have:

- Neurons for the input layer, $N_{input} = d$, where d represents the dimension of the features vector used to define samples corresponding to each window.
- Neurons for the output layer, N_{output}. It matches the number of classes, c, for which the network is going to be trained for a further classification process. In our particular case, $c = 3$, for classes are bone, cartilage and others.
- Activation function. It has been selected the sigmoidal function for being widely used in *backpropagation*-type networks, because it is optimal to develop the training rule through backpropagation error.
- Training algorithms. We have performed experiments with gradient-based training algorithms as well as methods aimed to accelerate the learning process, as explained in Sect. 6.3.
- Validation. We have used a cross-validation method [8], which consists of dividing the set of controlled samples into two parts: training set, used to determine the classifier parameters, and validation set, used to evaluate the designed classifier. For these two data sets, we have used 70 % and 30 % of the input samples, respectively.

4.2 Radial Basis Functions

Radial Basis Functions (RBF) are designed with neurons in the hidden layer activated through radial non-linear functions with their own gravitational center and in the output layer through linear functions. Unlike MLP, RBF is built with a

Fig. 4 A Radial Basis Functions (RBF) neural network

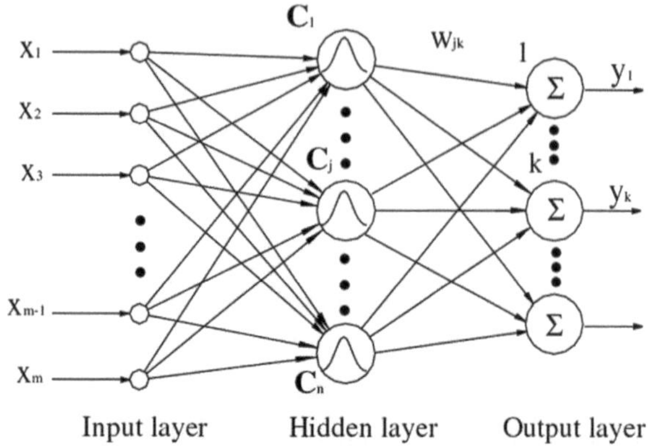

rigid architecture composed of three layers: input, hidden and output. This network is quite sensitive to the dispersion of the input parameters, so it is highly recommended to transform the input values to an specific scale in a preliminary stage.

$$y_i = g(\overline{x}, \overline{w}_i) = \sum_{j=0} w_{i,j} \exp\left(-\frac{(\overline{x} - \overline{C}_j)^T (\overline{x} - \overline{C}_j)}{2\sigma_j^2} \right) \tag{13}$$

RBF shares with MLP a similar structure of neurons as input layer plus an output layer consisting of as many processing units as classes to be distinguished by the classifier (three in our case). To study classification accuracy, we also use the cross-validation method.

Since our goal is to build a RBF with the minimum classification error, we will train the classifier until it reaches a minimum validation error. This way, we try to avoid an undesirable over training effect. The error will be calculated as the number of image tiles wrongly classified divided by the total number of input image tiles (Fig. 4).

4.3 Other Classification Methods

Our classification process was also enriched by studying a number of classifiers included in the WEKA (Waikato Environment for Knowledge Analysis) tool [4]. Among them, decision trees and association rules provide a general umbrella to generate assorted classifiers that we will meet later in this study.

4.3.1 Decision Tree

A decision tree is a predictive model used in the context of artificial intelligence. Given a database, diagrams of logical constructions are built very similar to those used in rule-based prediction systems, which are useful to represent and categorize a number of conditions that occur in a chained manner towards a problem resolution. A decision tree has inputs which may be an object or a situation described via a set of attributes, and taking this as a departure point, returns an answer in the form of a decision based on inputs [13].

4.3.2 Association Rules

Association rules are used to discover common facts that a given data set may have. Methods for learning association rules have been widely investigated, which have proven to be very effective to discover relationships between variables on large data sets [12]. Closer to our scope of application, association rules have been widely applied in areas like data mining and bioinformatics as well.

4.4 Postprocessing to Detect False Positives

In certain situations, the information contained within a single study window can be misleading and we need to lean on information provided by neighbor windows to perform a correct classification. For example, a classifier can determine that an image tile is 100 % bone, but looking at its neighborhood, we can see that it is in fact an accumulation of fibrous tissue.

One of the most interesting error filtering techniques is based on the KNN (k nearest neighbors) classifier, in fact one of the most frequently used in biomedical applications. In our particular case, we tailor this strategy to the 8 nearest neighbors as Fig. 5 illustrates. That way, whenever our classifier based on neural networks has analyzed the image and a tile is classified as bone but it is surrounded by tiles belonging to "other tissue", this tile will also be classified the same way.

5 Our Tool

We start building our tool in Matlab as a project decomposed into three main modules:

1. **Sample construction.** In this module, the user selects samples among our input images library, and, optionally, he may run a preliminar PCA (see Fig. 6).
2. **Window classification.** This module allows user to choose among a wide set of classifiers. We combine here Matlab and WEKA [4], an open source Java application which provides a rich set of classifiers such as decision trees, association rules and bayesian classifiers. The communication between Matlab and WEKA was established with the help of the Java virtual machine available

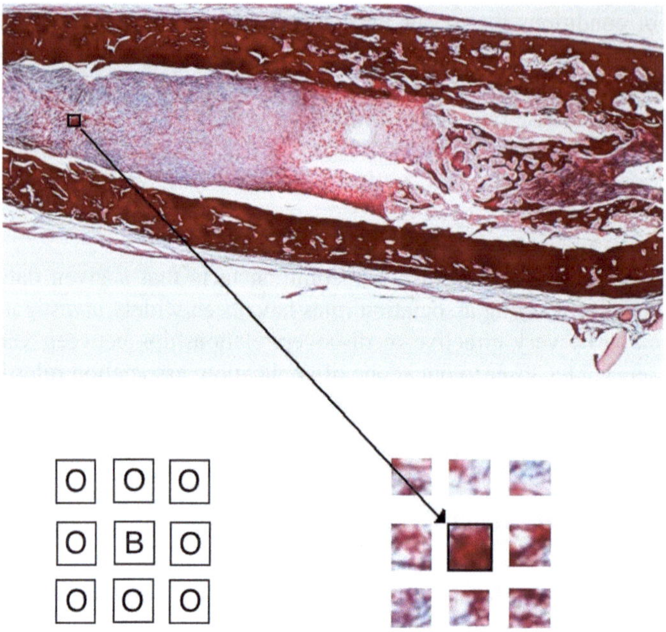

Fig. 5 Detection of false positive image tiles. *B* false bone, *O* other type of tissue

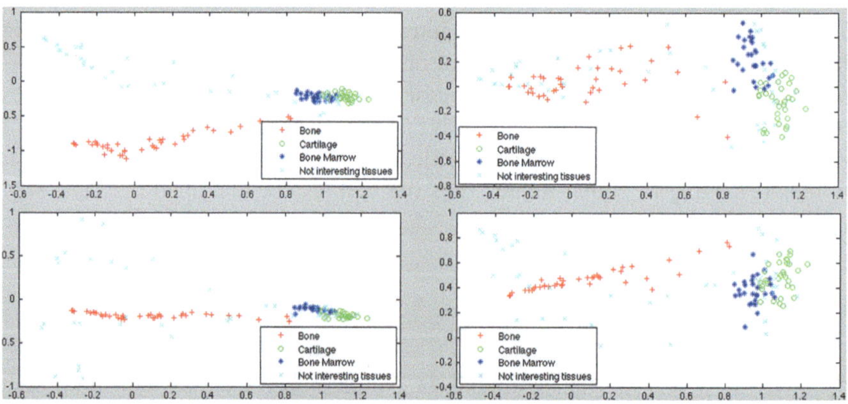

Fig. 6 Our tool for PCA. On the X-axis, we set the first principal component, and on the Y-axis, we represent the second, third, fourth and fifth principal component on the *upper left*, *upper right*, *lower left* and *lower right side*, respectively

in Matlab. Once the classifier is built, the user can display the results for a validation sample as Fig. 7 shows.

3. **Image analysis** The image analysis process can be decomposed into four major tasks connected through a pipeline as Fig. 8 shows. This module starts from an input image and a selected classifier. The first task decomposes the image into k

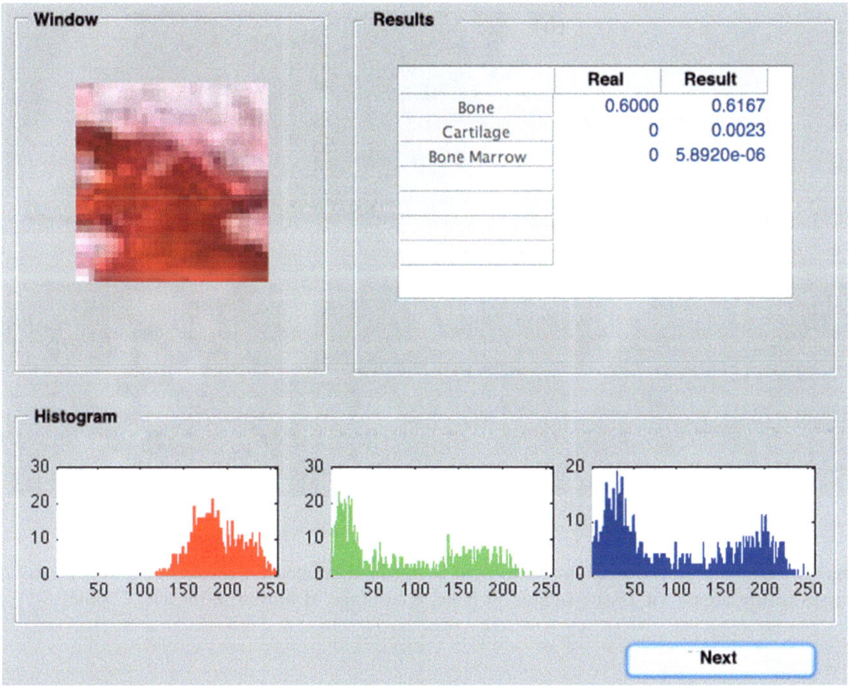

Fig. 7 Displaying the results for a validation sample

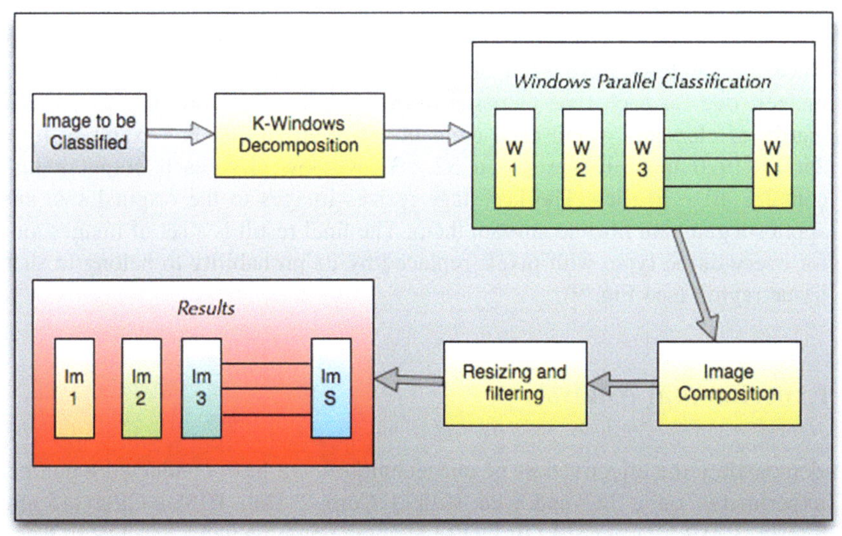

Fig. 8 Image analysis pipeline implemented within our biomedical image processing application

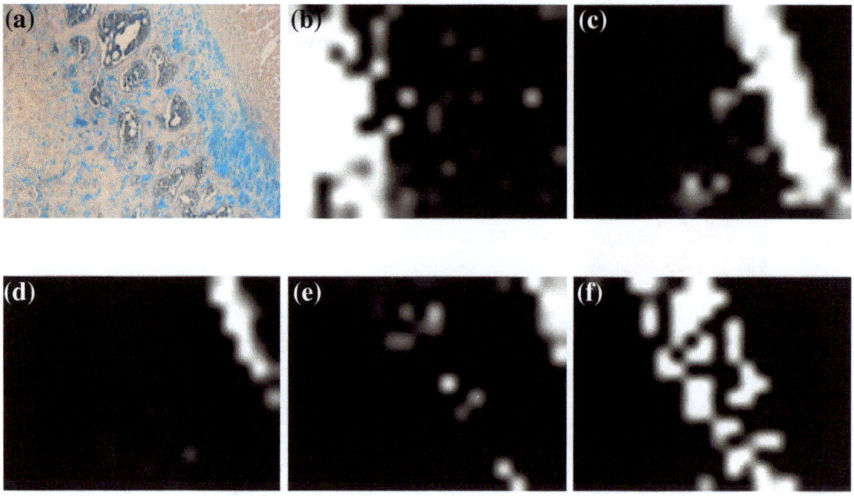

Fig. 9 Image classification example. **a** Input biomedical image, **b–f** regions classified as tissue classes (*white* areas). (**a** Tissue sample, **b** bone, **c** cartilage, **d** fibrous, **e** muscle, **f** spine)

windows (image tiles) and stores them in an array. The second task obtains the parameters vectors for each windows and classifies it. This is the bottleneck in our application, and because it is an embarrassingly parallel task, we have used the Parallel Computing Toolbox [14] to classify windows simultaneously, so the execution time depends on the number of active workers active in Matlab. Once all windows have been classified, a third stage composes the output images, one for each type of tissue to distinguish. Therefore, this output is a matrix of elements where each element represents a tile. For example, for a 2560×1920 input image and a 32×32 window size, each output matrix contains 40×30 tiles. The last stage resizes images to the original size and applies a gaussian filter to smooth them. The final result is a set of images, one for every tissue type, with pixels replaced by its probability to belong to such tissue region (see Fig. 9).

6 Experimental Analysis

To demonstrate the effectiveness of our techniques, we have conducted a number of experiments on a PC endowed with a Core 2 Duo P7550 CPU (45 nm, 2.26 GHz, 3 MB L2 Cache, 4 GB DDR3 memory) running under MacOS 10.6 and using Matlab R2009b.

Table 2 Error percentage incurred by each classifier

Learning algorithm	PCA applied?	Window size (image tiles) 16 × 16	32 × 32	64 × 64	128 × 128
		Error incurred by MLP classifier			
Gradient descent with adaptive learning rate backpropagation	No	8.35 %	3.91 %	10.93 %	18.56 %
	Yes	9.14 %	5.68 %	14.16 %	21.08 %
	Loss	+9.46 %	+45.26 %	+29.55 %	+13.57 %
Gradient descent with momentum and adaptive learning rate backpropagation	No	4.72 %	2.70 %	10.85 %	18.10 %
	Yes	6.71 %	5.24 %	12.76 %	18.85 %
	Loss	+42.16 %	+94.07 %	+17.60 %	+4.14 %
Resilient backpropagation	No	7.66 %	3.33 %	11.15 %	17.55 %
	Yes	9.40 %	4.41 %	12.25 %	19.15 %
	Loss	+22.71 %	+32.43 %	+9.86 %	+9.11 %
	PCA applied?	Error incurred by RBF classifier			
	No	14.50 %	9.12 %	15.73 %	25.92 %
	Yes	16.00 %	12.25 %	19.45 %	27.00 %
	Loss	+10.34 %	+34.32 %	+23.64 %	+4.16 %

6.1 Selection of the Window Size

Different window sizes were analyzed in a preliminary phase of our study. In particular, we tried windows composed of $4 \times 4, 8 \times 8, 16 \times 16$ and 32×32 pixels. We discarded 4×4 and 8×8 sizes soon for being little representative, and incorporate 64×64 and 128×128 instead.

In order to verify the accuracy of our classifier we took 30 samples of 128×128 pixels belonging to each of the three classes (cartilage, bone and remaining elements). The number of samples is four times higher on every downgraded size to produce 120 samples on 64×64 windows, 480 samples on 32×32 windows and 1,920 samples on 16×16 windows.

As demonstrated by results shown in Table 2, windows of 32×32 pixels achieve the best results, so we subscribe this window size from this moment on.

6.2 Tuning the Number of Neurons Used

The number of neurons to be used is specific of each problem, and most of the times it is determined by trial and error procedures. In general, fewer neurons simplify the model at the expense of being unable to retain information which is critical for the classification process. On the other hand, too many neurons may lead to over training, which basically means that training samples are precisely identified but the model is unable to extend this skill to the input samples.

Table 3 Number of neurons used by each classifier and savings when PCA is applied

Learning algorithm	PCA applied?	Window size (image tiles) 16 × 16	32 × 32	64 × 64	128 × 128
		Neurons used by MLP classifier			
Gradient descent with adaptive learning rate backpropagation	No	55	70	68	98
	Yes	12	20	35	78
	Savings	−43	−50	−33	−20
Gradient descent with momentum and adaptive learning rate backpropagation	No	35	42	45	104
	Yes	4	8	28	72
	Savings	−31	−34	−17	−32
Resilient backpropagation	No	40	65	83	90
	Yes	12	15	24	65
	Savings	−28	−50	−59	−25

PCA applied?	Neurons used by RBF classifier			
No	50	125	165	200
Yes	50	95	115	200
Savings	0	−30	−50	0

Many classifiers behave well on a wide interval of neurons, say between 10 and 100. Our findings in Table 3 demonstrate that more neurons are required on bigger image tiles and that PCA reduces these needs in a remarkable margin.

6.3 Classifying 3 Tissue Classes

Our first experiment tries to classify tissue tiles of size 32 × 32 pixels into three different classes: Bone, cartilage and all the remaining types of tissue (muscle, fiber and spine) grouped into a third and heterogeneous class.

Our training sample is composed of 30 representative windows for every class plus 36 windows of non interesting areas and 40 random (mixed) windows. A total of 166 windows were selected manually, all stained with picrosirius, whose distribution is shown in Fig. 10.

Among those 40 random windows, 20 were used for validation purposes, 10 were involved in the testing phase and 10 were used for training. The validation error was calculated using the k-cross-validation technique [8].

6.3.1 Using the MLP Classifier

This classifier was taken from the Neural Network Computing in Matlab, and samples were used to estimate the best configuration.

To accomplish this task, we vary the number of neurons in layer one, ranging from 10 until 100, and using three learning algorithms:

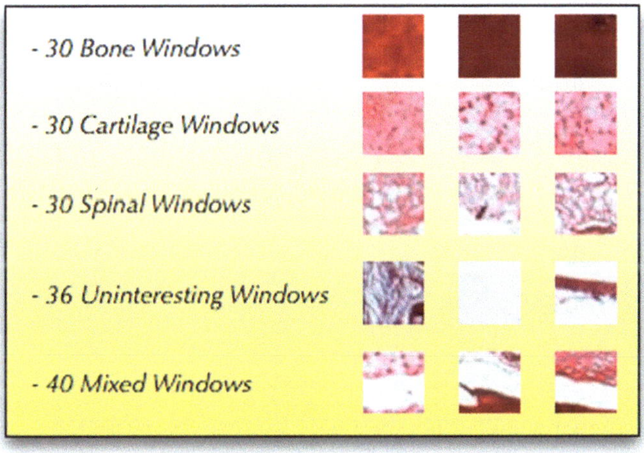

Fig. 10 Samples and validation test used with a biomedical image stained with picrosirius to classify windows into three tissue classes: bone, cartilage and others

- **traingda:** Gradient descent with adaptive learning rate backpropagation.
- **traingdx:** Gradient descent with momentum and adaptive learning rate backpropagation.
- **trainrp:** Resilient backpropagation.

Figure 11 shows the results obtained when using our T3 running test, where we can see that the last algorithm behaves better and reaches its peak (minimum error) when 30 neurons are used in the first layer. Consequently, we have chosen these parameters for building our MLP classifier, which later was applied to all seven running tests to proceed similarly under different feature vectors.

Experimental results are shown in Table 4, where we can see the effect of performing a preliminary PCA: Execution times are reduced up to 50 %, but at the expense of sacrificing accuracy (the error percentage goes up). We can also see how the error is reduced when input features are normalized, with the best results attained for the T3 test.

6.3.2 Using the RBF Classifier

For this classifier we have used the `newbr` function provided by the Network Toolbox in Matlab. which can be tuned through the `spread` parameter: When this value is too big, a great amount of neurons are forced to adapt to a function with steady changes, but the best way to tune this function is through a test and error loop. So, we vary `spread` from 1 to 20 to draw the chart we present in Fig. 12, which suggests the use of the T4 test together with a spread value of two. Under these settings, we repeat all runs already covered by the MLP in our benchmark,

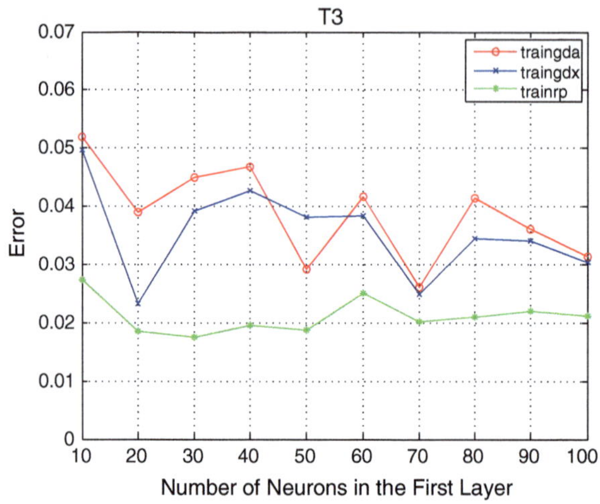

Fig. 11 Classification error for our T3 running test using the MLP classifier and three output tissue classes: bone, cartilage and others

Table 4 A comparison between MLP and RBF neural networks classifiers

Classifier	T1	T2	T3	T4	T5	T6	T7
	Error percentage (in %)						
MLP	3.25	1.86	1.83	1.94	1.98	2.28	1.85
MLP + PCA	3.74	2.91	2.95	3.22	2.69	2.45	3.66
RBF	14.26	5.58	8.31	4.38	5.89	5.73	4.50
RBF + PCA	14.26	11.25	9.67	5.52	6.58	6.55	5.62
	Execution times (in s)						
MLP	21.89	6.83	5.92	7.63	6.09	8.19	7.18
MLP + PCA	21.05	3.10	3.61	3.54	3.14	3.58	2.91
RBF	0.11	0.11	0.11	0.11	0.11	0.11	0.12
RBF + PCA	0.08	0.08	0.08	0.08	0.08	0.08	0.08

and experimental results are also shown in Table 4. This time, the normalization process improves accuracy by a wide margin, going down from 14 % to just 5 %. Accuracy remains better on the MLP side, but the execution is much faster on the RBF classifier. Therefore, precision comes along with MLP, but at the expense of computational performance.

6.3.3 Using WEKA

To provide a fair measurement of how good our classifiers behave, we compare our results with a broad set of classifiers existing in the popular WEKA tool [4]. WEKA is implemented in Java, and from a performance perspective, it suffer a severe slowdown of 14 s in computational times without using PCA and 9 s when

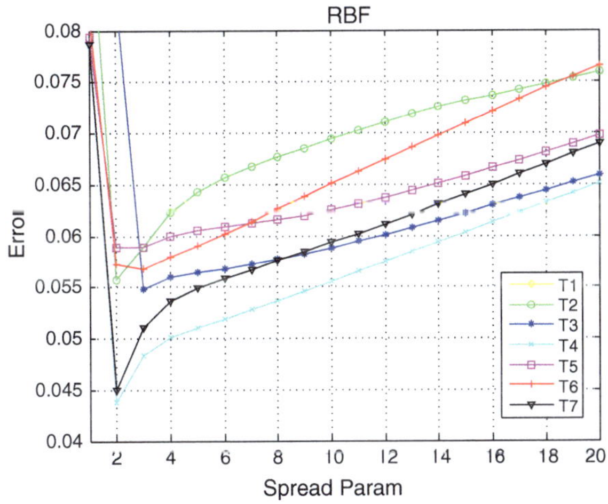

Fig. 12 Classification error depending of the spread factor for our test run using the RBF classifier and three output tissue classes: bone, cartilage and others

PCA is used (on average). In order to compare with previous analysis, we only take the T3 test, which provides the best results as far as classification accuracy is concerned. Experimental results are shown in Table 5.

Overall, the more accurate method implements base routines for generating M5 Model trees and rules. Error percentage is around 3–4 % in this best case scenario, and does not differ very much when PCA is enabled. We got errors below 2 % without PCA and below 3 % using PCA for a much faster execution time (see Table 4), so we can claim our implementation effort contributes to improve both accuracy and execution time in wide margins with respect to well established tools in our application area.

6.4 Selecting a Staining for an Optimal Bone Tissue Classification

Our last experiments aims to determine the best tissue staining to be used when handling biomedical images in clinical practice if we are interested on a automated classification. To run this experiment, we regenerated input samples from a broader set of image tiles (see [3] for a detailed description on a procedure we share here). Input parameters for the MLP have been 65 neurons in the first layer, together with the training algorithm `trainrp`. For the RBF case we have chosen a value of 0.83 for the `spread` parameter. In this case, parameters have been adjusted using a minimization algorithm [9]. The test used was again T3, this time without applying PCA beforehand.

Table 6 shows the results obtained, where we can see the error incurred by each of our two classifiers for each of the tissue stainings. Again, MLP performs better, but this time its behavior improves when picrosirius is used as tissue staining.

Table 5 Error percentage for different WEKA classifiers when three tissue classes are distinguished and the T3 vector of features is used

Classifier (WEKA name)	PCA disabled (%)	Rank	PCA enabled (%)	Rank
trees.M5P	3.23	3	4.17	1
trees.DecisionStump	4.62	7	4.83	3
trees.REPTree	3.08	2	6.12	9
functions.IsotonicRegression	3.34	4	5.31	6
functions.LeastMedSq	14.26	19	14.26	20
functions.LinearRegression	91.87	20	7.85	13
functions.PLSClassifier	5.25	11	5.22	5
functions.SimpleLinearRegr.	4.79	8	7.00	12
functions.SMOreg	12.23	18	6.07	8
lazy.IBk	5.68	14	12.08	19
lazy.LWL	3.65	5	6.26	11
meta.AdditiveRegression	5.17	9	7.85	14
meta.Bagging	2.36	1	4.72	2
meta.CVParameterSelection	11.10	15	11.10	16
meta.GridSearch	5.18	10	5.14	4
meta.MultiScheme	11.10	16	11.10	17
rules.ConjunctiveRule	5.39	12	6.16	10
rules.DecisionTable	5.59	13	8.38	15
rules.M5Rules	3.74	6	5.93	7
rules.ZeroR	11.10	17	11.10	18

A rank has been built based on classification accuracy for our testbed based on picrosirius staining tiles

Table 6 Error fraction incurred by the two classifiers proposed in this work when applied to three tissue stainings for distinguishing among three different tissue classes (bone, cartilage, others)

Our classifier	Tissue staining		
	Picrosirius (%)	Alcian blue (%)	Safranin blue (%)
MLP	2.70	12.61	14.10
RBF	9.12	17.82	19.67

T3 is used as feature vector and no PCA is applied

This result differs from those findings in [3], where safranin blue behaves better when we extend our classification coverage to five classes [3]: bone, cartilage, muscle, fiber and spine.

7 Conclusion

We have built a robust, multi-platform and easy to use tool for an automatic classification of bone tissue which achieves a remarkable success in the process of segmenting biomedical images, mostly extracting the amount of bone and cartilage that each image contains. This allows to assess the degree of bone tissue regeneration starting from stem cells in an automatic way, which allows an easy and fast method for evaluating those culture conditions that benefit the most.

The MLP classifier obtains the most accurate results with an error around 1–3 %, but at the expense of a higher computational complexity which derives in execution times around 6–8 s. When a quick response is required, RBF may be used instead as it reduces the execution time to just 0.11 s, with errors starting in 4.5 % and reaching even percentages of 14 %. PCA provides another way of reducing the computational burden in both classifiers, sometimes even more than 50 %, but again introducing penalties on classification accuracy.

We have also studied the influence of tissue staining, making an analysis for picrosirius, alcian blue and safranin blue. Our survey provides clear signs that the first reveals better those features which may act as effective biomarkers.

Acknowledgments This work was supported by the Junta de Andalucía of Spain, under Project of Excellence P06-TIC-02109. We want to thank Silvia Claros, José Antonio Andrades and José Becerra from the Cell Biology Department at the University of Malaga for providing us the biomedical images used as input to our experimental analysis.

References

1. Alegre Gutiérrez E, Sánchez González L, Alaiz Rodríguez R, Domínguez-Fernández Tejerina JC (2004) Utilización de Momentos Estadiísticos Y Redes Neuronales en la clasificación de Cabezas de Espermatozoides de Verraco (in spanish). XXV Jornadas de Automática
2. Andrades JA, Santamaría J, Nimni M, Becerra J (2001) Selection, amplification and induction of a bone marrow cell population to the chondro-osteogenic lineage by rhOP-1: an in vitro and in vivo study. Int J Dev Biol 45:683–693
3. Gil JE, Aranda JP, Mérida-Casermeiro E, Ujaldón M (2012) Efficient biomarkers for the characterization of bone tissue. Int J Numer Methods Biomed Eng (in press). doi:10.1002/cnm.2505
4. Hall M, Frank E, Holmes G, Pfahringer B, Witten IH (2009) The WEKA data mining software: an update. SIGKDD Explor 11(1):10–18
5. Haykin S (1999) Neural networks: a comprehensive foundation. IEEE Press, New York, pp 135–155
6. Hubert M, Engelen S (2004) Robust PCA and classification in biosciences. Bioinformatics 20(11):1728–1736
7. Hyvarinen A (1999) Survey on independent component analysis. Neural computing surveys, pp 94–128
8. Kohavi R (1995) A study of cross-validation and bootstrap for accuracy estimation and model selection. In: 14th international conference on joint artificial intelligence vol 2, pp 1137–1143
9. Kroon DJ (2010) Quasi Newton limited memory BFGS and steepest
10. Li Y (1992) Reforming the theory of invariant moments for pattern recognition. Pattern Recog 25(7):723–730
11. Martín-Requena MJ, Ujaldón M (2011) Leveraging graphics hardware for and automatic classification of bone tissue, Chap. 19. Computational methods in applied sciences. Computational vision and medical image processing—recent trends, pp 209–228

12. Piatetsky-Shapiro G (2007) Data mining and knowledge discovery 1996 to 2005: overcoming the hype and moving from university to business and analytics. Data Min Knowl Discov 15(1):99–105
13. Quinlan J (1988) Decision trees and multi-valued attributes. Mach Intell 11:305–319
14. Sharma G, Martín J (2009) Matlab: a language for parallel computing. Int J Parallel Program 37:3–36
15. Tuceryan M, Jain AK (1998) Texture analysis. World Scientific Publishing, Singapore

Colour Video Segmentation for the Quantification of Sweat Dynamic Function

J. L. Quintero-Morales, E. Nava-Baro, A. García-Linares, B. Camacho-García and M. S. Dawid-Milner

Abstract Our main objective is design and develop a system that assesses sudomotor function with spatial and temporal resolution through digital image processing techniques. Its evaluation has become significant in the diagnosis of several nerve diseases. The current methods to evaluate post-ganglionic sudomotor function are not very successful because they are too expensive or they do not give enough information. It will be desirable to achieve useful results with a low cost approach. In order to this, it can be used a pH indicator on the skin of patient that changes colour when it comes in contact with sweat and a digital image processing algorithm to quantify it. The sudomotor function of more than 20 patients, with a wide range of profiles, has been tested. There is a high correlation between our results and those of others kinds of sweat tests. From all of this it can conclude that it is possible to implement an evaluation system for sudomotor function using digital image processing with a low cost solution.

Keywords Cholinergic sudomotor function · Neurophysiology · Autonomic nervous system · Colour space · Image processing

J. L. Quintero-Morales (✉) · B. Camacho-García · M. S. Dawid-Milner
CIMES Autonomic Nervous System Unit, University of Malaga, Malaga, Spain
e-mail: jlquintero@uma.es

B. Camacho-García
e-mail: beacamacho@uma.es

M. S. Dawid-Milner
e-mail: msdawid@uma.es

E. Nava-Baro
Department of Communications Engineering, University of Malaga, Malaga, Spain
e-mail: en@uma.es

A. García-Linares
Brain-Dynamics S.L, Malaga, Spain
e-mail: antonio.linares@brain-dynamics.es

J. M. R. S. Tavares and R. M. Natal Jorge (eds.), *Topics in Medical Image Processing and Computational Vision*, Lecture Notes in Computational Vision and Biomechanics 8,
DOI: 10.1007/978-94-007-0726-9_11,

1 Introduction

Our study focus on the evaluation of eccrine sweat glands. They are very important in human thermoregulatory function, which is controlled by the sympathetic cholinergic nervous system, concretely by the hypothalamic regulatory center. Innervation is primarily by cholinergic fibers, each tract from the spinal cord to one gland is consisted of two neurons, one preganglionic fiber and one postganglionic. Therefore it can classify nervous lesions in connection with sudomotor function into two groups: pre- and postganglionic neuropathies [9].

There are several sweating disorders, which can be classified into hyperhidrotic or hypo/anhidrotic. But we are interesting not for these conditions, but for the associated neurologic diseases.

Nowadays, the assessment of sudomotor function has gain importance for the diagnosis of several diseases and disorders, specially diabetes and those associated with peripheral nerve disease. But high cost and complex equipment have prevented its widespread use [10].

Some of these disorders are: diabetic autonomic neuropathy, pure autonomic failure, distal small fiber neuropathy, amyloid neuropathy, multiple system atrophy, idiopathic neuropathy, reflex sympathetic dystrophy and Sjogren's syndrome [1].

The selected area for testing is the forearm. Because distal regions are the most sensitive to denervation of sweat glands and to other complications of the autonomic nervous system, and also forearm normally has a high concentration of glands. Feet and shins are also regions of interest, but they are not studied in this chapter. We will deal with them in subsequent researches.

We can find diverse techniques to characterize sudomotor function: silicone impressions, thermoregulatory sweat test (TST), sympathetic skin responses (SSR), acetylcholine sweat-spot test. There are also quantitative techniques: quantitative sudomotor axon reflex test (QSART) and quantitative direct and indirect axon reflex testing (QDIRT) which offer numerical data that can be useful in the assessment of disease progression or degree of recovery. These techniques have been widely reviewed and described, with testing methodology and limitations [6].

To sum up, QSART [14] evaluates post-ganglionic cholinergic sudomotor function with spatial and temporal resolution measuring changes in relative humidity inside a sweat capsule, which is located on the patient skin. First of all, a sudomotor response is induced by iontophoresis of an antagonist of acetylcholinesterase, then the hermetic capsule is placed on the stimulated area, and data about the humidity inside this capsule are collected with a hygrometer for 15 min. This test offers a thorough knowledge about the sudomotor function of the patient, but the equipment is very expensive and specific, particularly the capsule. Other techniques, like Silicone Imprint Method, are more affordable than QSART, however they are not quantitative but qualitative, and their results are not very useful.

A good technique would be an application allowing a dynamic and real-time quantification of sudomotor function, and computerized image analysis would be a natural choice. In addition, three more objectives can be addressed: process time should be satisfactorily short, the whole system should be economical, and it should insure the health and well-being of the patients [3].

2 Conceptual Model

The main goal of our system is to detect and to quantify the colour of a pH marker that changes when it comes in contact with sweat.

Applying modular design techniques, the whole task can be split into smaller subsystems, facing problems one by one, using a divide and conquer strategy. The structure of the proposed algorithm is presented in Fig. 1.

These blocks are:

- Image Acquisition. A video sequence is obtained and selected digital images are chosen, or these are directly taken. In any case information about sweating, which it will be processed later, is obtained.
- Conversion to colour Space YC_xC_y. Using a specifically designed adaptive colour space based on YC_bC_r for this application, the images are transformed to the new colour coordinates.
- Lighting Changes Correction. A subsystem to compensate temporal variations in the luminance of the images.
- Movements Correction. It compensates possible movements of the patients.
- Segmentation. Sweat area is detected, marked and quantified, using a simple two step thresholding technique.
- Results. Graphs of the dynamic evolution of sweat are computed and presented.

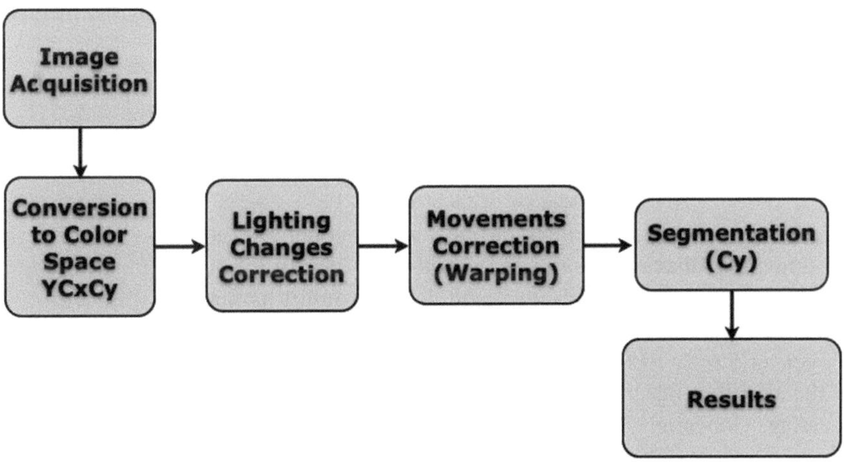

Fig. 1 Block diagram of the system

3 Analysis

We have tested the right forearm of twenty-eight selected patients with a wide range of sweat function (hyperhidrotic, normohidrotic and hypohidrotic) with also a wide range of features (age, skin colour…). Some cases, we have repeated the experiment with different set-up.

In a brief description, we can classify the patients under study as detailed below:

- Sex: 60 % men, 40 % women.
- Age: 30 % under 20 years old, 45 % 20–25 years old, 15 % 25–35 years old, 10 % upper 35 years old.
- Constitution: 40 % weak, 45 % average, 15 % strong
- Sudomotor Response: 35 % anhidrotic and hypohidrotic, 45 % normohidrotic, 20 % hyperhidrotic.

All of these patients constitute the control group to develop and to test our system, but they have not been subjected to statistical conditions, which are necessary for a clinical research. In the future, this statistic work should be carried out by medical staff.

This control group have not been subjected to statistical conditions, because they have been the volunteers to the develop and test phase of our system. For clinical use, an exhaustive statistical study is yet required, but we are working on it.

In fact, the number of tested patients continues growing every day, because our system has been included in routine tests to evaluate autonomic disorders in the Autonomic Nervous System Unit at CIMES (Medical and Health-Care Research Center of University of Málaga), which collaborates on our studies [12].

The different tasks and subsystems that form the sweat test are detailed below. Some are not really technical works, but they have to do correctly by the medical staff.

3.1 Sweating Stimulation and Preparation of Patients

Before the test, the forearm is cleaned with alcohol and acetone. We strongly recommend to shaving the arm of the patient in case of it has much hair, because the pH marker adheres easily to it and does not fulfill its function (Fig. 2).

The latency of sudomotor response is reduced by iontophoretic stimulation with Pilogel® (1.5 mA, 10 min) [5]. This technique consists in applying an electric field on the skin that injects a pharmacologic agent, i.e. pilocarpine, which stimulates sweating. Concretely, any cholinergic agonist that not be degraded by Acetyl-cholinesterase(AChE), an enzyme with a very high catalytic activity. In this way, the test duration can be reduced in comparison with thermal stimulation, and it gets

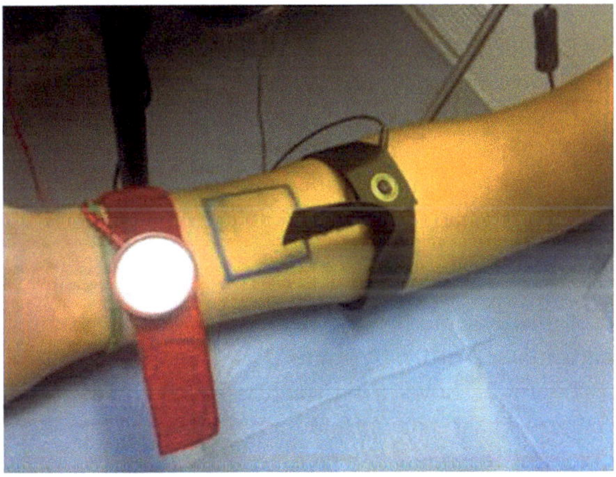

Fig. 2 Setup before iontophoresis sweat stimulation

a better response from the patient. The discs of pilocarpine and the iontophoresis stimulator can be purchased, but they can be self-made if it is necessary. The equipment is based in a controlled current source, with important safety specifications but widely known. And the discs have not a complex formulation, its basic components are agar (or agarose), pilocarpine nitrate and purified water, which are heated and mixed [15].

After iontophoresis, we apply a blue square mark around the stimulated area, and we cover this region of the patient skin with a pH indicator, which is compounded by alizarin red, cornstarch and sodium pyruvate. This mixture changes its colour when sweat is diluted in it, from light brown into red.

We have manufactured a rubber stamp to apply the blue square mark, with dimensions of $4 \times 4\,cm^2$. This stamp enables an easy and fast procedure and the mark is very useful to the movement corrections and to relate pixels with centimeters, working as a calibration reference.

3.2 Images Acquisition

We have decided to acquire the images with a conventional web-cam camera (Logitech® Webcam Pro 9000), which allows a low-cost solution and offers enough quality and resolution for our purposes.

With regard to the acquisition method, we have developed two different options. First idea was to record a video sequence of 10 min at standard rate (25 fps) for each test. This video sequence started just after the stimulation of sweat and images with sizes of 1200×768 pixels (probably, it can be used a lower resolution without sensible degradation of results) are extracted every 10 s to obtain a set of 60 images per test. Another method consisted in to register only the 60 images of the test, directly through an algorithm that control the webcam.

This method has given acceptable results, even with a low resolution of 320×240 pixels. Thus computational load and storage space are reduced significantly.

In practice, lower resolutions offer better performance specially in movement corrections. As it is described below, movement correction module is based in edge detection and warping techniques. For this reason, a reduction in number of little corners and singularities improves the performance of that module and so of the whole system.

Of course, an excessive reduction of the resolution entails loss of accuracy and usefulness of the results. We have to reach a compromise solution to get the best performance of the system.

Figure 3 shows a typical example of the obtained images. We can see the forearm of the patient upon a blue flat surface, the blue square mark and the red pixels in the middle, which correspond to the sweaty skin surface. All external elements are blue because this colour is unusual in human skin.

The choice of blue is important because, in that way, each part of the images could be clearly identified using colour information.

Additionally, the images are subjected to a preprocessing step that consists of decimate and filter operations, in order to reduce computational load, to keep safe the significant information, and to avoid some interference and aberration artifacts of the original pictures.

3.3 Colour Space

Given that the important information of the images is related to colour, the choice of the correct colour space is crucial. After trying several options with standard colour spaces, we have decided to design a specific one to this system, based on colour space YC_bC_r (ITU-R BT.601). We named the new colour space as YC_xC_y

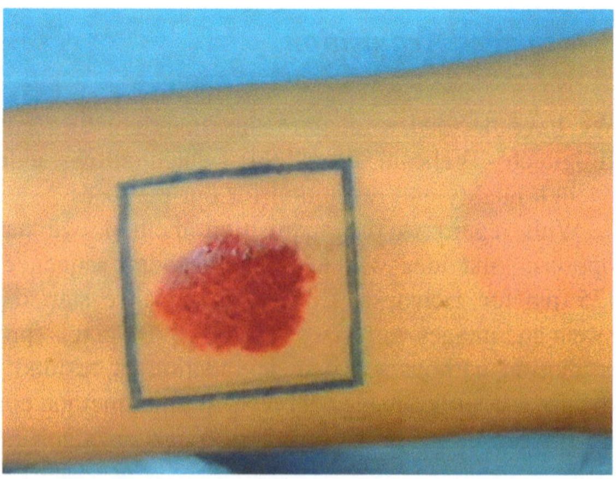

Fig. 3 Forearm with the marked work area

and it has three components: Y, the luminance component; C_x, a component with higher values for blue elements and skin; and C_y, the component with high values for red pixels, optimized for sweat response.

As can be seen in Fig. 4, the original colour space, RGB, showed histograms with no clear separations between different elements in images. Therefore it is not possible to segment these correctly for our purposes. Besides this space involve much inefficiency in representation of information, because it spend resources in irrelevant data for this application, i.e. green colour, which is unimportant in the image sequence of the patients.

In Fig. 5 it show the mean distribution of histograms for different components, based on results of our experiments. In this case, it is easier to determine an optimal combination of thresholds that divides any image of the sequence in its main parts: background, forearm, blue mark and sweated skin. All of three components are useful here, Y component to correct luminance variations, C_b component to localize blue background and mark, and C_r component to get the area affected by sweating. Despite this good performance, we have worked on improve it and design that specific colour space, YC_xC_y.

Our specific colour space adapts itself to the patient skin, defining the values of the transformation matrix for each particular test. Images are recorded and saved in RGB format and converted to YC_bC_r colour space using a standard methodology, the range of Y is [16,235] and chromatics components are between [16,240]. The equations to get the new base is described as

$$\begin{pmatrix} Y \\ C_b \\ C_r \end{pmatrix} = \begin{pmatrix} 65.481 & 128.553 & 24.966 \\ -37.797 & -74.203 & 112 \\ 112 & -93.786 & -18.214 \end{pmatrix} \begin{pmatrix} R \\ G \\ B \end{pmatrix} + \begin{pmatrix} 16 \\ 128 \\ 128 \end{pmatrix} \tag{1}$$

Then, a simple segmentation of blue background and free-sweat small areas is performed to compute C_b and C_r average values of the skin of the patient and background of the image. The values of red alizarin in the YC_bC_r colour space have been calculated only once time like the average of multiple realizations. The advantage of this approach is that the system can adapt to different skins and situations.

The new YC_xC_y coordinate system is defined as

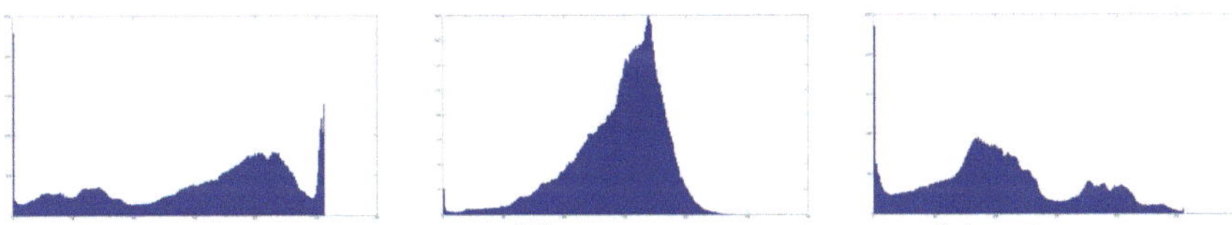

(a) R Component (b) G Component (c) B Component

Fig. 4 Mean values of histogram for RGB colour space

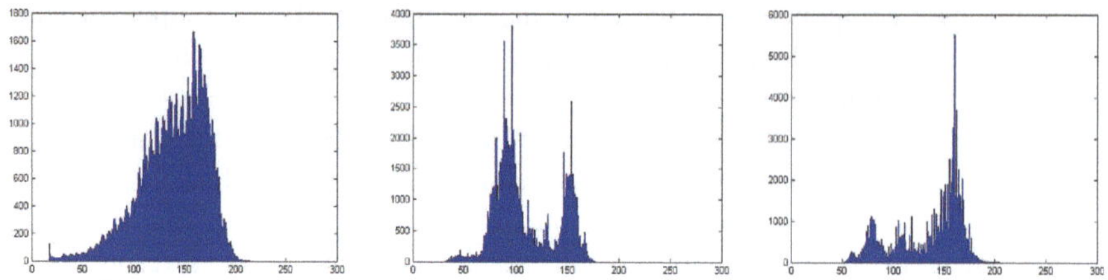

(a) Y Component **(b)** C_b Component **(c)** C_r Component

Fig. 5 Mean values of histogram for YC_bC_r colour space

$$\begin{pmatrix} Y \\ C_x \\ C_y \end{pmatrix} = \begin{pmatrix} 1 & 0 & 0 \\ 0 & a & b \\ 0 & c & d \end{pmatrix} \begin{pmatrix} Y \\ C_b \\ C_r \end{pmatrix} + \begin{pmatrix} 0 \\ e \\ f \end{pmatrix} \tag{2}$$

where the parameters $\{a, b, c, d, e, f\}$ model the skin of the patient and environmental conditions. To compute these parameters, the following two linear equations are solved

$$\begin{pmatrix} 255 \\ 0 \\ 0 \end{pmatrix} = \begin{pmatrix} B_{mark} & R_{mark} & 1 \\ B_{skin} & R_{skin} & 1 \\ B_{aliz} & R_{aliz} & 1 \end{pmatrix} \begin{pmatrix} a \\ b \\ e \end{pmatrix} \tag{3}$$

$$\begin{pmatrix} 0 \\ 100 \\ 255 \end{pmatrix} = \begin{pmatrix} B_{mark} & R_{mark} & 1 \\ B_{skin} & R_{skin} & 1 \\ B_{aliz} & R_{aliz} & 1 \end{pmatrix} \begin{pmatrix} c \\ d \\ f \end{pmatrix} \tag{4}$$

where B_{mark} and R_{mark} are the C_b and C_r components of blue mark, B_{skin} and R_{skin} of skin of the patient, and B_{aliz} and R_{aliz} of red alizarin, respectively. It is important to have a fixed reference for alizarin colour, and so to be able to compare results of different patients. For this reason, it has been performed a study with patients who show a significant amount of sweat and the experimental values of 100 for B_{aliz} and 190 for R_{aliz} were selected as adequate.

To obtain the C_b and C_r components of each patient, it is enough that we examine the histograms of these components for the first image of the patient. Any histogram has two main maximums corresponding to the blue elements and to the skin of the patient, in C_b the highest value of this component is assigned to the mark and the lowest to the skin and vice versa in C_r.

This homomorphism leads us to get histograms like those shown in Fig. 6. The Y component is the same that in YC_bC_r, and it is useful to correct possible lighting variations as we will see later. Two other components have taken a shape that be

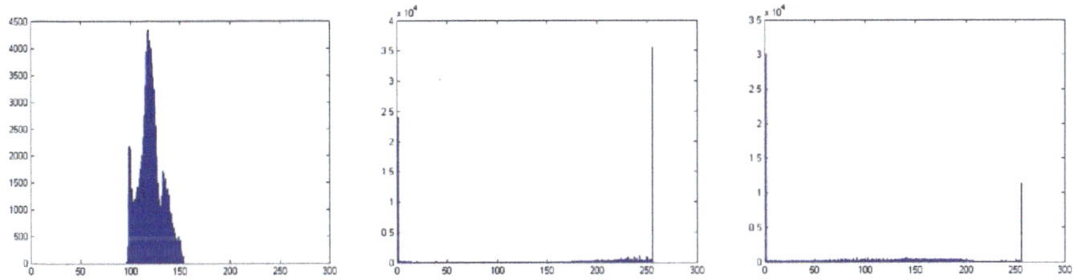

(a) Y Component **(b)** C_x Component **(c)** C_y Component

Fig. 6 Mean values of histogram for YC_xC_y colour space

better the reliability of thresholds selection and segmentation, so the probability of error has been minimized.

The C_x and C_y histograms are almost bimodal, as already described improving the segmentation. In C_x component, lowest values are corresponded with the skin of the patient and highest values with blue background and mark. While in C_y, all the elements present low values except the skin affected by sweating, with a characteristic red-brown colour.

These improvements result from the reduction in range of the colour space, covering less hues but representing with more resolution the colours really important for our purposes. Figure 7 compares a representation of YC_bC_r colour space with our YC_xC_y colour space, both with a fixed luminance Y equal to 120, their colour representation and the three components RGB, for black and white documents, of this representation are exposed. It is noteworthy that green colour become irrelevant in YC_xC_y colour space, focusing efforts in red and blue hues.

To end this topic, changes in the histograms of an initial and final image of a hyperhidrotic patient are considered. We can see this evolution using each of

(a) coloured - YC_bC_r **(b)** R Component- YC_bC_r **(c)** G Component - YC_bC_r **(d)** B Component - YC_bC_r

(e) coloured - YC_xC_y **(f)** R Component - YC_xC_y **(g)** G Component - YC_xC_y **(h)** B Component - YC_xC_y

Fig. 7 YC_bC_r and YC_xC_y colour space representations

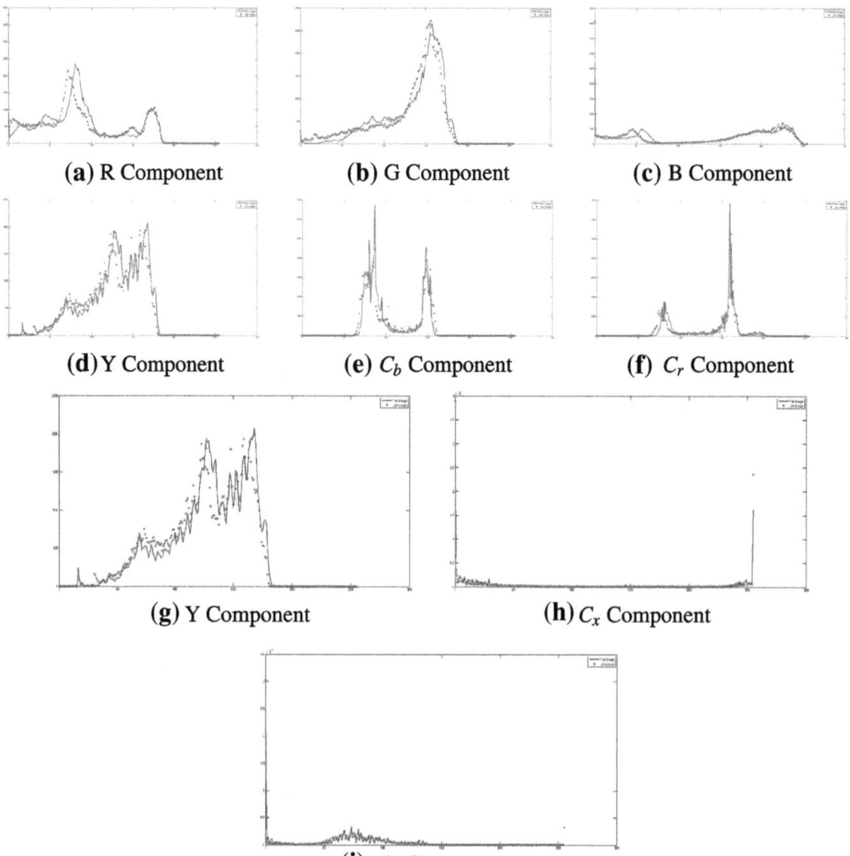

(a) R Component **(b)** G Component **(c)** B Component

(d) Y Component **(e)** C_b Component **(f)** C_r Component

(g) Y Component **(h)** C_x Component

(i) C_y Component

Fig. 8 Comparative between initial(−) and final(+) images histograms for each colour space and components: RGB, YC_bC_r and YC_xC_y

described colour spaces in Fig. 8. In RGB and YC_bC_r all the components changes slightly and it is hard to assign each graph to the correct image, in other words to recognize a histogram of a sweated forearm. However in YC_xC_y a significant change is observed in histograms of images with important amount of sweat, that is showed as the appearance of pixels with high value in C_y component.

We focus now on the YC_xC_y colour space, studying thoroughly its chromatics components. The C_x component has not significantly changes because it has been designed to identify blue elements and skin, and there are not differences between the initial and the final image for that matter, maybe only a little increase in some pixels due to red alizarin, because it has higher value for this component than the skin. Instead, the C_y component undergo an important raise in its maximum value (255) according to apparition of red coloured sweat drops, in this case around 5 % of the total image pixels.

3.4 Lighting Changes Correction

In the clinical practice, illumination is spatially non-uniform when conventional lighting is used, but these changes were not found significant in our work because of the small area displayed in the images. Their influence have nonetheless been studied and corrected by several spatial lighting and contrast correction techniques, getting poor improvements. But in addition to spatial variation, there are also temporal changes, due to flicking and small changes in the ambient illumination, which are typical of a clinical environment (i.e. the opening of the door where the test is under realization produces small changes in the mean illumination of the scene). These changes not only modify the luminance but also the chromatic components. Keep in mind that the connection between luminance and chromatism affects the system in two ways: to quantify the lighting change, an area that does not modify its colour is needed, and to correct the influence of luminance variation on final results.

We have developed a method to compensate the average lighting variations in the temporal domain, preventing error in our tests due to these changes in the lighting conditions. Our algorithm compute the mean value of a small area which is not stimulated with pilocarpine and this value is used to normalize the overall image. Chromatic components are strongly related to luminance, thus changes in one of them affects the measured mean luminance. The result is a sequence of images with little variations of luminance that scarcely distort important chromatic information.

Figure 9 shows a pair of comparisons before and after the lighting changes correction, we can see that the dynamic range of mean luminance has been strongly reduced. Then our system is less vulnerable to instant interferences, like in the right graph, and to stationary modifications caused by a new light source or permanent changes in the conditions, like in the other case shown.

The spatial changes of the illumination has not important effects over our system, as we said, to reach this conclusion some improving contrast techniques

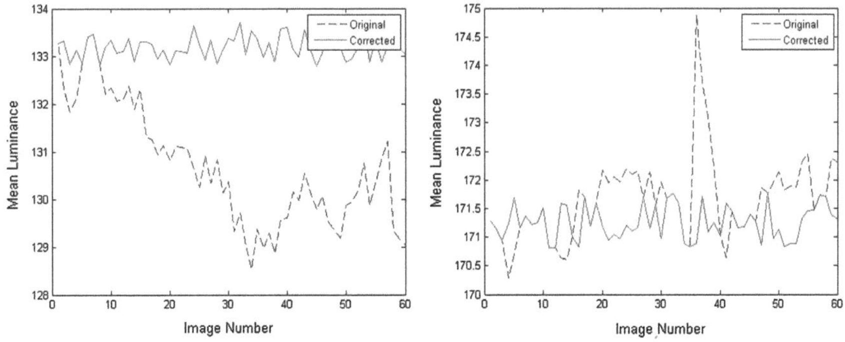

Fig. 9 Examples of lighting changes correction results

has been used like HMF, HDRC, WF, AHE… [13]. In all cases, the improvement is minimal in compare in compare with the increase of computational load. For that reason, this task has been ruled out.

3.5 Movement Correction

We must consider the difficult for the patient to be completely still during 10 min, although our test is very short in time in compare with other sudomotor function assessment systems. We discuss later about a device to reduce movements allowing a certain degree of comfort for the patient. But in technical plane a motion compensation algorithm has been implemented and developed, studying different viewpoints.

Due to the position of the forearm, rested on a flat surface, the dominant movement is the torsion around its own arm axis. From the point of view of the camera, the images suffer not only linear translations but also non-linear deformations. This problem can be addressed by applying warping techniques after finding the corners of the square that limits the work area and tracking them along the video sequence. This is the idea to use a blue square mark during the tests.

We have used a Harris and Stephens detector to find the four corners of the blue square [4]. But we had a lot of error in the thresholding phase selecting only four candidates, hence a set with more than four points were chosen as corner candidates. And later it has applied a very simple technique based in pattern recognition theory, selecting some geometric features of the relation between these candidates. Neural networks solutions have been ruled out, because it is important for us to hold a low computational load, using conventional or even domestic computer equipment.

By this way, to decide which quadruple of points in the set are the best ones, the following similarity measure $R = R_1 R_2$ is computed, where R_1 and R_2 are defined as

$$R_1 = |h^2 - a^2 - b^2| \tag{5}$$

$$R_2 = \sum_{i=1}^{4} |L_i - \overline{L}| \tag{6}$$

where R_1 is the Pythagoras theorem for the triangle defined by three of the points in the quadruple and R_2 is the L1—norm of the lengths of the four edges of the polygon L_i and $\overline{L}$ is its mean value

$$\overline{L} = \frac{1}{4}\sum_{i=1}^{4} L_i$$

The point quadruple with a minimum value of R is selected as the best four edge polygon. To compensate deformation, an affine transformation is used

$$\begin{pmatrix} x_f \\ y_f \end{pmatrix} = \begin{pmatrix} a & b \\ c & d \end{pmatrix} \begin{pmatrix} x_i \\ y_i \end{pmatrix} + \begin{pmatrix} e \\ f \end{pmatrix} \tag{7}$$

where (x_i, y_i) and (x_f, y_f) are the Cartesian coordinates of the corresponding pixels of the previous and actual images, respectively, a, b, c, d, e, f are a set of unknowns that can be solved using the Eq. 7 with the vertices of the four-points polygon and the diagonals cross point.

Figure 10 shows the superposition of the first image and the most displaced image in a sequence, concretely the Y luminance component of these, before and after warping. It can be seen how the squared mark remains in the same place when movement correction is applied. The goal of these geometrical corrections is to preserve the pixels inside the blue square, where important information is contained, allowing a simple tracking of the polygon.

Other methods and techniques for motion compensation [7] have been tested but the results are better using our warping technique. Figure 11 shows a comparative between some of them applied to a sequence: the original displacement of the image, normalize frequency cross-correlation technique [2], block-matching with exhaustive search [2], block-matching with 3 steps search [2], and our warping technique. The measured magnitude has been the cross-correlation between the first image and the evaluated image, along the complete sequence. In any case, our warping technique offers better performance than others, mainly as a result of non-linear deformations. A detailed comparison and discussion can be found in [13].

In a material plane, we have try some elements to reduce movements of the patients during the 10 min of the test, because the position of the forearm in not uncomfortable but neither anatomical. The best option was an airtight plastic bag with a contents of polysterol microspheres, which has a valve to evacuate air and so it results in a rigid close fitting cast [8]. This device allows to immobilize the forearm without hurting the patient, and it gets really significant reductions of movement.

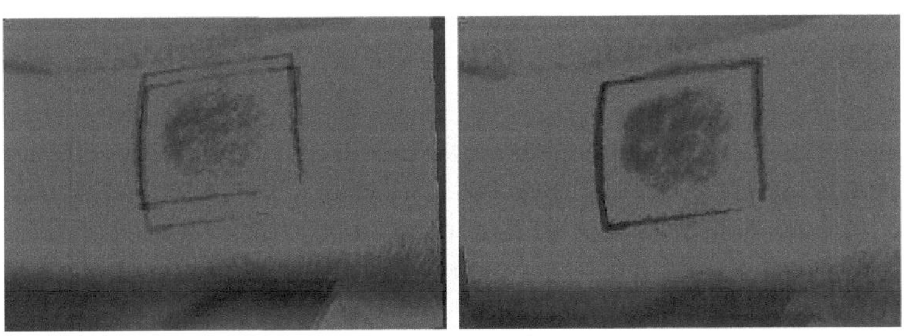

(a) Original images - not corrected **(b)** Warped images - corrected

Fig. 10 Superposition of worst case owing to movement

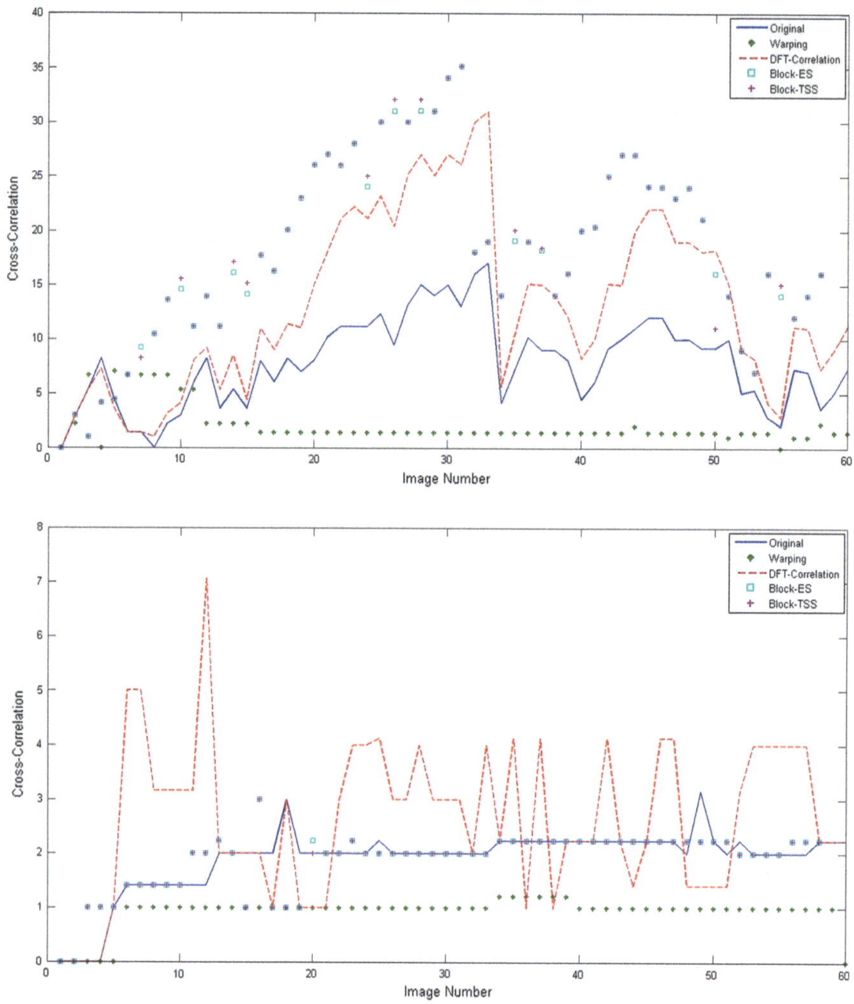

Fig. 11 Comparatives between different displacement correction techniques over two images sequences

3.6 Segmentation

After the correction of lighting temporal variations and movements of the arm, the sweat area is segmented using the proposed C_x and C_y components. To do that, the optimal thresholding method with minimum probability error proposed by Otsu [11] is used with both chromatic components. Using the C_x component, pixels are classified as skin or blue, and with C_y component, the skin pixels are classified as sweat and non sweat. The threshold values T_x and T_y, respectively, were found using the whole set of patient cases to optimize the best value for the T_x value and

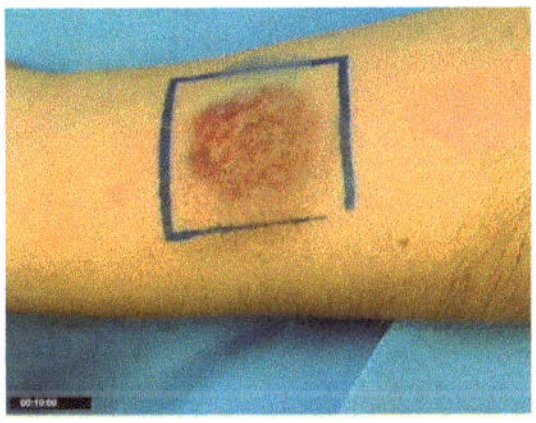

(a) Initial image

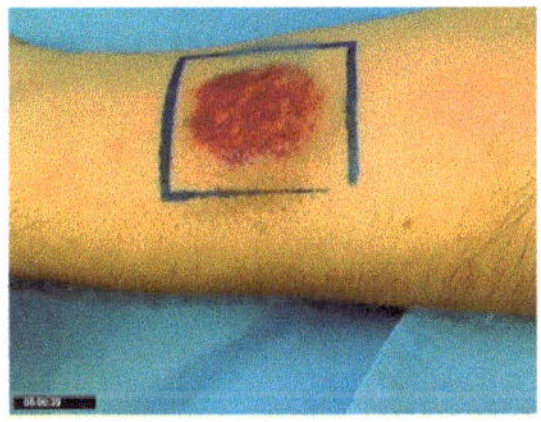

(b) After 5 minutes

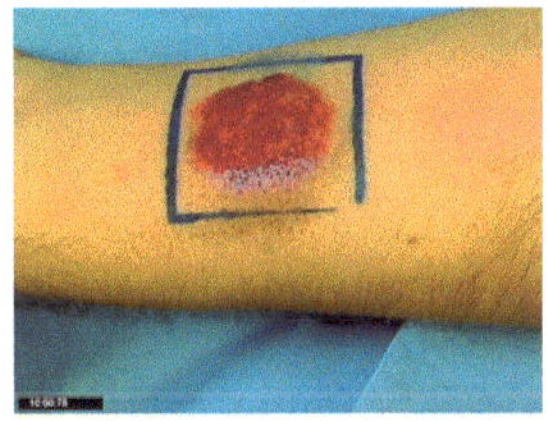

(c) After 10 minutes

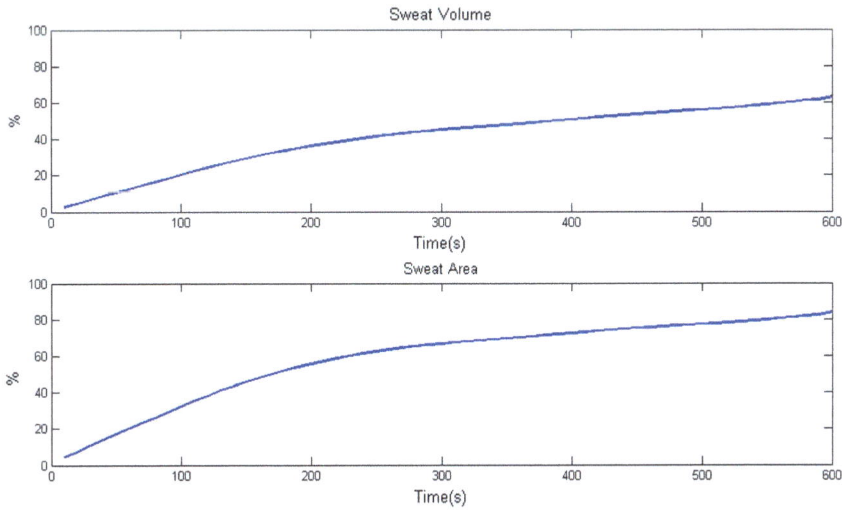

(d)

Fig. 12 Response of a normohidrotic patient

using the set of patients with high levels of sweat to determine the T_y value. In our work, obtained values were $T_x = 119$ and $T_y = 153$.

These thresholds have been checked with other methods, global basic and adaptive thresholding, obtaining values very close to the above-mentioned T_x and T_y.

3.7 Sweat Quantification

Subsequently, when we have finished all the corrections, lighting and movements, and we have decided the thresholds which define the sweat pixels, we only need to count these and offer the final results. Previously we have to standardize the number of pixels in relation with respect to the area of the blue square mark. So this mark is not only useful to correct the movements of the patients, but also it gives us a ratio between pixels in our images and centimeters in the real world.

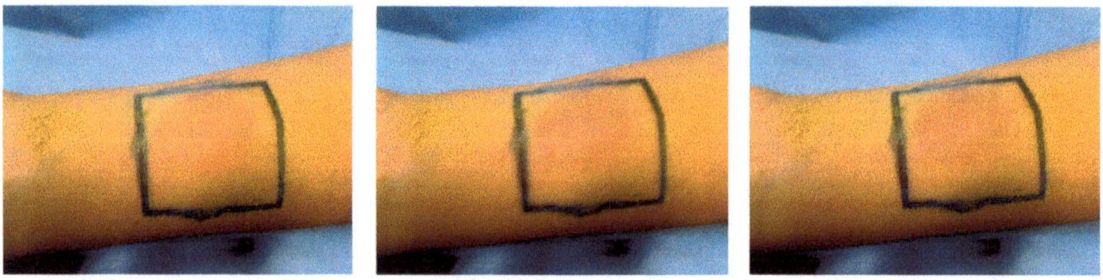

(a) Initial image **(b)** After 5 minutes **(c)** After 10 minutes

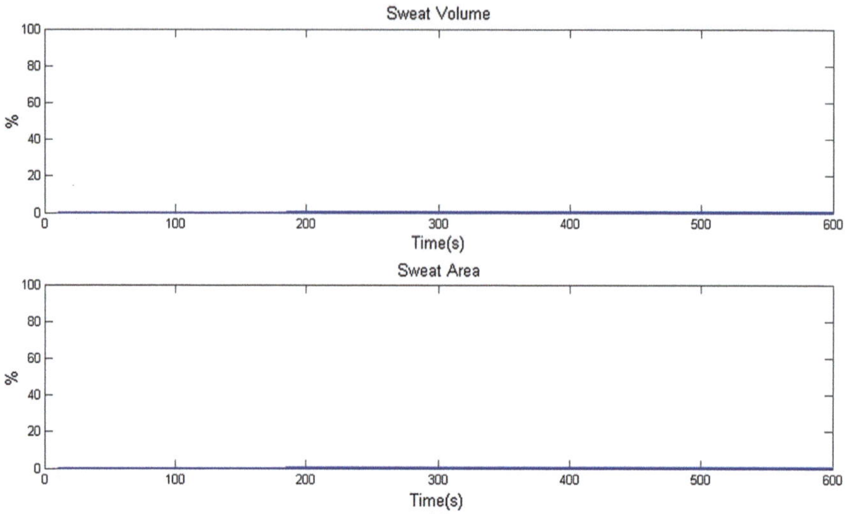

(d)

Fig. 13 Response of a hypohidrotic patient

Three examples of the three typical sweat responses are detailed below:

To start with, Fig. 12 shows a typical result for a normohidrotic patient, who presented a noticeable amount of sweat at the end, as it can be qualitatively seen in Fig. 12a, b, c, which correspond to three instants of the sequence, initial, in the middle of the sequence and final respectively. The pair of graphs presented in Fig. 12d are the dynamics of sweat area and virtual volume. In both cases, there is an initial steep slope, which levels off at the end. A measure of this gradient could be useful to define sweating response. One could say that this sort of patients shows a linear response.

In Fig. 13, the results and some image samples of a hypohidrotic patient are displayed. We have not a lot to say about this profile. As one can see, the patient hardly perspires and there are not red pixels to count, so the result graphs are nearly null.

On the other hand, Fig. 14 describes typical behavior of a hyperhidrotic patient. This kind of person corresponds with a significant amount of sweat to iontophoresis stimulation quickly. That is why the graphs have an important slope at the beginning, increasing affected area up to get an almost permanent final level.

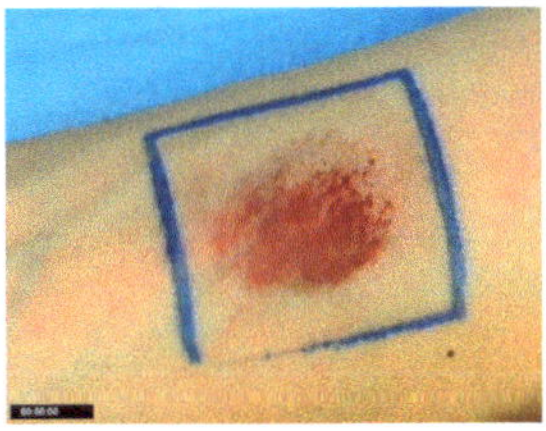

(a) Initial image

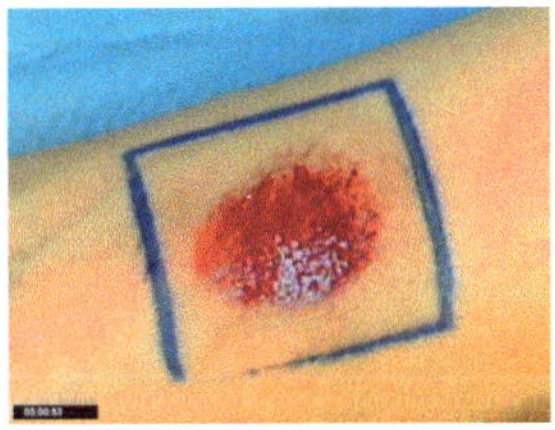

(b) After 5 minutes

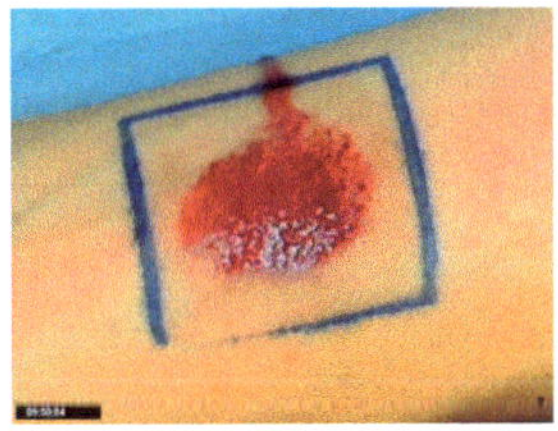

(c) After 10 minutes

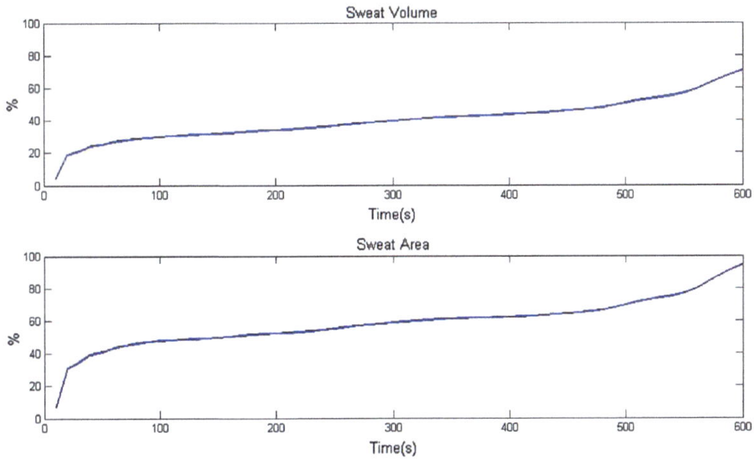

(d)

Fig. 14 Response of a hyperhidrotic patient

Sometimes, the sweat accumulation can lead to some errors and interferences that it can be seen at the end of the graphs presented in Fig. 14d, where an increase in the sweat area and virtual volume can be seen. This is due because a drop of sweat rolled down entering non stimulated surface of the skin.

As we can see, it is easy to tell the difference between these three profiles, so we can class people in accordance with the results of our test in hyperhidrotic, normohidrotic or hypohidrotic.

Mentioned virtual volume is product of the sweat area and the C_y component value of the pixels that compose it. It is just an approximation, but it describes a curve similar to analogous tests. Our research team is working to get a reliable conversion between these results and real volume of excreted sweat.

When the movement of the patient is not significant and lighting variations are small, the corrections subsystems can be omitted, as it is shown in Fig. 15, where the final result, in this case, is similar to the result of the complete system. In this case, the patient is a normohidrotic, exactly the same that is shown in Fig. 12. It can be easily seen that the use of the specific colour space is the key block of our system.

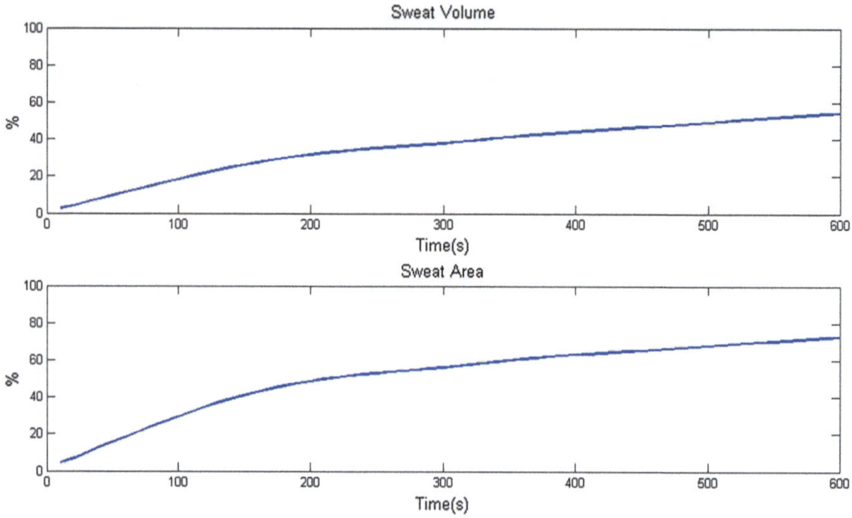

Fig. 15 Response of a normohidrotic patient using only colour space and segmentation subprocesses

4 Results

Using a training set of 28 patients to improve different algorithms for our system, it has been arrived at the final version that is described in this paper. The sudomotor function of 14 subjects (3 hyperhidrotic, 6 normohidrotic and 4 hypohidrotic) was assessed by this version of the test, up to this document has been written. The response of hyperhidrotic patients reached around 70 % sweat production area, its gradient moved higher to low till to get saturation status. In the case of normohidrotic subjects, final values were similar or a little lower, but the slope was nearly constant in the course of the test. The response of hypohidrotic patients hardly reached 5 %. Sweat response, measured with our system, was consistent with the results seen by other testing techniques.

Figure 16 shows the sweat area percentage of the three typical behaviors. The first line(−) corresponds to a hyperhidrotic patient, thus the graph increases fast from the beginning until it reaches saturation state. The next one(+) is a normohidrotic profile, its graph has almost linear performance during the experiment. Last, we can see a hypohidrotic result in the line(∗), which presents very low values all the time because the patient produces very little sweat.

The computational cost of the algorithm is less than 5 min in a typical PC computer (2.4 GHz Intel Core 2 Duo and 4 GB of memory). Because the acquisition of images needs 10 min, results could be ready a few seconds after the sudomotor test is finished. This good performance is due to an optimal code for warping and reconstruction process, more efficient that other techniques, and to the

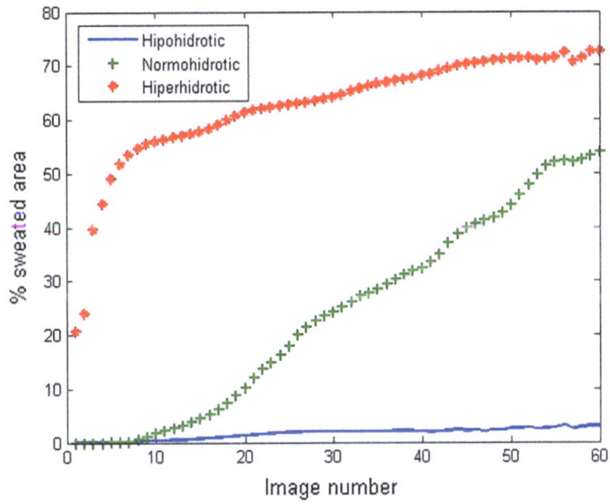

Fig. 16 Example of hyperhidrotic, normohidrotic and hypohidrotic results

reduced image resolution, enough to get good results, preserving the sweat information.

Table 1 shows some statistic values of the results of some patients. The classification is subject to clinical judgement and requires a more extensive and complete analysis, but it seems to be clear that hyperhidrotic behavior is associated with high slope and area values. So, in general terms, we can describe the different behaviors: A hyperhidrotic patient has a high mean and standard deviation of the sweated area and its slope is too high and variable. Normohidrotic patients have lower means of the sweated area and the slopes are less variable. And Hypohidrotic patients present lower values for all the statistics.

Table 1 Results of various kinds of patients

ID	Class	Mean	Std	Max	Slope mean	Slope std	Slope max
LGF	Hyperhidrotic	61.07	12.06	74.29	1.03	2.49	13.77
JMJ	Hyperhidrotic	47.49	13.72	61.62	1.04	1.93	13.41
JOS	Hyperhidrotic	60.95	34.23	99,82	1.73	1.41	5.62
JAM	Normo/Hyperhidrotic	48.60	14.59	64:55	0.99	1.05	5.75
WEN	Normo/Hyperhidrotic	43.90	13.78	64.89	0.90	0.70	5.32
JJG	Normo/Hyperhidrotic	45.34	24.58	84.9	1.40	0.82	4.73
RBV	Normohidrotic	61.45	27.53	93.12	1.57	1.14	4.77
SEB	Normohidrotic	26.82	19.87	47.73	0.70	1.46	5.09
MJT	Hypo/Normohidrotic	10.83	6.27	18.52	0.31	0.40	2.05
RDI	Hypohidrotic	17.66	7.70	30.50	0.45	0.29	1.35
JUL	Hypohidrotic	4.75	4.77	17.37	0.29	0.32	1.49
FMP	Hypohidrotic	6.59	3.39	11.91	0.19	0.13	0.62
FRA	Hypo/Anhidrotic	0.93	0.79	3.01	0.05	0.11	0.81
HAN	Hypo/Anhidrotic	2.01	1.46	4.33	0.05	0.23	0.52

5 Conclusions and Other Considerations

In general, we have met all the proposed objectives. But it can be interesting to consider one to one:

- To design an effective and reliable assessment system of sudomotor function, through digital image processing, with spatial and temporal resolution. Our qualitative results obtained with the proposed system correlate well with silicone impression and other sweating tests, and they are complied with clinical predictions, quantitative results seem to be similar to QSART technique.
- Reduce implementation and maintenance costs, and so to be common in the autonomic evaluation routines. We are especially pleased with the results in this matter, because the required equipment is inexpensive and not specialized. Except the iontophoretic stimulation, all the task can be carrying out with conventional systems (personal computer, webcam…)
- Respect the comfort and well-being of the patients. They only have to keep as still as possible for 10 min, that is easier with some additional means of immobilization like vacuum cushion, and wash their forearms when the experiment have finished to remove blue ink and alizarin rests, both of them are washable.

Our system requires a specific set-up, which the personal staff must know and be able to do it correctly. However, we have design the system to be robust against little errors and technical defects. We are still working to reduce the training time for the doctors and nurses.

Showing the results in real time can be interesting also. So the medical staff can detect immediately any circumstance or problem, and make instantaneous decisions to improve the clinical experience. For example, reducing the test time of patients with a clear diagnosis. Our block design, with clearly separated tasks, is compatible with the needed modifications to calculate partial results each 10 s with minimal delay. So sweating response can be observed live during the test, and software operations seem immediate in the eyes of the medical staff.

With what we have seen so far, it can evaluate and quantify the sudomotor function, but we still working on this system, searching enhancements and extending its applications. An important research line is focused on the whole body evaluation through a sweating chamber, as we can see in Fig. 17. Where patients are brought in, and sweating is stimulated by heat convection. As well, we are working on modify the setup of our sweat test to adapt it to other body zones, like shins and feet.

In summary, sweat response can be assessed with spatial and temporal resolution using digital image processing, and this solution does not need complicated equipment or a large economic investment. In this way, it has been developed a simple and inexpensive tool for the research of the sudomotor function that can be used in neurophysiology diagnosis and other disciplines.

Fig. 17 Sweat evaluation chamber

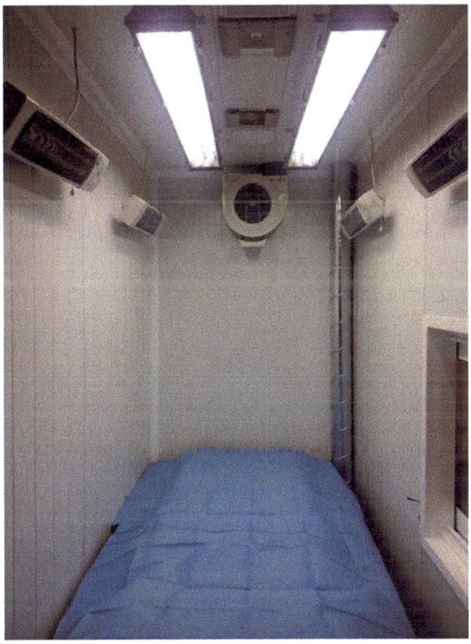

References

1. AAN (1996) Assessment: clinical autonomic testing report of the therapeutics and technology assessment subcommittee of the american academy of neurology. Neurology 46(3): 873–880
2. Barjatya A (2004) Block matching algorithms for motion estimation. DIP 6620 Spring 2004 Final Project Paper (Utah State University, USA), pp 1–6
3. Gibbons CH, Illigens BMW, Centi J, Freeman R (2008) Quantitative direct and indirect test of sudomotor function. Neurology 24:2299–2304
4. Harris C, Stephens M (1988) A combined corner and edge detector. In: Proceedings of the fourth Alvey vision conference, pp 147–151
5. Hjortskov N, Jepsen LT, Nielsen B, Juul A, Skakkebk NE (1995) Pilocarpine iontophoresis test: an index of physiological sweat secretion? Clin Physiol 15(4):409–414. doi:10.1111/j.1475-097X.1995.tb00530.x. http://dx.doi.org/10.1111/j.1475-097X.1995.tb00530.x
6. Illigens BMW, Gibbons CH (2009) Sweat testing to evaluate autonomic function. Clin Auton Res 19(2):79–87
7. Jain J, Jain A (1981) Displacement measurement and its application in interframe image coding. IEEE Trans Commun 29(12):1799–1808
8. Jakobsen A, Iversen P, Gadeberg C, Hansen JL, Hjelm-Hansen M (1987) A new system for patient fixation in radiotherapy. Radiother Oncol 8(2):145–151. doi:10.1016/S0167-8140(87)80168-8. http://www.sciencedirect.com/science/article/pii/S0167814087801688
9. Low P, Benarroch E (2008) Clinical autonomic disorders. Lippincott Williams & Wilkins, Philadelphia
10. Low VA, Sandroni P, Fealey RD, Low PA (2006) Detection of small-fiber neuropathy by sudomotor testing. Muscle Nerve 34(1):57–61
11. Otsu N (1979) A threshold selection method from gray-level histograms. IEEE Trans Syst Man Cybern 9(1):62–66

12. Quintero J, Nava E, Dawid M (2011) Analysis system of sudomotor function using digital image processing. In: Computational vision and medical image processing: VipIMAGE 2011, pp 291–296
13. Quintero JL (2011) Sistema de análisis de la función sudomotora mediante la aplicación del tratamiento digital de imágenes. Universidad de Málaga (Master thesis, in Spanish)
14. Riedel A, Braune S, Kerum G, Schulte-Mnting J, Lcking C (1999) Quantitative sudomotor axon reflex test (qsart): a new approach for testing distal sites. Muscle Nerve 22(9):1257–1264
15. Webster HL (1982) Improved pilocarpine reservoir for use in sweat testing. Clin Chem 28:2182–2183

Current Issues in Medical Thermography

Ricardo Vardasca and Ricardo Simoes

Abstract Digital Medical Thermal Imaging (DMTI) is a modality of medical imaging for monitoring the surface of the skin temperature. The technology evolution over the last 50 years contributed for more accuracy in the measurements and to significantly decrease the size of the equipment making them portable today. The applications of this technique in medicine are on the peripheral vascular, neurological and musculoskeletal conditions assessing and monitoring, in such areas like: cardiology, chronic diseases, dermatology, dentistry, obstetrics, occupational medicine, oncology, physiotherapy, public health, surgery and veterinary medicine. In this chapter the technique is introduced, with its historical perspective, the fundamental physics, the human physiology concepts, the equipment characterization, the existing proposals for examination protocols, the used image processing techniques, the latest developments and applications and the current limitations and challenges.

R. Vardasca · R. Simoes (✉)
Institute for Polymers and Composites–IPC/I3 N, University of Minho,
Campus de Azurém, 4800-058 Guimarães, Portugal
e-mail: rsimoes@dep.uminho.pt; rsimoes@ipca.pt

R. Vardasca
e-mail: rvardasca@dep.uminho.pt

R. Simoes
Life and Health Sciences Research Institute (ICVS/3B's—PT Government Associate Laboratory), School of Health Sciences, University of Minho, Campus de Gualtar, 4710-057 Braga, Portugal

R. Simoes
Polytechnic Institute of Cávado and Ave, 4750-810 Barcelos, Portugal

J. M. R. S. Tavares and R. M. Natal Jorge (eds.), *Topics in Medical Image Processing and Computational Vision*, Lecture Notes in Computational Vision and Biomechanics 8,
DOI: 10.1007/978-94-007-0726-9_12,

1 Introduction

Temperature has been defined by the National Physics Laboratory in UK as the measurement of the average energy of the microscopic components of which an object is made. Temperature is a physical propriety of human body and it is related with healthy equilibrium of its physiology [1].

In 1800 Sir William Herschel, based on the Newton experiment in using white light exposed to a glass prism generating a colored rainbow, decided to measure the temperatures of such colors with thermometers and found that the color presenting the higher temperature was the red and at the outer side of this color there an invisible light with a much higher temperature, discovering the infrared [2].

Carl Wunderlich in 1868 has published his work in "On the Temperature in Diseases", where he characterized the temperature in several pathologies and introduced the usage of clinical thermometers and temperature charts in the clinical practice [2].

The bolometer was invented in 1880 by the American astronomer Samuel Langley. This instrument is used to measure infrared or heat radiation, and he claimed it could measure the heat irradiated by a cow at 400 m distance [3]. This sensor had particular importance to the development of the thermal cameras. In 1929, Tihanyi invented the first infrared (IR) camera in Britain for usage in anti-aircraft defense as night vision [4]. The first conventional IR camera, the Evaporograph, was developed in the 30 s by Czerny for military use only [5].

The first usage of a thermographic system to look at temperature distribution on the human body was made by Ray Lawson in 1956 when he used an evaporograph system to look at temperature distribution of a breast cancer malignant tumor [6].

2 Thermal Physics

The non-contact temperature measurement of an object is made based on the temperature of a blackbody, where the microscopic components are the photons which make up the electromagnetic field within the blackbody cavity. The temperature difference between two points, hotter and cooler, can be expressed by the rate of heat transfer. The transfer of energy from a hotter object to a cooler object is called heat flux. When two close objects present similar level of thermal energy they are in thermal equilibrium [7].

The electromagnetic spectrum is a representation of the characteristic distribution of electromagnetic radiation emitted or absorbed by a particular object in wavelength (Fig. 1).

All matter at a temperature above absolute zero emits electromagnetic radiation, which is thermal radiation. Objects in the electromagnetic spectrum have the ability to emit and absorb electromagnetic radiation; a physical object that absorb all incident electromagnetic radiation is called a blackbody, which is also the best

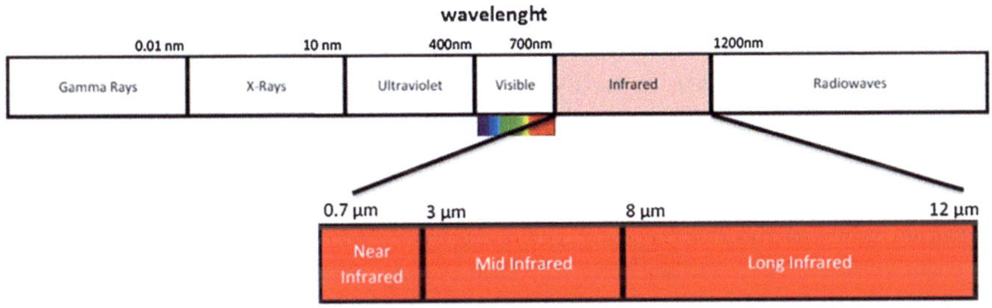

Fig. 1 The electromagnetic spectrum by wavelength with emphasis in the infrared region

possible thermal radiator based on the Kirchoff's Law, where the amount of absorption will equal the amount of emission [7].

To some degree all matter also absorbs electromagnetic radiation. A blackbody, which is an idealized object, absorbs all radiation falling on it, at all wavelengths, and at a uniform temperature, its emission also called blackbody radiation has a characteristic frequency distribution that depends on the temperature. There are three equations that describe the radiation emitted from a blackbody: Planck's radiation law, Win's displacement law and Stefan-Boltzmann formula. The amount of energy emitted by a black body in radiation of a certain wavelength or frequency is given by the Planck's law. However the Planck's law predicts that a black body will radiate energy at all frequencies; its intensity rapidly tends to zero at both high and low frequencies or short and long wavelengths. This means that a black body at room temperature does not emit in the visible range. The Wien's displacement law exemplifies how the spectrum of black body radiation at any temperature is related to the spectrum at any other temperature. Knowing the shape of the spectrum at one temperature, the shape at any other temperature can be calculated. The Stefan-Boltzmann equation expresses the total radiated energy from a blackbody, per unit area and per unit time, which is proportional to the fourth power of its absolute temperature. Most of the radiation thermometers are based upon it [7].

The most important factor in non-contact temperature measurement is the object emissivity, which is the ratio between the radiant emittance produced by an object to that of a blackbody at a specific temperature. This factor affects the accuracy of the measurement. A perfect blackbody has an emissivity value of 1 and is considered a perfect emitting surface. For highly reflective materials the emissivity value approaches zero [7].

3 Thermal Physiology

The human body needs an internal temperature at constant value (36–37.5 °C) to maintain its normal functions. Outside of that interval some functional activities would be compromised. A variation of more than 7 °C can be fatal [8]. However, this vital parameter may be affected due to several factors such as: internal homeostatic or disease processes and external environment. The largest organ in the human body is the skin. It involves the other structures of the body and acts as an interface with the external environment, isolating the human body and contains thermoreceptors, which have an important role in the human thermoregulation. Heat can be transferred from the body to the external environment through four physical mechanisms [9]:

Conduction: in the human body this heat is dissipated between the structures of the body from the internal organs to the skin. In an unclothed resting state about 3 % of body heat is dissipated by this mean.

Convection: through the blood circulation and urine. At a steady state the amount of percentage of heat lost from an unclothed human body by convection is about 15 %.

Radiation: the body loses heat by radiating more infrared waves than it absorbs from cooler objects; however, when surrounded by warm objects, the opposite happens. In an unclothed steady state about 60 % of heat loss occurs by radiation.

Evaporation: certain amounts of water are lost through the skin, mucous membranes and breathe. The amount of evaporation is directly related to the relative humidity of the air. The relative humidity is inversely proportional to the evaporation rate. In a situation of 100 % relative humidity heat may be gained by the body through condensation of water on the skin as fast as heat is lost by evaporation. For an unclothed human body under resting conditions, about 22 % of heat loss occurs by evaporation.

Thermoregulation is the capacity of a body to maintain and regulate its temperature within a limited range of values. That temperature is regulated by the autonomic nervous system and by behavioral means. When a decrease in temperature is perceived the heat gain mechanisms are activated such as: vasoconstriction, shivering and a slow increase of metabolism rate. If a temperature increase is perceived, the body temperature decrease mechanisms such as: vasodilatation and sweat glands stimulation are activated. Factors such as age, body mass index and gender affect the thermoregulation, and this is a reason why they should be taken into consideration [9].

Microcirculation is the name given to the smallest blood vessels (<100 μm in diameter) with thin muscular walls in the vasculature. Its components are arterioles, capillaries and venules. The increase of total peripheral resistance of the arterioles may lead to hypertension, this resistance affects directly affects the peripheral temperature. Arterioles are composed of vascular smooth muscle and endothelium that have direct communication between them. These cells are involved in several vascular aspects such as the control of blood pressure by vasoconstriction or vasodilation. The endothelium produces nitric oxide and any deregulation in this function may be a sign of a pathological state, which may be reflected in the peripheral temperature. The regulation of blood flow into capillaries is provided by pre-capillary sphincters that answer to nitric oxide. The blood flow influences the peripheral temperature, which is transferred to the external environment through infrared emission. This emission can be recorded by an infrared imaging system and used to monitor pathological states indicated by deficient nitric oxide regulation [9]. There are health causes for internal temperature increase and decrease, from which the peripheral skin temperature effect can be observed with medical thermal imaging [8].

4 Equipment

Thermal cameras are the instruments used in thermography to capture and monitor object temperature through surface irradiated heat.

The main components of a thermal camera are: the optics, that focus the infrared energy onto the detector, the infrared detector array, which converts the infrared energy into a proportional electrical signal, the shutter system, that performs an image correction whenever the auto adjust button is depressed and the Digital Signal Processing (DSP) unit, which is the electronic component that process the electrical signal to produce a radiometric picture and perform temperature calculations [7].

The IR camera optics are mainly made of Silicon (Si) or Germanium (Ge). Germanium lenses are used for long-wavelength (7–14 μm) cameras and Silicon for short-wavelength (3–5 μm) cameras. The internal design of the optics system is also very important. It should be adequate for the system to transmit close to 100 % of incident radiation [10, 11].

The method of constructing the images has been the aspect of the infrared cameras that has evolved with time. The scanning mode was the first imaging systems and it was composed of one sensor element, which scans the whole scene starting column by column and jumping from line to line until finishing the whole image. This system has been preceded by another scanning system which was composed of an array of sensor elements capable of scan a whole line of a scene completing the image line by line. The most recent system is based on a matrix of sensor elements, called Focal Plane Array (FPA), which is capable of record the whole scene at once, being faster and producing images of better quality [7].

There are two families of infrared detectors, the cooled and the uncooled. The cooled require cooling and normally operate at cryogenic temperatures. Old models of thermal cameras were cooled through liquid nitrogen and argon gas. More recent cooled detectors are refrigerated using thermoelectric (e.g. Peltier) or Stirling coolers and have an limited operational life (typically from 8–15 h) with expensive back-to factory repair. The cooled systems normally operate in the range of 60–100 K, below the environmental temperature, to reduce the thermally-induced noise to a level below that of the signal from the scene being imaged. These detectors are more expensive to produce and use than uncooled sensors. The need of cooling is power and time consuming and the cooling apparatus of the whole system is bulky and expensive. This type of detectors is based on detecting and converting light and designed to operate mainly in the 3–5 μm wavelength range. The lenses for the uncooled systems are more costly due to the needed focal length. The cooled detectors provide a superior image quality and a greater sensitivity to small differences in the scene temperatures than the uncooled detectors [12].

The uncooled detectors operate at ambient temperature or stabilized at temperature close to ambient using temperature control elements to reduce image noise. This type of system operates based on changes in resistance, voltage or current when heated with infrared radiation. These changes are measured and compared with the values of the operating temperature of the detector. These detectors produce images of lower quality and sensitivity to differences in the scene temperatures when compared with the cooled detectors. They are limited by the currently available technology and operate mainly in the 7–12 μm wavelength range, which is where most of the terrestrial temperature targets emit most of their infrared energy. Cameras using uncooled detectors are smaller, easy to use and less costly due to being manufactured in fewer steps and built in less expensive vacuum packaging than the cooled ones. In comparison with the cooled detector cameras the uncooled have fewer moving parts, cheaper lenses (require smaller focal length) and have more longevity in usage time [12].

The two main groups of infrared detectors are the thermal detectors and the photon detectors. The thermal detectors are used by uncooled cameras and photon detector by the cooled cameras [12].

When choosing a camera, from the aspects of portability, size and weight there are a few parameters to have in consideration such as: mode of operation, type of sensor, dynamic range, thermal resolution, spatial resolution, Noise Equivalent Temperature Difference (NETD), Minimal Resolvable Temperature Difference (MRTD), accuracy, precision, responsiveness and dwell [7].

Despite of many models available in the market, none of them have been conceived for medical use, so in order to choose which camera is recommended for a specific situation a guideline to specify and test a thermal camera for medical use was presented in 2009 by Howell and Smith [13].

5 Proposals of Examination Protocols

There are no reference values of temperature distribution on the human body surface in the existing literature, so DMTI does not have a generally accepted range of standardized positions to improve the quality of temperature recordings. Standardization of the technique allows repeatability, facilitates understanding and knowledge exchange and reduces the amount and influence of variables. This is a relevant aspect as some past errors were made due to the lack of using a standard image capturing methodology which contributed to a decreased application in medicine and considerable loss of credibility [14, 15].

Environmental conditions such as temperature, humidity and air circulation affect the measurements as well as laboratory. A patient having medication, meals, drinks, drugs and physiotherapy before the appointment, and having ointments and clothing over the skin during examination will have influence in the recordings. The duration and thermal conditions of the subject pre-examination acclimatization period affects the results. Using an imaging system that is not in conformity with the quality assurance requirements will affect the process and quality of acquiring the image. The usage of standardized regions of interest (ROI) enforces the quality of the recording by facilitating correct subject positioning and distance from the camera as well as the size and position of the ROI itself. All these variables have to be taken into consideration in order to homogenize the capture and analysis process and to allow comparisons and the generation of reference data [16].

Guidelines have been proposed on how this technique should be conducted in terms of: patient communication and preparation, patient assessment, usage of standard views with correspondent indication of reliability, thermal provocation tests, examination room conditions, equipment preparation and operation, examination procedure, reporting and continuing professional education. The objective of these documents is to standardize the technique, offering the opportunity for multi-center data exchange and modality improvement [17, 18].

6 Infrared Image Processing

Medical thermal images can be evaluated both subjectively and quantitatively. In infrared cameras the focal plane array (FPA) typically captures a frame (image) every 16 ms. Pixels are usually digitalized with 12 or 14 bits. The temperature range for studying the human body is normally from 25° to 35 °C, a 10 °C difference. For this range as with an 8-bit pixel resolution it is possible to represent 256 levels of temperature. This represents a thermal resolution of slightly more than 0.1 °C over the 10 °C range and similar to the thermal resolution limit of most microbolometer based cameras [19].

During capture the usual processing is an image non-uniformity correction, made by the imager itself. After capture, most cameras perform some degree of simple pre-processing. This can be low pass filtering, thinning and binarization. More complex functions are then executed by computer based software [19].

After an image is captured three stages typically describe the subsequent operations: processing, analysis and understanding. The image processing can be divided in two different phases: segmentation and registration. Segmentation normally involves image enhancing techniques to reduce or minimize the noise effect (thermal images by their nature are very affected by noise) and techniques to delineate and identify the objects of the scene such as: edge detectors, gap bridging techniques, fill area operations, histogram equalization, and Hough transforms (for shape detection) [20].

Common post-processing techniques in thermal imaging, used in the image analysis, are high-pass filters (to detect hot or cold spots), temperature averaging and computing spatial, temporal or frequency variations of temperature.

Temperature analysis on defined regions of interest are the most common operations to absolute or relative temperature measurements with interpretation of the pixels. Other auxiliary thermal imaging analysis tools are: isotherms, line profiling, histograms and cross section [19].

The final phase in infrared images processing is the understanding that can be divided in two different applications: static or dynamic. Static is when only an image is interpreted; dynamic when several images from different examinations or a sequence of the same examination are analyzed. For the dynamic understanding artificial intelligence techniques can be employed such as: Artificial Neural Networks, Bayesian Belief Networks, Linear Discriminate Analysis and Fuzzy Logic, or high order statistical classifiers such as: variance, skewness and kurtosis to assess equal detected regions of interest [19, 21]. Due to the anatomical shapes and sizes differ from individual to individual and in the same examination, the difficulty of a subject remain still, it is hard to compare or average objects temperature values if these objects are placed differently in the images or differ in size. To solve this problem there are image warping techniques to translate object temperature values to a reference object image using vector, mesh or triangle based transformations implementing interpolations to correct the final result [22].

The use of digital imaging in medicine brought several improvements such as: the ability to post-process images improving the results, the development of permanent record systems that lead to better pathological understanding and improved treatments and clinician knowledge, and the possibility to send images to third parties over networks increases the spread of knowledge and understanding, allowing advice from remote specialists and the establishment of reference information based on image comparison, and consequently reducing human error [19].

7 Recent Development and Applications

Digital medical thermal imaging (DMTI) has already been successfully applied in: skin oncology, pain management and control, assessment and characterization of vascular disorder, diabetes vascular peripheral circulation assessment, rheumatic arthritis, nerve entrapments assessment, open heart and transplant surgeries, cataract removal, burn assessment, assessment and characterization of dermatological disorders, monitoring efficacy of drugs and therapies, thyroid monitoring, dentistry, respiratory allergies, and sports and rehabilitation medicine [23].

DMTI has proved itself scientifically as a good technique for diagnosing and monitoring diseases such as: Paget's bone disease, soft tissue rheumatic conditions (muscle spasm and injury, sprains and strains, enthesopathies: tennis elbow, golfer elbow and periarthropathia of the shoulder, and fibromyalgia), peripheral nerve injury (nerve entrapment: radiculopathy, thoracic outlet syndrome, and carpal tunnel syndrome, and peripheral nerve paresis: brachial plexus paresis, facial nerve and peroneal nerve), and Complex Regional Pain Syndrome (neurological condition) [24]. Raynaud's phenomena and scleroderma are clinical conditions where functional DMTI proved to be a relevant diagnostic method [25].

In cardiovascular applications, DTMI has been successfully used for assessment of vascular dysfunction of coronary heart disease [26] and for monitoring hand temperature changes during hemodialysis preventing ischemia [27, 28]. It has been proven a recommended technique for evaluating occupational conditions affecting the upper limbs [29–31]. DTMI has assisted with relevance in laser [32] and laparoscopic [33, 34] surgical procedures, it has been demonstrated to be a powerful assistive technique in combination with a thermal challenge for assisting flap tissue transplant from the abdomen to correct a removed breast, in identifying the perforated blood vessels, facilitating the tissue vascular irrigation and the restoration of circulation in the tissues, and it was also important in the post-surgical following in assessing the recovery [35].

In dermatology, DTMI was found useful in the assessment of skin lesions [36], pressure ulcers [37], melanomas [38] and allergies [39]. In diabetics, the technique has been applied with success in the evaluation of tissue viability and peripheral circulation to prevent lesions [40, 41] and treatment monitoring [41].

The modality has been tested and validated for massive fever screening in case of possible pandemic influenza [42–44]. It was found that the best localization in the face to monitor core temperature is the inner canthus of the eyes [43, 44]. Standard documentation was produced for minimal requirements, concern and guidelines [45, 46].

Hyperbaric oxygen therapy was successfully monitored with DMTI [47]. It has shown relevance in identifying back pain [48] and severity of pain caused by the implant of artificial knee joints [49]. In dentistry the modality proved efficient in assessing nerves, pain and tissue vitality [50, 51].

None of many proposed approaches to diagnose breast cancer with DTMI to date has shown scientific evidence of applicability, it is unable to localize a lesion or tumor, it can be concluded that the technique is not indicated for the primary evolution of symptomatic patients nor should it be used on a routine basis as screening test for breast cancer [52, 53]. Regulatory actions are been taken against companies who continue to mislead the public to ensure patient safety looking to exploit them in providing breast cancer diagnosis with thermography [54]. However, DTMI has proved to be a good tool to evaluate sarcoma and leukemia treatments [55, 56].

The use of DMTI in acupuncture was reliable in identifying the needle points [57] and to demonstrate the visual effect of the treatment [58].

Thermal symmetry of the human body has been defined and the discriminant value of 0.5 ± 0.3 °C can be used to access abnormalities in specific pathological states at the limbs [59].

In veterinary medicine the use of DMTI was useful to assess clinical signs of dermatome patterns, peripheral neurovascular conditions (Horner's syndrome, neurectomies, and vascular occlusions and compressions), joint disease, tendonitis and other musculoskeletal problems in various animal species. It also proved its value in monitoring healing processes after surgery and on screening to prevent severe injuries, particularly on competition horses, which prevented financial losses associated with delayed diagnosis and treatment [60].

A combination of IR image with visible 3D image had accurately and quantitatively detected inflammation in diabetic foot disease [61]. Despite the different image formats for thermal images, it has been demonstrated that the best method to store and communicate IR images in using the JPEG-LS standard lossless compression algorithm embedded in the current form of the standard DICOM, enforcing security, privacy, availability, efficiency and efficacy [62, 63].

The combination of thermal and visual images was useful either to see which part of the anatomy is affected by a certain disease or to judge the efficacy of the treatment [64].

The recommended method for improving medical thermal images are the Median, Mean and Wiener filters; however noise filtering should only be applied when specifically needed [65]. Probability-based edge operators produce the best outcome in delineating objects in a thermographic scene especially after preprocessing with a noise homomorphic removal filter [66]. In reconstructing thermal images the recommended interpolation method for scaling images following the standard capture protocol is the Nearest Neighborhood, although an error is introduced [67]. Thermal images can be standardized using geometrical barycentric based warping method with high accuracy in a change of scale of less than 10 %, eliminating human error. Comparison and/or averaging of images are then possible [68].

8 Technique Limitations and Challenges

Digital Medical Thermal Imaging (DMTI) has some limitations such as: high quality cameras are expensive and can easily get damaged, image interpretation often requires training and experience, accurate temperature measurements at an outside environment is difficult to perform due to the existence of different emissivities, presence of casts, bandages or other technical factors can limit the exposure skin to a temperature equilibration environment, high dependency in the patient cooperation and low penetration of the technique (2.5 mm) [17]. Static DMTI only demonstrates local vasodilation and vasoconstriction [51]. Static DMTI is a passive measurement and the individual variability combined with the complex character of thermoregulation limits the thermographic interpretation. The lack of specificity makes it necessary to combine its measurements with other modalities that give structural information of the human body (CT, MRI and ultrasound); on other hand this technique is highly operator dependent [69]. The unique way for addressing these limitations is through a standardized procedure for DMTI.

The current challenges for IR detector are: size reduction of the uncooled detectors maintaining or reducing the NETD for consequently reducing the Signal to Noise Ratio; in the electronics: faster digital signal processing with internal memory; and in optics, the reduction of lenses size to improve the required field of view. The so called third generation cooled imagers are expect to have a reduction on chip size (pixel <20 μm) and, consequently, cost; introduce the two color pixel; a change on the sensor format for a wide field of view and high space resolution; and a reduction on the temperature cycling fatigue in order to extend the equipment usage and life [70].

Research is required, in terms of structuring specific guidelines and protocols, for DTMI to become an accurate and reliable method of collecting skin temperature data following cryotherapy [71]. Two projects have been proposed to build a medical reference database of the distribution of temperature surface of the human body attending gender, age and different body mass index (BMI) classes, which would significantly improve the gap of medical reference data for regular examinations [16].

A biometric method based on face recognition in thermal images using unique and time invariant physiological information and regarding nonlinear deformations of the vascular network is proposed. A Bayesian segmentation method is suggested for separating the face tissue from the background, and a white top-hat segmentation preceded by anisotropic diffusion is the recommended technique to extract the vascular network of the skin face [72]. Automatic discovery of the anatomic control points, which delimitate the geometrical model of regions of interest, in order to produce a fully automated solution for standardizing medical thermal images, would be of great interest [68]. Novel methods for calibration and acquisition processes are required in order to enhance real-time acquisition of 3D thermograms [73]. Improvement of the reliability and reproducibility of hot spot identification is needed and has to be investigated through software assisted identification of hot spots [74]. An automated discovery and measure method of the temperature parameters of the inner canthus of the eyes is needed for real time fever screening detection [44]. A globally accepted false color scale is needed to standardize the qualitative aspect of evaluating an image [75].

The thermal camera manufacturers have not produced yet thermographic equipment exclusively for medical use. There is an absence of an updated software package to record and analyze medical thermograms in a standardized way incorporating the current edge thermal image processing techniques. However, technology in general for DMTI has evolved considerably over the past decades, and it is recommended that some of the studies performed in the 1960 and 1970s be reproduced with current technology (high resolution cameras and advanced image processing techniques) and standard procedures be set for prospective findings.

Acknowledgments Foundation for Science and Technology, Lisbon, through the 3° Quadro Comunitário de Apoio, the POCTI and FEDER programs, and project PEst-C/CTM/LA0025/2011 (Strategic Project—LA 25—2011–2012). Projects "AAL4ALL—Padrão de Cuidados Primários para Serviços de AAL" (n° 13852) and "Do-IT—Desenvolvimento e Operacionalização da Investigação de Translação" (n° 13853), co-financed by European Community Fund through COMPETE—Programa Operacional Factores de Competitividade. We thank the Hospital de Braga (Portugal) and the collaboration from its staff in the Department of Obstetrics and Gynecology.

References

1. NPL (2012) Thermal frequent asked questions page. URL: http://www.npl.co.uk/engineering-measurements/thermal/temperature/faqs/what-is-temperature-(faq-thermal) Accessed 27 Jan 2012
2. Ring EFJ (2007) The historical development of temperature measurement in medicine. Infrared Phys Technol 49:297–301
3. Richards PL (1994) Bolometers for infrared and millimeter waves. J Appl Phys 76:1–36
4. Lisowska-Lis A, Mitkowski SA, Augusty J (2011) Infrared technique and its application in science and engineering in the study plans of students in electrical engineering and electronics. In: Proceedings of 2nd world conference on technology and engineering education (WIETE 2011), pp 104–108
5. Lloyd JM (1975) Thermal Imaging Systems. Plenum, New York
6. Lawson RN (1956) Implications of surface temperatures in the diagnosis of breast cancer. Can Med Assoc J 75:309–331
7. Thomas RA (1999) The thermography monitoring handbook. Coxmoor Publishing, Oxford
8. Houdas Y, Ring EFJ (1982) Human body temperature. Plenum Press, New York
9. Tortora GJ, Grabowski SR (2003) Principles of anatomy and physiology, 10th edn. Wiley, New York
10. Rogalski A, Chrzanowski K (2002) Infrared detection and devices. Opto-Electron Rev 10(2):111–136
11. FLIR (2011) FLIR R&D Handbook, Institutional webpage. http://www1.flir.com/l/5392/2011-12-05/2YFPK
12. Rogalski A (2010) Infrared detectors, 2nd edn. CRC Press, Boca Raton
13. Howell KJ, Smith RE (2009) Guidelines for specifying and testing a thermal camera for medical applications. Thermology Int 19(1):5–14
14. Ammer K (2003) Need for standardisation of measurements in thermal imaging. In: Wiecek B (ed) Thermography and lasers in medicine. Akademickie Centrum, Lodz, pp 13–17
15. Ring EFJ, Ammer K, Jung A, Murawski P, Wiecek B, Zuber J, Zwolenik S, Plassmann P, Jones CD, Jones BF (2004) Standardization of infrared imaging. In: Conference proceedings of the IEEE engineering in medicine biology, vol 2, pp 1183–1185
16. Ring EFJ, Ammer K, Wiecek B, Plassmann P (2005) Technical challenges for the construction of a medical IR digital image database. In: Chatard, JP, Dennis PNJ (eds) Proceedings of SPIE, detectors and associated signal processing II vol 5964, pp 191–198
17. Schwartz RG (2006) Guidelines for neuromusculoskeletal thermography. Thermol Int 16(1):5–9
18. Ammer K (2008) Standard procedures for recording and evaluation of thermal images of the human body: the Glamorgan protocol. Thermol Int 18(4):125–144
19. Jones BF, Plassmann P (2002) Digital infrared thermal imaging of human skin. IEEE Eng Med Biol 21:41–48
20. Gonzales RC, Woods RE (2009) Digital image processing, 3rd edn. Pearson education, Prenctice Hall, New Jersey
21. Jiang LJ, Ng EYK, Yeo ACB, Wu S, Pan F, Yau WY, Chen JH, Yang Y (2005) A perspective on medical infrared imaging. J Med Eng Technol 29(6):257–267
22. Gomes J, Darsa L, Costa B, Velho L (1999) Warping and morphing of graphical objects. Morgan Kaufmann, San Francisco
23. Diakides NA, Diakides M, Lupo JC, Paul JL, Balcerak R (2008) Advances in medical infrared imaging. In: Diakides NA, Bronzino JD (eds) Medical infrared imaging. CRC Press, Boca Raton, pp 1–13
24. Ring EFJ, Ammer K (2008) Thermal imaging in diseases of the skeletal and neuromuscular systems. In: Diakides NA, Bronzino JD (eds) Medical infrared imaging. CRC Press, Boca Raton, pp 1–13

25. Merla A, Romani GL (2008) Biomedical applications of functional infrared imaging. In: Diakides NA, Bronzino JD, (eds) Medical infrared imaging. CRC Press, Boca Raton, pp 15.1–15.20
26. Gul KM, Ahmadi N, Wang Z, Jamieson C, Nasir K, Metcalfe R, Hecht HS, Hartley CJ, Naghavi M (2009) Digital thermal monitoring of vascular function: a novel tool to improve cardiovascular risk assessment. Vasc Med 14(2):143–148
27. Kalicki B, Jung A, Ring EFJ, Saracyn M, Niemczy S (2011) Monitoring renal dialysis patients by hand thermography. Thermol Int 21(4):116–117
28. Novljan G, Rus RR, Koren-Jeverica A, Avčin T, Ponikvar R, Buturović-Ponikvar J (2011) Detection of dialysis access induced limb ischemia by infrared thermography in children. Ther Apher Dial 15(3):298–305
29. Vardasca R, Ring EFJ, Plassmann P, Jones CD (2008) Thermal monitoring of hand stress during keyboard typing. In: Proceedings of 9th international conference on quantitative infrared thermography, pp 169–174
30. Vardasca R (2011) The use of medical thermography as a complementary examination for occupational conditions affecting the upper limbs. Thermol Int 21(4):146
31. Govindu NK, Babski-Reeves K (2012) Reliability of thermal readings of the skin surface over the anterior deltoid during intermittent, overhead tapping tasks. Int J Ind Ergon 42(1):136–142
32. Campbell P, Thomas R (2008) Thermal imaging in surgery. In: Diakides NA, Bronzino JD (eds) Medical infrared imaging. CRC Press, Boca Raton, pp 19.1–19.18
33. Song C, Tang B, Campbell PA, Cuschieri A (2009) Thermal spread and heat absorbance differences between open and laparoscopic surgeries during energized dissections by electrosurgical instruments. Surg Endosc 23(11):2480–2487
34. Steiner G, Sobottka SB, Koch E, Schackert G, Kirsch M (2011) Intraoperative imaging of cortical cerebral perfusion by time-resolved thermography and multivariate data analysis. J Biomed Opt 16(1):016001
35. Mercer JB, De Weerd L, Miland AO, Wuem S (2010) Pre-, intra- and postoperative use of dynamic infrared thermography (DIRT) provides valuable information on skin perfusion in perforator flaps during reconstructive surgery. In: Proceedings of inflammation, vol 11, pp 313–320
36. Mikulska D (2008) Dermatoscopy and thermal imaging: a comparative investigation of melanocytic nevi of the skin. Thermol Int 18(3):101–106
37. Burton C, Judy D, Brooks B, Fennie K, Lyder C (2011) Improving the detection of pressure ulcers using the TMI image med system. Adv Skin Wound Care 24(1):18–24
38. Di Carlo A (2011) Telethermography assisted by thermal stimulation an innovative method to improve the accuracy of the technique. Thermol Int 21(4):114–115
39. Laino L, Di Carlo A (2010) Telethermography: an objective method for evaluating patch test reactions. Eur J Dermatol 20(2):175–180
40. Roback K (2010) An overview of temperature monitoring devices for early detection of diabetic foot disorders. Expert Rev Med Devices 7(5):711–718
41. Bagavathiappan S, Philip J, Jayakumar T, Raj B, Rao PN, Varalakshmi M, Mohan V (2010) Correlation between plantar foot temperature and diabetic neuropathy: a case study by using an infrared thermal imaging technique. J Diabetes Sci Technol 4(6):1386–1392
42. Hewlett A, Kalil A, Strum R, Zeger W, Smith P (2011) Evaluation of an infrared thermal detection system for fever recognition during the H1N1 influenza pandemic. Infect Control Hosp Epidemiol 32(5):504–506
43. Howell KJ, Smith RE (2011) Temperature of the face in children and fever screening by thermography. Thermol Int 21(3):85–89
44. Ring EFJ, Jung A, Kalicki B, Zuber J, Rustecka A, Vardasca R (2011) Infrared thermal imaging for fever detection in children. Thermol Int 21(4): 122
45. Mercer JB, Ring EFJ (2009) Fever screening and infrared thermal imaging: concerns and guidelines. Thermol Int 19(3):67–69

46. Ring EFJ, Machin G, Jung A (2011) New standards for infrared thermal imaging and applications for fever detection. Thermology Int 21(4):118–119
47. Jedrusik-Pawłowska M, Niedzielska I, Bogucki R, Kajewski B (2010) Effectiveness of hyperbaric oxygen therapy in mandibular osteoradionecrosis shown by thermography monitoring. Med Sci Monit 16(2): MT1–8
48. Wu CL, Yu KL, Chuang HY, Huang MH, Chen TW, Chen CH (2009) The application of infrared thermography in the assessment of patients with coccygodynia before and after manual therapy combined with diathermy. J Manip Physiol Ther 32(4):287–293
49. Glehr M, Stibor A, Sadoghi P, Schuster C, Quehenberger F, Gruber G, Leithner A, Windhager R (2011) Thermal imaging as a noninvasive diagnostic tool for anterior knee pain following implantation of artificial knee joints. Int J Thermodyn 14:71
50. Gratt B (2008) Infrared imaging applied to dentristy. In: Diakides NA, Bronzino JD (eds) Medical infrared imaging, vol 20. CRC Press, Boca Raton, pp 1–8
51. Jafarzadeh H, Udoye CI, Kinoshita J (2008) The application of tooth temperature measurement in endodontic diagnosis: a review. J Endod 34:1435–1440
52. Kennedy DA, Lee T, Seely D (2009) A comparative review of thermography as a breast cancer screening technique. Integr Cancer Ther 8:9–16
53. Ammer K (2011) Screening for breast carcinoma: what is the place of infrared thermal imaging? Thermol Int 21(3):81–84
54. Lovett KM, Liang BA (2011) Risks of online advertisement of direct-to-consumer thermography for breast cancer screening. Nat Rev Cancer 11:827–828
55. Craciunescu OI, Stauffer PR, Soher BJ, Wyatt CR, Arabe O, Maccarini P, Das SK, Cheng KS, Wong TZ, Jones EL (2009) Accuracy of real time noninvasive temperature measurements using magnetic resonance thermal imaging in patients treated for high grade extremity soft tissue sarcomas. Med Phys 36(11):4848–4858
56. Păunică SC, Dumitriu A, Mogoş M, Georgescu O, Mogoş I (2009) The evaluation of the periodontium in patients with leukemia using thermographic imaging. Hematology 14(6):341–346
57. Agarwal-Kozlowski K, Large AC, Beck H (2009) Contact- free infrared thermography for assessing effects during acupuncture: a randomized, single-blinded, placebo-controlled crossover clinical trial. Anesthesiology 111(3):632–639
58. Wang L, Litscher G (2010) Modern technology for acupuncture research: a short review from the medical university of graz. Chin Med 1:59–62
59. Vardasca R (2011) Thermal symmetry of the limbs in healthy subjects. Thermol Int 21(4):146
60. Purohit R (2008) Use of infrared imaging in veterinary medicine. In: Diakides NA, Bronzino JD (eds) Medical infrared imaging, vol 21. CRC Press, Boca Raton, pp 1–8
61. Barone S, Paoli A, Razionale AV (2006) A biomedical application combining visible and thermal 3D imaging, XVIII Congreso internactional de Ingenieria Grafica, Barcelona, pp 1–9
62. Schaefer G, Huguet J, Zhu SY, Plassmann P, Ring EFJ (2006) Adopting the DICOM standard for medical infrared images In: Proceedings of the 28th Annual International conference of the IEEE—engineering in medicine and biology society, New York, pp 236–239
63. Schaefer G (2008) Storage and retrieval of medical thermograms. In: Diakides NA, Bronzino JD (eds) Medical infrared imaging, vol 23. CRC Press, Boca Raton, pp 1–15
64. Schaefer G, Tait RJ, Howell K, Hopgood AA, Woo P, Harper J (2008) Automated overlay of infrared and visual medical images. In: Dong F, Ghinea G, Chen SY (eds). User centered design for medical visualization, pp 174–183
65. Vardasca R, Bajwa UI (2008) Impact of noise removal techniques on measurement of medical thermal images. Thermol Int 18(4):153
66. Bajwa UI, Vardasca R, Ring EFJ, Plassmann P (2010) Comparison of boundary detection techniques to improve image analysis in medical thermography. Imaging Sci J 58:12–19
67. Vardasca R (2008) Template based alignment and interpolation methods comparison of regions of interest in thermal images. In: Proceedings of the 3rd research student workshop, faculty of advanced technology, University of Glamorgan, South Wales, pp 21–24

68. Vardasca R (2009) Hand thermogram standardisation with barycentric warp model. In: Proceedings of the 4th research student workshop, faculty of advanced technology. University of Glamorgan, South Wales, pp 73–75
69. Hildebrandt C, Raschner C, Ammer K (2010) An overview of recent application of medical infrared thermography in sports medicine in austria. Sensors 10:4700–4715
70. Norton PR, Horn SB, Pellegrino JG, Perconti P (2008) Infrared detectors and detector arrays.In: Diakides NA, Bronzino JD (eds) Medical infrared imaging, vol 3. CRC Press, Boca Raton, pp 1–26
71. Costello JT, McInerney CD, Bleakley CM, Selfe J, Donnelly AE (2011) The use of thermal imaging in assessing skin temperature following cryotherapy: a review. J Therm Biol 37(2):103–110
72. Buddharaju P, Pavlidis I (2008) Physiology-based face recognition in the thermal infrared spectrum. In: Diakides NA, Bronzino JD (eds) Medical infrared imaging, vol 13. CRC Press, Boca Raton, pp 1–16
73. Grubisic I, Gjenero L, Lipic T, Sovic I, Skala T (2011) Active 3D scanning based 3D thermography system and medical applications. In: Proceedings of the 34th International Convention MIPRO, pp 269–273
74. Ammer K (2011) Repeatability of identification of hot spots in thermal images is influenced by image processing. Thermol Int 21(2):40–46
75. Vardasca R (2010) The need of a standard false colour scale for medical thermography analysis. Thermol Int 20(4):145

Detection of Anatomic Structures in Retinal Images

José Pinão, Carlos Manta Oliveira, André Mora and João Dias

Abstract A retinal image presents three important structures in a healthy eye: optic disk, fovea and blood vessels. These are diseases associated with changes in each of these structures. Some parameters should be extracted in order to evaluate if an eye is healthy. For example, the level of imperfection of the optic disk's circle contour is related with glaucoma. Furthermore, the proximity of the lesion in the retina to the fovea (structure responsible for the central vision) induces loss of vision. Advanced stages of diabetic retinopathy cause the formation of micro blood vessels that increase the risk of detachment of the retina or prevent light from reaching the fovea. On the other hand, the arterio-venous ratio calculated through the thickness of the central vein and artery of the retina, is a parameter extracted from the vessels segmentation. In image processing, each structure detected has special importance to detect the others, since each one can be used as a landmark to the others. Moreover, often masking the optic disk is crucial to reach good results with algorithms to detect other structures. The performance of the detection algorithms is highly related with the quality of the image and with the existence of lesions. These issues are discussed below.

J. Pinão (✉) · C. M. Oliveira
Critical Health, Coimbra, Portugal
e-mail: jm-pinao@critical-health.com; josemnpinao@gmail.com

C. M. Oliveira
e-mail: caoliveira@critical-health.com

A. Mora
Universidade Nova de Lisboa, Lisbon, Portugal
e-mail: atm@uninova.pt

J. Dias
Universidade de Coimbra, Coimbra, Portugal
e-mail: uc2007102438@student.fis.uc.pt

J. M. R. S. Tavares and R. M. Natal Jorge (eds.), *Topics in Medical Image Processing and Computational Vision*, Lecture Notes in Computational Vision and Biomechanics 8,
DOI: 10.1007/978-94-007-0726-9_13,

1 Retinal Image Quality Assessment

Beyond lesions detection, there are some key features that an automated retinal images analysis system must possess. From those, integration of results from various images of the same patient and image quality assessment stand out [1]. This section is focused on the last one, trying to prove how important it is and to present a brief state of the art description.

One can think retinal image quality assessment as a process which main mission is to analyse some images parameters and based on them classify the image in terms of its potential usage to evaluate a patient's health. Hence, this quality classification allows one to understand to what extent the patient's health appraisal is reliable. Moreover, in a telemedicine environment, a real-time retinal image quality assessment is a plus, since transmitting ungradable images might mean the need to call back patients in order to repeat the retinal exams, with time and monetary costs. Even regarding longitudinal studies, quality assessment during image acquisition is very important, as an image "lost" due to quality problems may result in exclusion of that patient from the study or a decrease in the statistical power of the results [2]. Therefore, quality assessment is mandatory to develop complete and trusty automated retinal images analysis software.

The importance of image quality assessment is even greater due to a considerably large prevalence percentage of retinal images with insufficient quality to be graded (by humans or software). In fact, the reported percentage of ungradable images is usually between 4.85 and 17.3 %, as the following table confirms (Table 1).

This "ungradability" may result from a series of impaired image features. A study (Atherosclerotic Risk in Communities—ARIC) performed by the Fundus Photograph Reading Centre from the Deptartment of Ophthalmology & Visual Sciences of the University of Wisconsin–Madison [10] allowed realising the importance of some critical parameters when evaluating retinal image quality. In this study, beyond the identification of characteristic lesions of diabetic retinopathy (DR) and age-related macular degeneration (AMD) in 45° field of view (FOV) images, graders were also asked to analyse and classify some image aspects which most affect their quality. These were: focus and clarity, field definition, visibility of the optic disc, visibility of the macula, and artefacts. (1) Focus and clarity relates itself with the grader's capacity on detection and assessment of

Table 1 Reported ungradable image prevalence in a set of articles

Ungradable image prevalence
11.3 % (from 1039 images) of images were ungradable [3]
17.3 % (from 98 patients) of patients had an ungradable image in at least one eye [4]
4.85 % (from 10000 exams) of exams had at least an ungradable image [5]
11 % (from 2771 patients) of patients had an ungradable images [6]
11.9 % (from 5575 patients) of patients had an ungradable image in at least one eye [7]
8.8 % (from 981 patients) of patients had an ungradable image in at least one eye [8]
12.0 % (from 1676 patients) of patients had ungradable images [9]

abnormalities (e.g., retinal microaneurysms or focal narrowing of arterioles). This reduction on the image quality may be due to haze which can be a consequence from eye lens opacity. A retinal image example with poor focus and clarity is Fig. 1. (2) Field definition evaluates the position of the two most relevant retinal landmarks: optic disc and macula. In a 45° FOV retinal image with perfect field definition, the optic disc must be between 1.5 ODD (optic disc diameter) to 2.5 ODD from nasal edge and be vertically centred. In this situation, is practically taken for granted that macula is within image. An example of a retinal image with poor field definition is Fig. 2. (3) Optic disc and macula visibility is related with the previous parameter. However, in addition to not being present due to poor field definition, optic disc and/or macula can be not visible if they are obscured by artefacts (e.g., dark shadow or blink). Examples of retinal images with poor optic disc visibility and poor macula visibility are, respectively, Figs. 3 and 4. (4) Finally, artefacts are all the remainder parameters which may affect retinal image quality and some of them can be thought as the causes for improper quality of the previous ones. In the ARIC study were considered the following artefacts: haze, dust and dirt, lashes, arcs, uneven illumination over macula, uneven illumination over optic disc, uneven illumination over image edge, and total blink. (4a) Haze is an artefact that causes the decrease of retinal image clarity and makes it seems yellower. In the ARIC study it was divided into two groups: overall and edge haze. Examples of retinal image with overall haze and edge haze are, respectively, Figs. 1 and 2. (4b) Dust and dirt are artefacts that may result from an unclean camera lens. They are characterized by small gray-white soft-edged circular spots and seem to be defocused due to being in a different plane of focus than retina. A retinal image example with dust and dirt is Fig. 4. (4c) Lashes are artefacts which have some resemblance with total blink due to their bright yellow-white appearance. However, these artefacts partially affect the image and are frequently seen as in Fig. 6. As the case of dust and dirt, also lashes are out of focus. (4d) Arcs are circular shaped artefacts which frequently result from improperly camera lens cleaning. (4e) Uneven illumination over macula, optic disc or image edge are artefacts that impair the visibility of these landmarks. These artefacts can be thought as the causes behind optic disc and macula poor visibility, and they frequently occur when pupillary dilation is less than optimal. An example of retinal image with uneven illumination over macula is Fig. 4. (4f) The last one, total blink is a bright yellow-white artefact which obscures all or most of the field, making the retinal image ungradable. A retinal image example showing a total blink is Fig. 3.

As one can easily conclude, it may be considered that these parameters falls into two categories: generic criteria (focus and clarity, and artefacts, except uneven illumination over macula, optic disc or image edge) and structural criteria (field definition, visibility of the optic disc, and visibility of the macula). It is on these criteria that the state of the art of image quality assessment is based.

Regarding generic criteria, the main objective is to apply simple image measurements in order to obtain a good image quality classification, while avoiding eye structure segmentation. Thereby, in 1999, Lee et al. [11] proposed a method

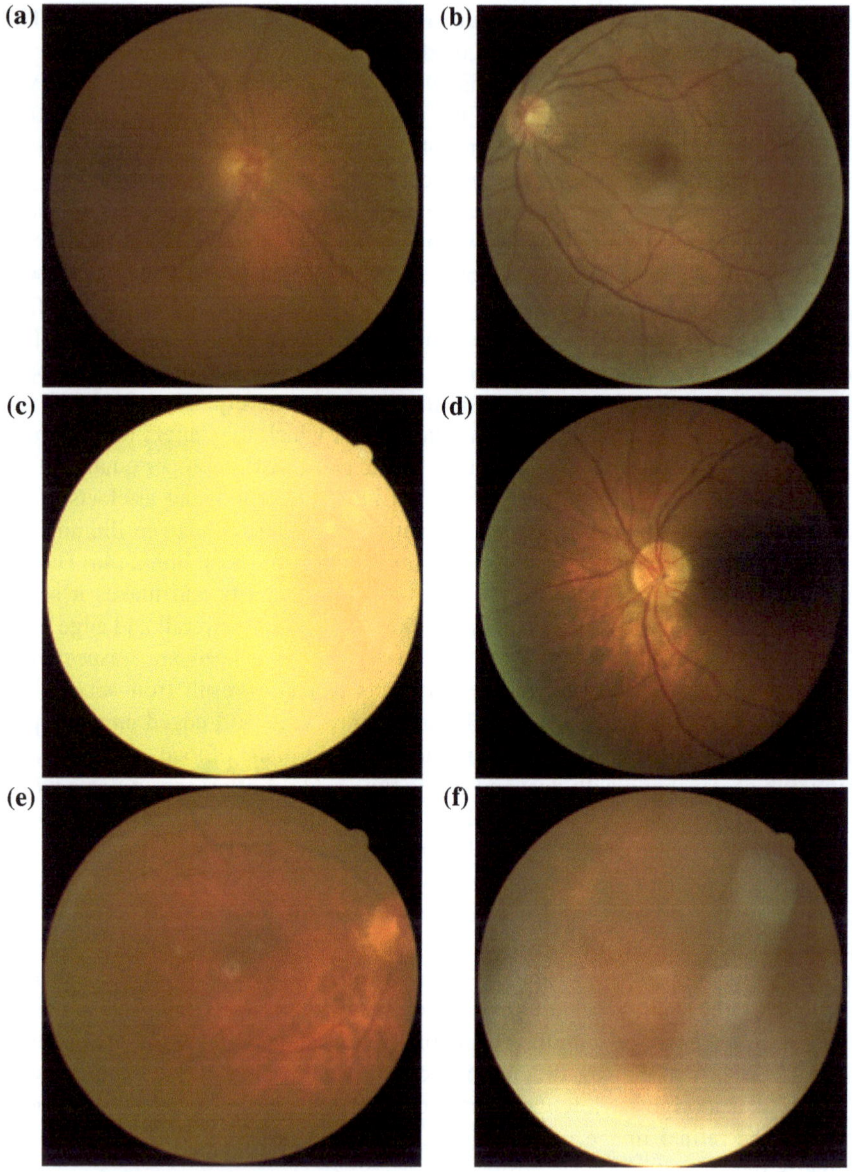

Fig. 1 Examples of impaired/ungradable images. **a** Poor focus and clarity due to overall haze. **b** Poor field definition and edge haze. **c** Poor optic disc visibility due to total blink. **d** Poor macula visibility due to uneven illumination over it. **e** Dust and dirt artefacts (at the *centre*). **f** Lash artefact

based on the resemblance between a template histogram, defined by the analysis of 20 excellent quality images, and the histogram of the retinal image to be classified. Two years later, in 2001, Lalonde et al. [12] stated that the connection between

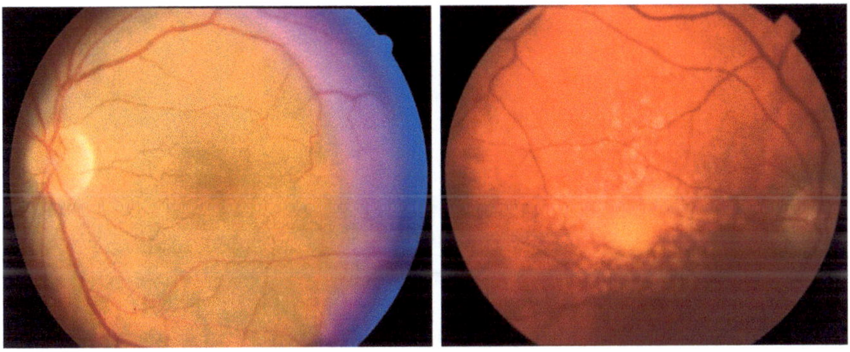

Fig. 2 Examples of fundus images containing uneven illumination and contrast. The image on the *left* is from a healthy person, while the *right* one contains confluent drusen

image quality and histogram similarity is not as strong as Lee et al. had proved. Hence, they proposed a new method based on the distribution of the edge magnitudes in the image, using a global histogram analysis, and on intensity distribution, employing a local histogram analysis. With these analyses, Lalonde et al. tried to evaluate image focus and illumination. Only eight years later, in 2009, a new generic image quality approach arose. Bartling et al. [13] focused their quality assessment algorithm on image sharpness and illumination, the latter being measured through retinal image contrast and brightness. In order to do it, the authors divided the original image into smaller squares and analyse each one separately. They achieved a concordance between computed and human quality score, following a kappa value approach and using 1000 images, within a range of 0.52—0.68 with a median kappa value of 0.64. In the same year, Davis et al. [2] published an article about retinal image quality assessment which relies on a total of seventeen simple features calculated for each colour channel in the CIELab space (CIELab is a colour model that represents colour perception qualities of the human eye; for further information consult [14]) and for each one of seven regions within the retinal image. This huge set of measures attempt to assess image colour, luminance and contrast. With their new method, the authors achieved 100 % of sensitivity and 96 % of specificity in identifying ungradable images in a dataset composed by 200 images.

With this brief description, it is possible to state that the greatest advantage of these generic image quality based methods is their relative simplicity and therefore, computation "lightness". However, this simplicity may have costs once the retinal image quality assessment relies only on generic criteria which might not be enough to perform a complete evaluation.

On the other hand, in the case of structural criteria, all methods require anatomical landmarks segmentation in order to withdraw meaningful information from the retinal image. The first ever proposed method based on eye structure criteria was published in 2003 by Usher et al. (*Automated assessment of digital fundus image quality using detected vessel area*). The authors followed a quality

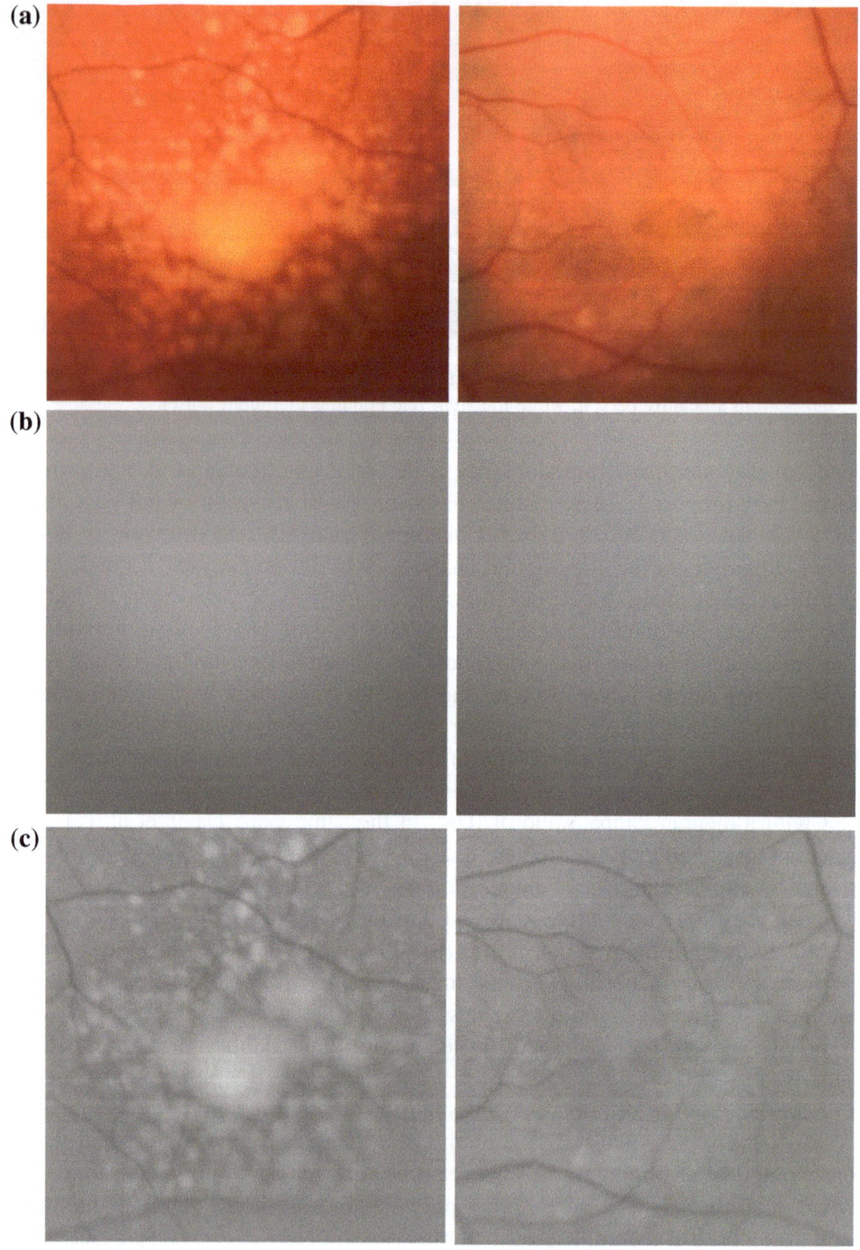

Fig. 3 Examples of non-uniform illumination correction by smoothing splines fitting; **a** original images; **b** estimated illumination pattern; **c** corrected images

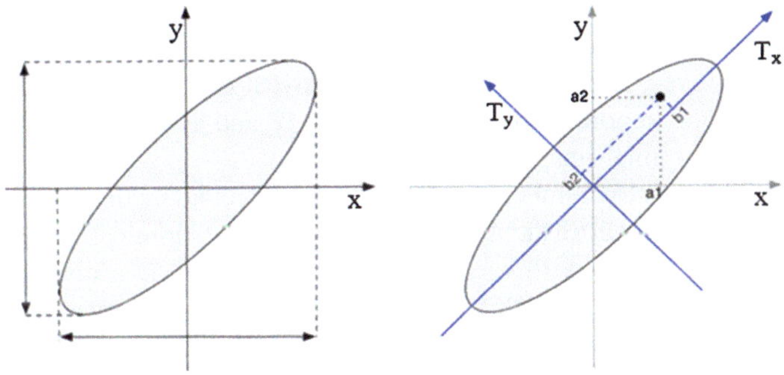

Fig. 4 Original and transformation axis in the data distribution

assessment based on the clarity and area of the detected eye vasculature, which was tested in a dataset of 1746 images, achieving a sensitivity of 84.3 % and a specificity of 95.0 % in detecting patients with at least one ungradable image. [3, 15, 16], Two years later, in 2005, Lowell et al. (*Automated Quantification of Fundus Image Quality*) proposed a new algorithm also based on blood vessels, but focused on a circular area around the macula, which needs to be automatically identified [17]. In the following year, 2006, Niemeijer et al. [17] proposed a much more complex method to classify image quality. Their approach begins with an Image Structure Clustering (ISC), whose purpose is to obtain a set of clusters (each one represents pixels on identical image structures) using a multiscale filterbank. Based on the obtained clusters, the next step is to set up a feature vector, which is composed by the 5 bins of the normalized histogram of the ISC clustered pixels and the 15 bins of the normalized histograms of the red, green and blue image plan (5 bins for each channel). Finally, an image quality classification is computed using the extracted features. The authors reported an area under ROC (receiver operating characteristic) of 0.9968 in a series of tests with different training and test sets using a total of 2000 images. In the same year, Fleming et al. [3] took the work produced by Usher et al. and Lowell et al. to a whole new level. The authors tried to assess retinal image clarity by analysing the detected vasculature within a region centred on the automatically detected, using Hough transform, fovea. They also evaluated field definition by defining a group of constrains including optic disc diameter, distance between optic disc and fovea, arcade vessels length and vertical image alignment. The authors achieved 99.1 % sensitivity and 89.4 % specificity for detection of ungradable retinal images on a dataset of 1039 images. After them, in 2008, Giancardo et al. [18] proposed a new method inspired in the work of Niemeijer et al., but only focused on eye vasculature and not on the entire eye structure. Thereby, based on the detected blood vessels, a set of features was withdrawn, which include vessels density within each one of a group of delimited regions, and 5 bins of the normalized zero mean and unit variance histogram for each RGB colour channel. The proposed method achieved an accuracy of 100 % on the identification of "Good" images, 83 % on "Fair" images, 0 % on "Poor" images and 11 % on "Outlier" images in a dataset with a total of 84 retinal images. Three years later, in 2011, Hunter et al. [15] proposed a new retinal image quality assessment focused on contrast and quantity of visible blood vessels within 1 ODD of the fovea, and on contrast between foveal core region and background retina. The authors reported a sensitivity of 100 % and a specificity of 93 % in a dataset with 200 retinal images.

This summary of structural criteria based methods found on the literature allows one to conclude that all of them imply some sort of anatomical landmarks segmentation. As it is known, this step is error prone, which is a major drawback. However, once correctly done, this segmentation phase can be very useful on image quality assessment and on later DR or AMD automatic detection algorithms.

The two aforementioned criteria were firstly joined together in 2010 by Paulus et al. [19] to give rise to a third group of state of the art approaches, which evaluates image quality based on both criteria. Thereby, in order to analyse eye anatomical landmarks, the authors followed an approach similar to ISC introduced by Niemeijer et al., although incorporating global information instead of local gradient information only. Furthermore, also sharpness, homogeneity and contrast measures were employed by Paulus et al. in order to evaluate generic image quality, achieving 96.9 % sensitivity and 80.0 % specificity in a dataset composed by 301 retinal images.

This third kind of methods combines the best features of generic and structural approaches while trying to avoid or eliminate those approaches' drawbacks. Thus, a more robust and complete method is expected to be developed, and yet keeping low computational time. However, segmentation phases are always FOV dependent which is a major drawback once a unique "screening" FOV has not yet been established. Proving this lack of a single and worldwide accepted FOV for screening purposes, are the national guidelines for DR screening settled by some different countries, such as Australia, Scotland, United Kingdom and United States of America [19].

Therefore, as it was discussed above, there are already a considerable number of methods to assess retinal image quality. In screening initiatives, a retinal image quality assessment algorithm is an important goal to be fulfilled. In order to satisfy the needs, the quality evaluation system must be fast enough to allow real-time analysis and should give information regarding the image characteristics with lower quality than a perfect retinal image.

2 Lesions Illumination Correction

The non-uniformity of illumination is very common in retinal images (Fig. 2). It can result from the different reflecting characteristics of the retinal surface, from problems of the eye lens, from the equipment vignetting and from poor patient collaboration in the image capture. The patient's voluntary and involuntary eye movements during the image capture can cause misalignment and interfere on the image quality. The consequences are different illumination and contrast areas over the image, which make it difficult for image interpretation and processing and should be corrected before any further processing.

The major difficulty in non-uniform correction algorithms is to accurately separate illumination from the reflectance. The illumination can be a constant value when illumination is uniform, but commonly it is composed by low frequency components that exhibit a complex pattern. However, not all the non-uniformities are random; it is known that the macula has a lower reflectance than the other parts of the retina (Fig. 2). This is due to the higher concentration of photoreceptors in this region, which have a higher absorption of visible light.

In the work of Smith et al. [20] the authors studied the reflecting properties of the macula and described the lower reflectance with a series of multiplicative factors gradually decreasing when they move away from the centre. Then they applied to the Green channel these multiplicative factors, a method which was entitled as *luteal pigment correction*.

Another approach to correct the non-uniformity of illumination is low-pass filtering. The major problem of this technique is to define the filter's cut-off frequency, in order to remove the non-uniformity of the illumination and maintain the image details. The mostly used technique is a convolution filter with a Gaussian kernel to estimate the image's illumination pattern and then normalize it accordingly [21–23]. The kernel used varied in size between these works but the criterion was to have a compromise between being larger than the abnormalities and smaller enough to detect local variations. The kernel values were generated using the Eq. (1), in which σ is related to the frequency interval, a value determined empirically. The output from the convolution is a smoothed image without any details, which is then divided by the original image, in order to normalize the illumination and the contrast.

$$G(x,y) = \exp\left(-\frac{x^2 + y^2}{2 \cdot \sigma^2}\right) \tag{1}$$

Homomorphic filtering is also a technique used to correct non-uniform illumination in retinal images [24]. It belongs to the family of frequency filtering techniques and it is usually applied on signals composed by multiplicative factors. The technique [25] is based on the fact that an image is roughly the product of illumination and reflectance (not considering the incidence angle) and converting the image to the logarithmic scale, where the multiplicative factors are converted into additive ones, as shown in Eq. (2). It is followed by a high-pass filter in the Fourier domain that amplifies the image reflectance (the higher frequencies) and attenuates the non-uniform illumination (the lower frequencies). It finishes by converting the image to the spatial domain and linear scale again, where it presents a higher contrasted image with normalized illumination.

$$\begin{aligned} f(x,y) &= i(x,y) \cdot r(x,y) \\ \ln(f(x,y)) &= \ln(i(x,y) \cdot r(x,y)) \\ &= \ln(i(x,y)) + \ln(r(r,y)) \end{aligned} \tag{2}$$

Other solution to correct uneven illumination is to estimate a model of the illumination pattern and correct it accordingly [26]. One of the analytical models that is adequate to model illumination is Cubic Smoothing Spline [27]. This is a special class of Splines that can capture the low frequencies characterizing the non-uniformity of the illumination. The fitting objective is to minimize the Eq. (3).

$$M = p \cdot \sum_{y=1}^{m} \sum_{x=1}^{n} (f(x,y) - S(x,y))^2 + (1-p) \iint (S''(x,y))^2 dxdy \qquad (3)$$

This equation contains two terms: the summation term (weighed by the smoothing factor p) that measures how close the spline is to the data, and the integral term (weighed by $(1 - p)$) that measures the spline smoothness using its second derivative. The smoothing factor p, controls the balance between being an interpolating spline crossing all data points (with $p = 1$) and being a strictly smooth Spline (with $p = 0$). A too high p value will tend to produce, after the normalization, a flatter image, flattening also the retina structures, which is a clearly unwanted side-effect. A too low p value will maintain the structures, but will not correct the uneven illumination.

In this fitting process, the large bright lesions influence negatively the illumination estimation, by being frequently evaluated as illumination. To overcome this, an iterative estimation process which masks these lesions was implemented. It is based on the method proposed by Smith et al. [28], applied to the whole region of interest using two clusters.

It is composed by the following steps that were repeated a predefined number of times, 5 (obtained empirically):

- estimation of the illumination pattern;
- division of the original image by the estimated illumination pattern;
- binarization of the image (using Otsu thresholding) to cluster the pixels into two classes: bright area and background; and
- replacement of the pixels belonging to the bright area class by the estimated spline in the original image, creating an image without these brighter areas.

This process progressively reduces the influence of higher intensity pixels on the next iteration. As result a corrected image with uniform illumination and without lost of contrast between the background and the bright areas is obtained (Fig. 3c).

3 Anatomical Structures Detection

A preprocessing is commonly implemented before the main approach followed to detect the interested structure. The majority of the implementation consists in low-level operations that performed the reduction of noise or enhance the contrast. These operations maximize the accuracy of the detection algorithms. The following section explains several methods of preprocessing operations.

3.1 Pre-Processing

Commonly, the first segmentation is done between the red foreground and the dark background of a retinal image. This operation is performed to reduce the area where the algorithm is implemented. Furthermore, it avoids the high transition between the background and the foreground.

The quality of the image is highly improved using Principal Component Analysis (PCA) [29], local contrast enhancement [30], the retinex algorithm [31–33] and the histogram equalization [25].

PCA consists in an orthogonal linear transformation that transforms the data to a new coordinates system which has the higher variance comes from the first coordinate (first principal component). This consists in transform a number of correlated variables in a number of uncorrelated variables—the principal components. This methodology provides a roadmap for how to reduce an image to a lower dimension to reveal hidden details (Fig. 4).

Local contrast enhancement, on other hand, use a point transformation dependent of an area bigger enough to contain a statistical representative distribution of the local variation of gray levels. However, the area needs to be small to be unaffected by the gradual change of contrast between the center and the periphery of the fundus image. Local contrast enhancement depends of the mean and variance of the intensity within each local area. The local contrast is enhanced only if the variance of the intensity is not high. This preserves some retinal and pathological features which change the local contrast. This method has as limitation also increase the noise, therefore is desirable before apply a smooth filter in the image (Fig. 5).

Retinex, initially proposed by Land [33], is a technique of image enhancement inspired in the human perception of colors. The nonlinear feature becomes this time domain algorithm a powerful tool for image processing. The dynamic range

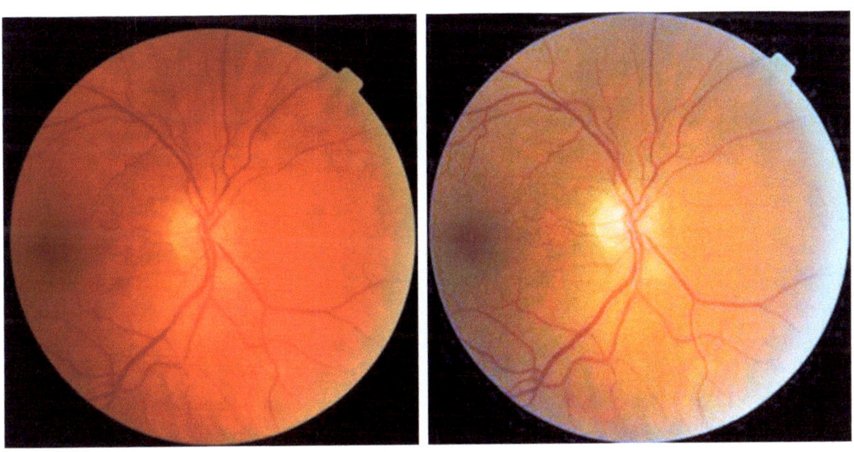

Fig. 5 Contrast improvement using the local contrast enhancement

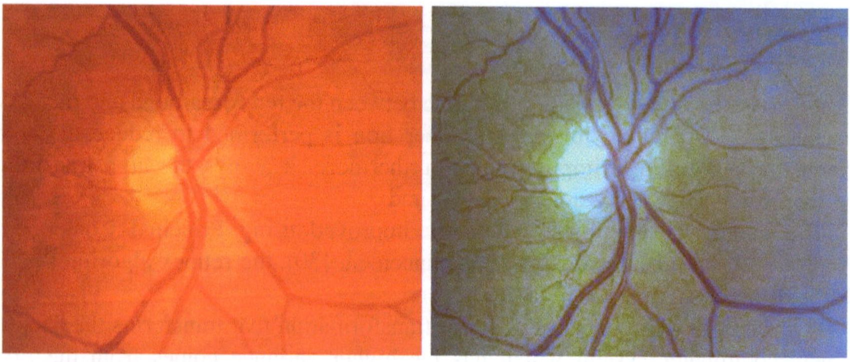

Fig. 6 Image enhancement using the multiscale retinex without color restoration

of a scene is the ratio between the darkest and the brightest part. The human system support a dynamic range around 10 000:1. However, an imaging system has a restricted dynamic range [32]. The Retinex had several stages of evolution until reach the multiscale stage which combines a dynamic range compression and tonal rendition to produce an output with better quality (Fig. 6).

A histogram describes the intensities distribution of an image counting the pixels between specified ranges. The histogram equalization enhances an image adjusting the distribution of the intensities. All the intensities are redistributed with equal probability over the intensities range. This method is particularly efficient in images with close contrast values. However, in some cases the contrast of the noise can be improved instead of the signal captured in the image decreased (Fig. 7).

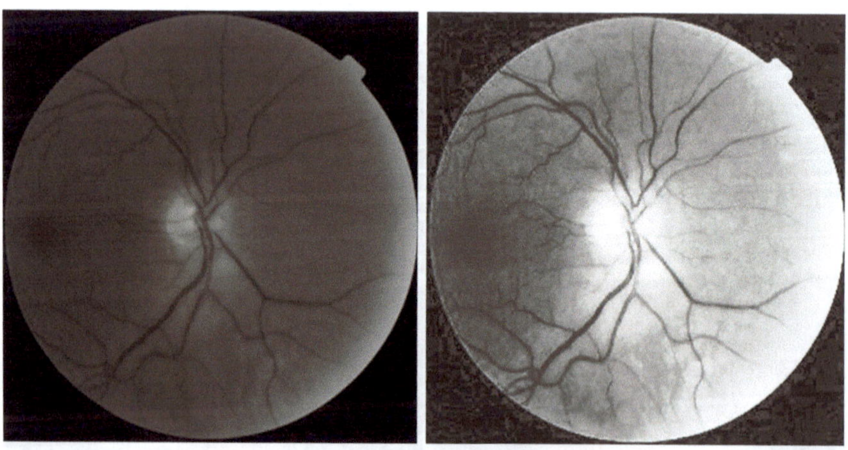

Fig. 7 Histogram equalization of a green channel of a retinal image

3.2 Main Approaches

The optic disk, fovea and blood vessels can be detected following several approaches. Fovea is located at 2.5 optic disks radius from its center. Commonly, fovea is detected using the optic disk as landmark finding the darkest region at the mention distance. There are six main approaches that allow reliable results:

- Blood vessels tracing [34, 35].
- Template matching [36, 37].
- Active contour or snake [38, 39].
- Machine learning [40, 41].
- Multilevel thresholding [42].
- Shape detection [43, 44].

Blood vessels tracing takes advantage of some anatomic features of the relative position between the existent structures. Blood vessels always cross the optic disk vertically. The arcades describe two inverted parabolas which intersect in a position near the optic disk center. This kind of methodologies do not need to segment all the blood vessels but only estimate the global direction of the gradient caused the presence of them to find the convergence point. Therefore, large blood vessels count with a higher weight than thinner ones. This approach is particularly reliable in case of lesions present caused by advance stage of pathology. Other techniques commonly fail the detection due the high gradient caused by lesions (Fig. 8).

Template matching is the classification of images comparing them with templates. This process consists in finding occurrences of one or more templates in an

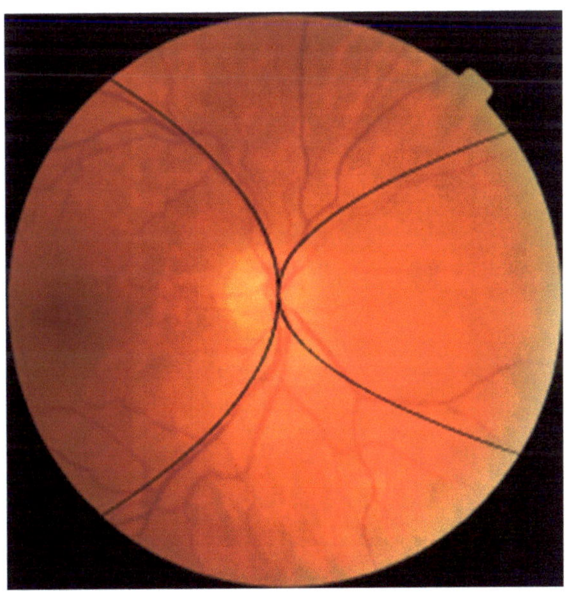

Fig. 8 Parabolic model of the blood vessels

image of interest. The application of this approach has several modalities for the building of a matching filter. A matching filter is designed to give the maximal response in the region of the image which matches with the template. However, each retina has unique features which makes impossible happens a perfect match between a region of the image and a general template. In retinal images it is mandatory to define a level of confidence for admitting that a position within the image is a potential region of interest. This approach was implemented by Youssif et al. [37] to detect the optic disk in retinal images. Sometimes the generation of multiple candidates is an issue hard to resolve. Lalond et al. [36] crossed the position of each candidate of the optic disk with the bright parts of the retinal image extracted using a pyramidal decomposition (Fig. 9).

Active contours or snakes are edge based algorithms built on complex mathematical models typically slow algorithms due to being iterative. The contour tries to fit the curve boundary of an object represented in an image space adjusting its position on each iteration of the algorithm. The contour will stop moving when equilibrium in the image space is reached or if there is defined a maximum number of iterations. The initial position and the velocity of the contour are crucial parameters to find the edge of interest. A good preprocessing is mandatory to reach good results with this approach. Remodelling the image space is necessary to generate favorable forces to shape the contour to adapt its position to the interested boundary.

Mendel et al. [38] developed a mathematical framework to run a contour to detect optic disks. This contour only reaches interesting results when there is a removal of the blood vessels crossing the optic disk boundary. The fully automatically contours need to have a previous process to estimate the best initial position to begin the process. Osareh et al. [39] used a simple template matching approach to calculate the initial position of the contour in the image space. The initial position needs to be located inside the optic disk boundary.

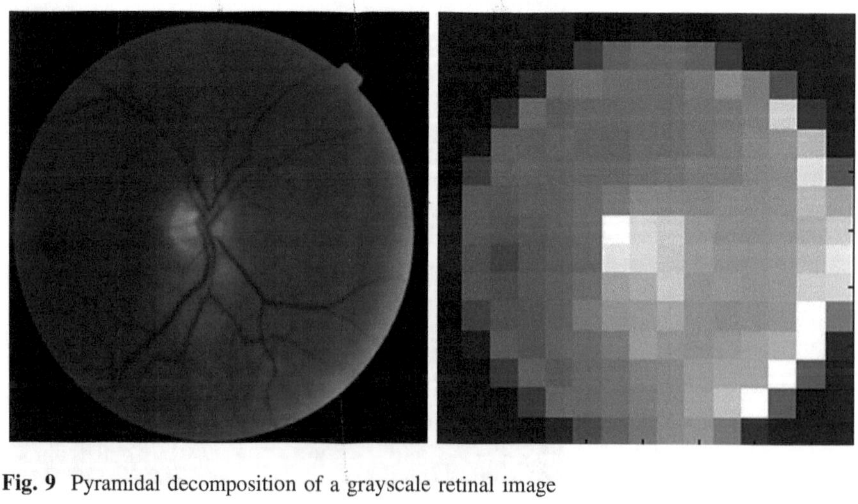

Fig. 9 Pyramidal decomposition of a grayscale retinal image

Similar contours are also applied in image processing in MRI brain images and 3D segmentation.

Machine learning approaches are methods where there is a learning of the computer to classify the data of interest. Neural networks are the most popular methodology to implement machine learning. Neural networks are a powerful data modeling tool that can understand the relationship between the input and output data. These networks work as similar way as the human brain due two points:

1. Acquire knowledge from learning.
2. The training effect is reflected in the synaptic weights.

There are some models of neural networks but the most commonly used is the multilayer percetron. The neural networks based in the multilayer perceptron learning using the back propagation algorithm. The back propagation consists in the weight adjustment considering the error generated when the input is comparing with the desired output during the training (Fig. 10).

The blood vessels network originates from the optic disk and is progressively branched and thinner presenting a dark red or orange red color. Sinthanayothin et al. [40] modeled a neural network to detect the blood vessels after a preprocessing of the image. Firstly, a Canny edge operator is applied in the principal component of the image to enhance the vessels. Then, a multilayer perceptron classify each pixel using the blood vessels features of the retinal image in vessel or non-vessel. The first principal component and edge strength values from a sub image of 10 × 10 were used as input in the neural network. The training of the network was done using a dataset of 25094 examples created and checked by clinicians. Sinthanayothin used 5/6 of the data for training and 1/6 for validation.

Active shape models (ASM) is another methodology of machine learning. Initially proposed by Cootes et al. [45], this model has similarities with the snakes. However, the active shape models only deform to fit with a way consistent with the training set. Therefore, active shapes consist in smart snakes. The training set consists in group of points surrounding the structure of interest. All the objects need to be labeled with the same number of points where each point always represents a particular part of the boundary. When all the images are manually labeled, the overlap of the marks shows that some of them have little variability and others generate clouds. Cootes assumed that each cloud is an ellipsoid and calculated its center. After estimates an initial position, the linear formulation of

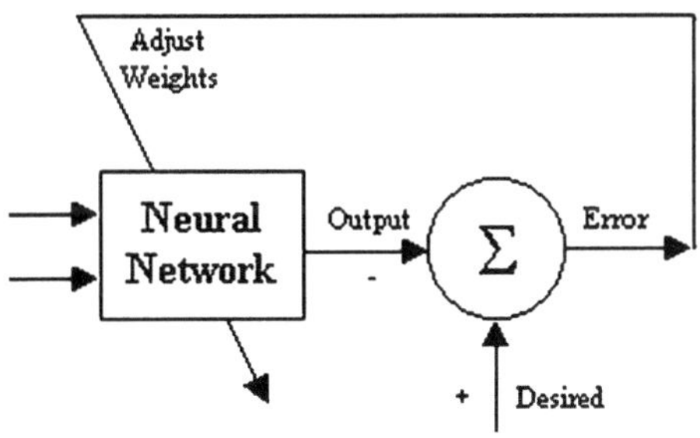

Fig. 10 Scheme of back propagation algorithm

the point distribution model (PDM) is exploited in an iterative search able to locate the modeled structures in images. In a first step is done an approximation to bending using the fitting straight lines to the clouds of points. The second step adjusts the bending due the linear approximation to be poor. The third does a second order adjustment. Li et al. [41] adapted an active shape model to detect the optic disk. The initial position of the ASM was calculated using a PCA methodology. Li generated a training dataset where each optic disk was labeled by 48 landmarks. Thirty five retinal images were tested with eight ware used for training to compare this modified ASM method and the ASM proposed by Cooted. This new method converges faster and is more robust when comparing with the ASM proposed by Cootes due to needing a lesser number of iterations and reaching better results even in case of strong blood vessels traces.

Thresholding is an image segmentation technique used to extract objects from the background of an image. The key is the definition of the threshold value. The simpler methods are a mean or median. Others complex methods consist in the analysis of the histogram to find the value of a peak or valley or using clustering to group the object and the background in different agregates. The Otsu's method [46] is an way to find a threshold value widely used it thresholding techniques. This non-parametric method select the value that maximize the separability the classes of grey levels using the zeroth- and the first order cumulative moments. Otsu's method is specially efficient in case of images with a bi-modal histogram. Kavitha et al. [42] developed a multilevel thresholding method to extract the optic disk and exudates from retinal images. Retinal images present a multimodal histogram due the existence of a variety of structures. This feature implicates that the application of the Otsu's method is not enough to extract the brighter structures. The valley-seeking method proposed by Kavitha seeks the local minima in a histogram as thresholds. After smoothing the histogram, the smaller valleys are removed and the last one is defined as the threshold to be used. This method was tested with five healthy images and fourteen images with traces of disease with a size of 256 × 256. The results were generated considering the probability of a pixel being correctly marked as exudate. For the healthy images the accuracy was 89.43 % and for the images with traces of disease 81.24 %.

Shape detection approaches are used in image processing to detect predefined shapes of objects in images. Hough transform [47] is the most popular way of shape detection in image processing. This transform is commonly used to detect lines or circles. Hough transform uses the mathematical equation of the structure of interest: $y = ax + b$ for lines and $(x - a)^2 + (y - b)^2 = r^2$ for circles. However, for the circles's case, the equation is used in polar coordinates: $x.\cos(\theta) + y.\sin(\theta) = \rho$ to reduce the number variables from 3 to 2 and reduce the computational weight. Infinite lines or circles pass in a generic point (x, y) satisfying its equation even varying the a and b values. The parameter space is divided in an accumulator (Fig. 11).

where (a_{min}, a_{max}) and (b_{min}, b_{max}) are the range of tested values for lines and (ρ_{min}, ρ_{max}) and $(\theta_{min}, \theta_{max})$ for circles. Initially, all cells of accumulator are set to zero. The number of subdivision of the accumulator scale is related with the

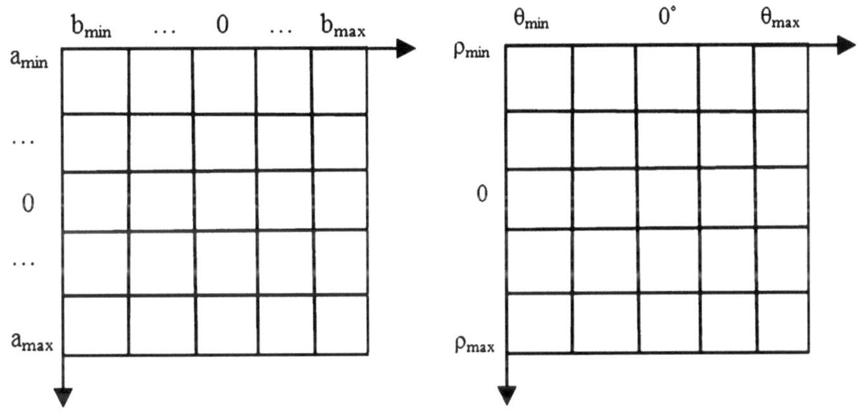

Fig. 11 Accumulator space scheme for lines and circles

accuracy of the points. Then, for every line or circle that match the point (x, y) of the image, counts as more a unity in the accumulator. The peaks in the accumulator are the geometric shape better represented in the image. The preprocessing of the retinal image is the key for the success for the application of the Hough transform.

Sekhar et al. [43] used the green component of the retinal image preprocessed with some morphological operations and select the region of interest basing in the brighter region to apply the Hough transform to detect the circular optic disk. On the other hand, Xiaolu et al. [44] developed a similar shape detection method using the Hough transform but a different preprocessing methodology. Xiaolu converted the retinal images to grayscale attributing weighs to each channel $Y = 0.299R + 0.587G + 0.114B$ and a median filter of 5×5 removes some artifacts of the image. Than, a Sobel operator [47] calculates the horizontal and vertical magnitude of the image to enhance the optic disk boundary. The Canny operator [48] reaches the binary edge map to apply the Hough transform.

An alternative shape detection model proposed by Pinão et al. [49]. The optic disk is located in a part of the image where the blood vessels and even the optic disk contribute for the presence of a strong vertical gradient. The vertical sobel operator was applied to detect the image parte where this kind of gradient is stronger and select the region of interest (Fig. 12).

The Gaussian operator is then used to calculate the gradient and binarize the image and isolate the boundaries of the structures. The image is binarized using a threshold reached using the Otsu's method and applied in the image with the Gaussian gradient (Fig. 13).

The wide vessels crossing the optic disk boundary are than occluded using a median filter of 31×31 from the image in grayscale to improve the accuracy of the Hough transform. The output image is then subtracted to the image in grayscale and the vessels are detected. After a binarization, the vessels are removed from the image reached from the binarization of the Gaussian gradient image.

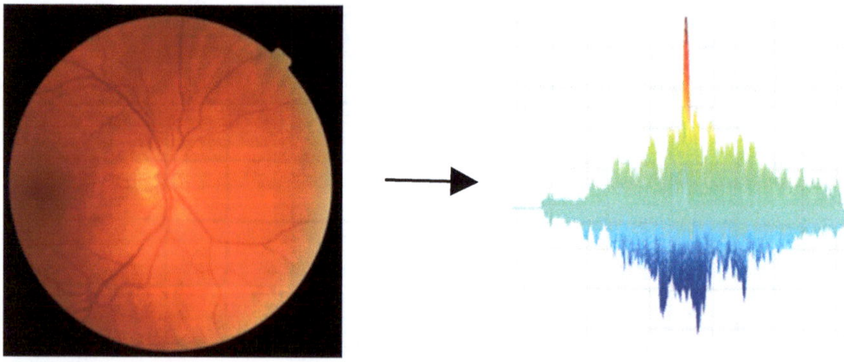

Fig. 12 Sobel application

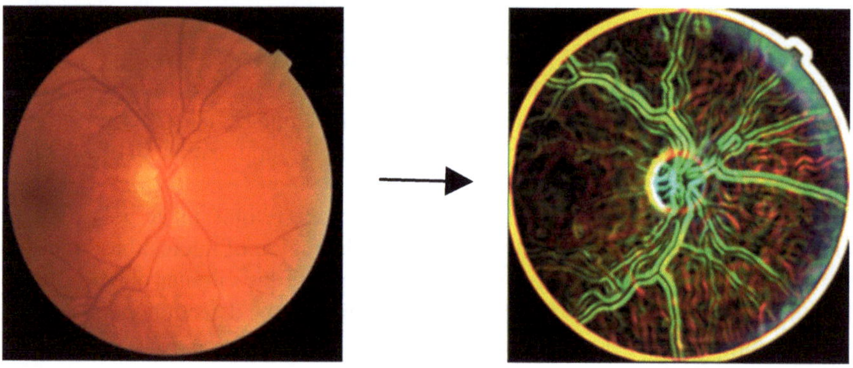

Fig. 13 Gaussian gradient calculation

The Hough transform is than applied in the region of interest after some morphologic operations to find the circular shape of the optic disk boundary (Fig. 14).

3.3 Comparative Analysis

None of the methodologies described above is perfect. All of them present some limitations. Shape detection and some template matching are the fastest to reach the results. Hough transform is computationally very attractive except in case of ellipses detection. However, in case of diseases tracing in the source images, these ones are also which present the worse accuracy. Analyzing the Table 2 is observed that the method proposed by Pinão et al. [49] reaches the best results of the shape model approaches in images with pathologies. On the other side, blood vessels tracing are practically immune to the presence of symptom due to diseases but

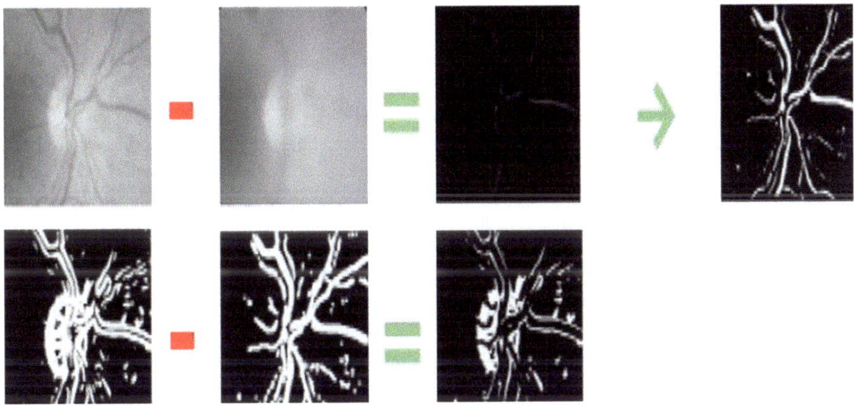

Fig. 14 Exclusion of the blood vessels

Table 2 Accuracy of several algorithms with Stare dataset (images traces of pathologies)

Optic disk detection method	Stare dataset (%)
Hausdorff—based template matching, piramidal decomposition [36]	71.6
Hough transform applied only to pixels close to the retinal vasculature [50]	71.6
Shape detection developed algorithm [49]	74.1
Fuzzy convergence [35]	89.0
A geometrical model of the vessel structure structure using 2 parabolas [34]	97.5
Vessels direction matched filter [37]	98.8

presents one of the higher processing time in average. The optic disk presents an irregular shape in case of pathology. Active contours or snakes are the better approaches in this case due can adjust to the shape of the optic disk boundary although presenting a slow processing time due of the iterative nature. Machine learning needs a huge training sample to cover an acceptable level of the real possibilities.

References

1. Jelinek HF, Cree MJ (2009) Automated image detection of retinal pathology. CRC Press, Boca Raton
2. Davis H, Russell S, Barriga E, Abràmoff MD, Soliz P (2009) Vision-based, real-time retinal image quality assessment. Russell J Bertrand Russell Archives, pp 1–6
3. Fleming AD, Philip S, Goatman KA, Olson JA, Sharp PF (2006) Automated assessment of diabetic retinal image quality based on clarity and field definition. Invest Ophthalmol Vis Sci 47:1120–1125
4. Boucher MCC, Gresset JA, Angioi K, Olivier S (2003) Effectiveness and safety of screening for diabetic retinopathy with two nonmydriatic digital images compared with the seven

standard stereoscopic photographic fields. Can J Ophthalmol. J canadien d'ophtalmologie. 38:557–568
5. Olson JA, Sharp PF, Fleming AD, Philip S (2008) Evaluation of a System for automatic detection of diabetic retinopathy from color fundus photographs in a large population of patients with diabetes. Diabetes Care 31:e63
6. Zimmer-Galler I, Zeimer R (2006) Results of implementation of the DigiScope for diabetic retinopathy assessment in the primary care environment. Telemed J e-health Off J Am Telemed Assoc 12:89–98
7. Philip S, Cowie LM, Olson JA (2005) The impact of the health technology board for Scotland's grading model on referrals to ophthalmology services. Br J ophthalmol 89:891–896
8. Heaven CJ, Cansfield J, Shaw KM (1993) The quality of photographs produced by the non-mydriatic fundus camera in a screening programme for diabetic retinopathy: a 1 year prospective study. Eye London England 7(Pt 6):787–790
9. Abràmoff MD, Suttorp-Schulten MSA (2005) Web-based screening for diabetic retinopathy in a primary care population: the EyeCheck project. Telemed J ehealth Off J Am Telemed Assoc 11:668–674
10. Department of Ophthalmology and Visual Sciences of the University of Wisconsin-Madison, F.P.R.C.: ARIC Grading Protocol. http://eyephoto.ophth.wisc.edu/researchareas/hypertension/lbox/LTBXPROT_995.html
11. Lee SC, Wang Y (1999) Automatic retinal image quality assessment and enhancement. In: Proceedings of SPIE, p 1581
12. Lalonde M, Gagnon L, Boucher MCC (2001) Automatic visual quality assessment in optical fundus images. In: Proceedings of Vision Interface 2001, pp 259–264
13. Bartling H, Wanger P, Martin L (2009) Automated quality evaluation of digital fundus photographs. Acta Ophthalmol 87:643–647
14. Acharya T, Ray AK (2005) Image processing: principles and applications. Wiley, Hoboken
15. Hunter A, Lowell JA, Habib M, Ryder B, Basu A, Steel D (2011) An automated retinal image quality grading algorithm. In: Proceedings of the annual international conference of the IEEE engineering in medicine and biology society conference, pp 5955–5958
16. Nirmala SR, Dandapat S, Bora PK (2011) Performance evaluation of distortion measures for retinal images. Int J Comput Appl 17:17
17. Niemeijer M, Abràmoff MD, van Ginneken B (2006) Image structure clustering for image quality verification of color retina images in diabetic retinopathy screening. Med Image Anal 10:888–898
18. Giancardo L, Abràmoff MD, Chaum E, Karnowski TP, Meriaudeau F, Tobin KW (2008) Elliptical local vessel density: a fast and robust quality metric for retinal images. In: Proceedings of the international conference on IEEE engineering in medicine and biology society, pp 3534–3537
19. Paulus J, Meier J, Bock R, Hornegger J, Michelson G (2010) Automated quality assessment of retinal fundus photos. Int J Comput Assist Radiol Surg 5:557–564
20. Smith RT, Nagasaki T, Sparrow JR, Barbazetto I, Klaver CC, Chan JK (2003) A method of drusen measurement based on the geometry of fundus reflectance. Biomed Eng Online 2:10
21. Soliz P, Wilson MP, Nemeth SC, Nguyen P (2002) Computer-aided methods for quantitative assessment of longitudinal changes in retinal images presenting with maculopathy. In: Medical Imaging 2002: visualization, image-guided procedures, and display, SPIE, San Diego, pp 159–170
22. Phillips RP, Spencer T, Ross PG, Sharp PF, Forrester JV (1991) Quantification of diabetic maculopathy by digital imaging of the fundus. Eye 5(Pt 1):130–137
23. Jagoe JR, Blauth CI, Smith PL, Arnold JV, Taylor KM, Wootton R (1990) Quantification of retinal damage during cardiopulmonary bypass: comparison of computer and human assessment. In: Proceedings of the IEE communications, speech and vision I(137):170–175

24. Rapantzikos K, Zervakis M, Balas K (2003) Detection and segmentation of drusen deposits on human retina: potential in the diagnosis of age-related macular degeneration. Med Image Anal 7:95–108
25. Gonzalez R, Woods R (1993) Digital image processing. Addison Wesley Publishing, New York
26. Mora AD, Vieira PM, Manivannan A, Fonseca JM (2011) Automated drusen detection in retinal images using analytical modelling algorithms. Biomed Eng Online 10:59
27. Culpin D (1986) Calculation of cubic smoothing splines for equally spaced data. Numer Math 48:627–638
28. Smith RT, Chan JK, Nagasaki T, Ahmad UF, Barbazetto I, Sparrow J, Figueroa M, Merriam J (2005) Automated detection of macular drusen using geometric background leveling and threshold selection. Arch Ophthalmol 123:200–206
29. Shlens J (2005) A tutorial on principal component analysis. Measurement 51:52
30. Newsom RS, Sinthanayothin C, Boyce J, Casswell AG, Williamson TH (2000) Clinical evaluation of "local contrast enhancement" for oral fluorescein angiograms. Eye (London, England) 14 (Pt 3A):318–23
31. Jobson DJ, Rahman Z, Woodell GA (1997) A multiscale retinex for bridging the gap between color images and the human observation of scenes. IEEE Trans Image Process Publ IEEE Signal Process Soc 6:965–976
32. Majumdar J, Nandi M, Nagabhushan P (2011) Retinex algorithm with reduced halo artifacts. Def Sci J 61:559–566
33. Land EH, McCann JJ (1971) Lightness and retinex theory. J Opt Soc Am 61:1–11
34. Foracchia M, Grisan E, Ruggeri A, Member S (2004) Detection of optic disc in retinal images by means of a geometrical model of vessel structure. IEEE Trans Med Imaging 2004(23):1189–1195
35. Hoover A, Goldbaum M (2003) Locating the optic nerve in a retinal image using the fuzzy convergence of the blood vessels. IEEE Trans Med Imaging 22:951–958
36. Lalonde M, Beaulieu M, Gagnon L (2001) Fast and robust optic disc detection using pyramidal decomposition and Hausdorff-based template matching. IEEE Trans Med Imaging 20:1193–1200
37. Youssif AR, Ghalwash AZ, Ghoneim AR (2008) Optic disc detection from normalized digital fundus images by means of a vessels' direction matched filter. IEEE Trans Med Imaging 27:11–18
38. Mendels F, Heneghan C, Thiran JP (1999) Identification of the optic disk boundary in retinal images using active contours. In: Proceedings of the Irish machine vision and image processing conference. Citeseer, pp 103–115
39. Osareh A, Mirmehdi M, Thomas B, Markham R (2002) Colour morphology and snakes for optic disc localisation. In: Proceedings of the 6th medical image understanding and analysis conference, pp 21–24
40. Sinthanayothin C, Boyce JF, Cook HL, Williamson TH (1999) Automated localisation of the optic disc, fovea, and retinal blood vessels from digital colour fundus images. Br J Ophthalmol 83:902–910
41. Li H (2003) Boundary detection of optic disk by a modified ASM method. Pattern Recogn 36:2093–2104
42. Kavitha D, Devi SS (2005) Automatic detection of optic disc and exudates in retinal images. In: Proceedings of 2005 international conference on intelligent sensing and information processing, pp 501–506
43. Sekhar S, Al-Nuaimy W, Nandi A (2008) Automated localisation of retinal optic disk using hough transform. In: Proceedings of the 5th IEEE international symposium on biomedical imaging from Nano to Macro. ISBI 2008, pp 1577–1580
44. Zhu X, Rangayyan RM (2008) Detection of the optic disc in images of the retina using the Hough transform. In: Proceedings of the Annual International Conference on the IEEE engineering in medicine and biology society, pp 3546–3549

45. Cootes T (1995) Active shape models-their training and application. Comput Vis Image Underst 61:38–59
46. Otsu N (1979) A threshold selection method from gray-level histograms. IEEE Trans Syst Man Cybern 9:62–66
47. Gonzalez R, Woods R (2002) Digital image processing. Prentice Hall, Upper Saddle River
48. Canny J (1986) A computational approach to edge detection. IEEE Trans Pattern Anal Mach Intell PAMI-8:679–698
49. Pinão J, Oliveira CM (2011) Fovea and optic disc detection in retinal images. In: Tavares JM, Natal Jorge RS (eds) Computational vision and medical image processing VIPIMAGE 2011. CRC Press, pp 149–153
50. ter Haar F (2005) Automatic localization of the optic disc in digital colour images of the human retina. Utrecht University, The Netherlands

Database System for Clinical and Computer Assisted Diagnosis of Dermoscopy Images

B. S. R. Amorim and T. F. Mendonça

Abstract Dermoscopy is a non-invasive diagnosis technique for in vivo observation of pigmented skin lesions used in dermatology. There is currently a great interest in the development of computer assisted diagnosis systems, given their great potential to this area of medicine. The standard approach in automatic dermoscopic image analysis can be divided in three stages: image segmentation, feature extraction/selection and lesion classification. In order to validate the algorithms developed for each stage, a great number of reliable images and clinical diagnosis are required. This paper presents a software tool to collect and organize dermoscopic data from hospital databases. It is suitable for clinical daily routine and simultaneously has a data structure to support the development and validation of algorithms created by the researchers to construct the computer assisted diagnosis system. This tool is composed by a database with three related but independent modules: Clinical Module, Processing Module and Statistical Module.

1 Introduction

Dermoscopy is a non-invasive diagnostic technique for in vivo observation of pigmented skin lesions used in dermatology (Fig. 1). This diagnostic tool allows the clinicians to have a better visualization of subsurface structures (Fig. 2) and permits the recognition and evaluation of important morphologic characteristics not distinguishable by the human naked eye [2]. The use of this procedure in daily

B. S. R. Amorim (✉) · T. F. Mendonça
Faculdade de Ciências da, Universidade do Porto, Rua do Campo Alegre s/n,
4169-007 Porto, Portugal
e-mail: barbarasofia7@gmail.com

T. F. Mendonça
e-mail: tmendo@fc.up.pt

J. M. R. S. Tavares and R. M. Natal Jorge (eds.), *Topics in Medical Image Processing and Computational Vision*, Lecture Notes in Computational Vision and Biomechanics 8,
DOI: 10.1007/978-94-007-0726-9_14,

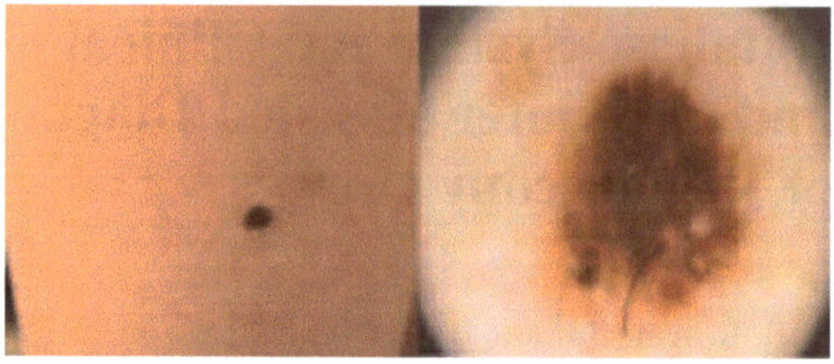

Fig. 1 Real image and corresponding dermoscopic visualization of a pigmented skin lesion. Dermoscopic image from hospital pedro hispano database

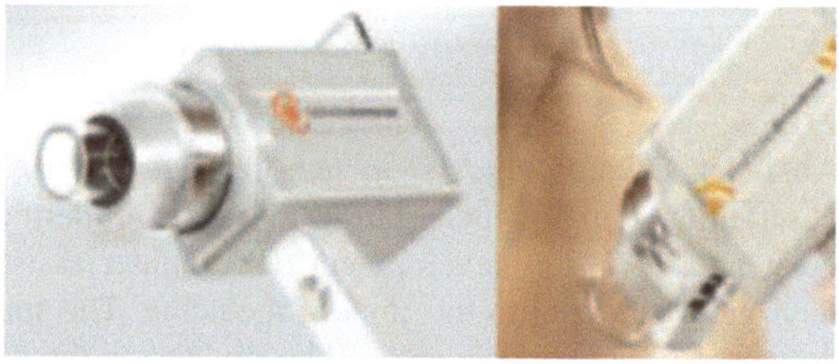

Fig. 2 Example of a dermoscopic imaging system, namely FotoFinder

clinical routine conducts to an improved accuracy and robustness of clinical diagnosis, along with an overall progress of the global health care system. For example, concerning to melanoma, the use of dermoscopy by trained observers is associated with an increase in both sensitivity (percentage of melanoma recognized over the total number of melanomas examined) and specificity (percentage of non-melanoma lesions recognized over the total number of non-melanoma lesions examined) compared with that expected by examination using the naked eye [2].

Several other benefits can be derived from dermoscopy, namely the earlier screening diagnosis, the restrain on the number of selected cases for exeresis, consequently driving to a decrease of unnecessary surgeries. All of this can be translated into human resources optimization, economical thrift and time effectiveness [9].

In the last few years a number of independent screening clinical tests have been proposed. These procedures are suitable for health care personal with a minimum clinical training and can reduce the number of cases that need to be analyzed by specialists. The screening methods, such as the pattern analysis method [7], the ABCD Rule algorithm [7], the 7 point checklist algorithm [2], the Menzies'method [3], the Cash algorithm [5] and the 3 point checklist [6], are based on an human interpretation of dermoscopic images. The common denominator of all these diagnostic methods is particular dermoscopic criteria that represent the backbone for the morphologic diagnosis of pigmented skin lesions. Nevertheless, none of these criteria is widely accepted for fitting the mental dermatologists' model for diagnosis. Furthermore, it is widely accepted and recognized that there is still considerable work to be done in order to translate the human based criteria into methodologies and algorithms capable to be implemented on Computer assisted diagnosis system (CADS).

2 ADDI Project

The ADDI project is a multidisciplinary project that joins medical doctors from Hospital Pedro Hispano (HPH) and academic researchers from different fields of engineering and mathematics from the University of Porto, University of Aveiro and Instituto Superior Técnico of Lisboa. The driving force behind of this project was several years of experience in dermoscopy, teledermoscopy and telemedicine at the HPH Service of Dermatology, and the lack of an efficient automatic image analysis system for dermoscopic images. The HPH database is a valuable resource including over 4000 clinical cases using dermoscopic images. One of project goals is to enrich the database, both through normalization and by the inclusion of the performance of selected cases on standard dermoscopy early screening methods. The purpose of the work presented here is the development of a data-base system to support the implementation of a CADS for dermoscopy. Existing commercial clinical software available and used in a daily basis in the Dermatology Service of HPH and the large database of dermoscopic images available were considered as the starting point for this work. A software tool was developed to collect and organize dermoscopic data, suitable for the daily clinical routine use, but also fulfilling the need for data structures and consistency required to support the development and validation of algorithms created for future CADS. The complete platform is currently being prepared so that it can be widely applied to other care centers and hospitals with minimal modifications. It will first perform the automatic identification of the skin lesion on a dermoscopic image, using image segmentation techniques. Then extract a number of features from the lesion, which will be used, together with the knowledge gathered on the existing database of clinical cases, to perform a simplified lesion classification. We believe that the key for a reliable and accurate lesion classification is the successful establishment of a link between the features used on human based early screening diagnosis methods and those produced by an algorithm implemented on a computer based system. The software prototype, together with the enriched database will also support the development of an educational tools suitable for clinicians and health-care staff, as well as researchers in the image processing area, in order to increase their familiarity with dermoscopy and teledermoscopy.

3 Information System for Dermoscopy

Taking into account the advantages of dermoscopy, there is currently a crescent interest in the development of automatic decision support systems given their great potential in this area. They should provide meaningful quantitative information to assist the clinical evaluation and perform the desired diagnosis accurately. There are several things to consider before the development of an information system for dermoscopy.

3.1 Dermoscopic Analyses and Algorithms

3.1.1 Pattern Analyses

All the dermoscopy analysis algorithms of pigmented skin lesions are based on pattern analysis [8]. Its basic principle is that pigmented skin lesions are characterized by global patterns and combinations of local features. This procedure takes in account all of the well-established dermoscopy features and it has the best diagnostic accuracy of all algorithms, being able to classify both melanocytic and non-melanocytic lesions. The five most common patterns of melanocytic lesions are reticular pattern, globular pattern, homogeneous pattern, starburst pattern and nonspecific pattern. When evaluating a non-melanocytic the features to have in account are: blue-grey blotches, arborizing vessels, milia-like cysts, comed-like openings, red-blue lacunas and central white patch [6]. The two algorithms presented next, ABCD Rule and 7 Point Checklist, are only valid to classify melanocytic lesions. They are the most used in dermoscopy due to their quantitative structure.

Table 1 ABCD criterion to classify a melanocytic lesion.

Criterion	Score
Asymmetry	0 for biaxial symmetry, 1 for monaxial symmetry and 2 for biaxial asymmetry
Border	1 for each abrupt cut-off in the periphery of the lesion (value between 0 and 8)
Color	1 for each color present in the lesion (value between 1 and 6)
Differential structures	1 for each dermoscopic structure present in the lesion (value between 1 and 5)

3.1.2 ABCD Rule

The ABCD Rule of dermoscopy is based on a semi quantitative analysis of asymmetry, border, color and some important dermoscopic structures of the given melanocytic lesion (see Table 1). Note that this algorithm only works on melanocytic lesions, so before this rule may be applied the given pigmented lesion must be classified as melanocytic or non-melanocytic [7]:

- Asymmetry (A)—the lesion is bisected by two axes. The first one is positioned over the larger distance between two borderers point of the lesion. The second axe makes a 90 angle with the first one. The axes intersect each other in the centroid of the lesion. Asymmetry is evaluated in terms of colors and dermoscopic structures.
- Border (B)—the lesion is divided into eight parts. Every zone with an abrupt cut-off of pigmented pattern at the periphery has to be considered to TDS.

In contrast, a gradual indistinct cut-off of pigmented pattern is not considered to the calculation of TDS.

- Color (C)—a total of six different colors are counted to determine the total color score, namely, white, red, light brown, dark brown, greyish blue and black. White color is only considered in total score if the area is lighter than the adjacent skin tone.
- Dermoscopic structures (D)—pigmented network, structureless or homogeneous areas, streaks, dots and globules are the five structural features considered here.

Table 2 Total dermoscopy score

Total dermoscopy score	Interpretation
Lower than 4.75	Benign melanocytic lesion
From 4.8 to 5.45	Suspicious lesion follow-up or excision
Higher than 5.45	Lesion highly suspicious for melanoma

The higher the number of these structures, the higher the probability of the lesion being a melanoma. The calculation of Total Dermoscopic Score (TDS) is done using the following formula (1). The interpretation of the result is done using Table 2.

$$TDS = [(A * 1.3) + (B * 0.1) + (C * 0.5) + (D * 0.5)] \tag{1}$$

3.1.3 Seven Point Checklist

This procedure is based in the evaluation of seven features frequently associated to melanomas. The seven features selected are divided in two groups—major criteria and minor criteria—since not all of them have the same influence in the diagnosis of melanoma. Three features have the most important part: atypical pigment network, blue-whitish veil and irregular vascular pattern. The remaining four (irregular streaks, irregular dots/globules, regression areas and irregular pigmentation) play a secondary role in the diagnosis of melanoma [2].

Major criteria:

- Atypical pigment network—pigment network is a grid-like or honey-comb-like structure consisting of round pigmented lines and lighter hypo-pigmented holes.
- Blue-whitish veil—blue-whitish veil is the name given to an indistinct, transparent, confluent gray-blue to whitish-blue diffuse pigmentation that may extend over almost all the area of the lesion.
- Atypical vascular pattern—atypical vascular pattern is a linear-irregular red structure or dotted vessels not clearly combined with regression structures and associated with pigment network alterations, dots/globules and/or streaks.

Minor criteria:

- Irregular streaks—streaks are brownish-black linear structures of variable thickness. They are typically found at the periphery of a lesion and are not necessarily connected to the lines of pigmented network. Linear-irregular streaks with variable thickness are a strong indicator of malignancy.
- Irregular dots/globules—dots are formed when pigment or cells occur in clumps. These nests of cells appear as small uniform dark dots in benign lesions. Large groups of pigmented cells in the dermis form large dots called globules. Irregular dots/globules tend to vary in size and shape and are frequently found in the periphery of lesions in tones of grey, black or dark brown.
- Irregular pigmentation—the structureless pigmented areas have irregular shape and/or distribution.

To get the TDS using Seven point checklist we assign a value of 2 to the three major criteria and a value of 1 to each of the minor criteria. Then, if the feature is present in the lesion its value is summed to the final score, else 0 is summed. In case the TDS of the lesion is higher than 3 it is classified as melanoma; otherwise it is classified as nevi. So, in order to have a lesion classified as melanoma, it has to present at least one major and one minor criteria or three minor criteria.

3.2 *System and Local Environment Analysis*

One of the most important aspects required before developing clinical software is to analyze the local environment and study the daily clinical routine and procedures. Better understanding of the clinicians work allows researchers to develop more efficient computational tools. In HPH, dermatologists use a device named dermatoscope to collect images of pigmented skin lesions (Fig. 3). Those images

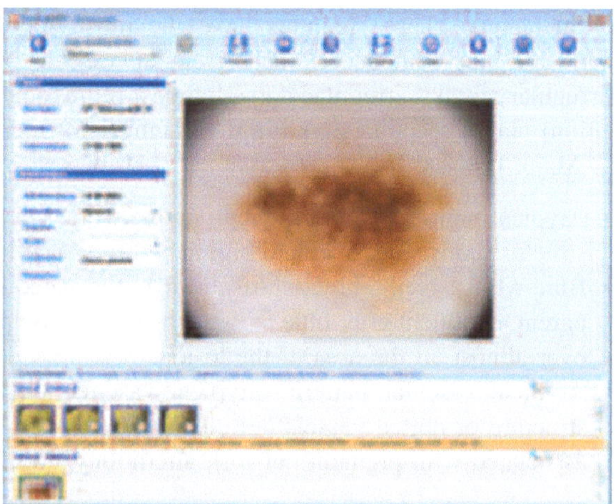

Fig. 3 Example of the FotoFinder software interface

are then storage in FotoFinder database software, the commercial software installed in HPH Dermatology Service. Clinicians use this software both in hospital and in teledermoscopy consulting in health care centers.

3.3 *Processing Dermoscopic Images*

The standard approach for processing dermoscopic images is usually composed of three different stages: image segmentation, feature extraction and selection and lesion classification. Several research groups have developed automated analysis procedures and algorithms for those tasks. However in all of these distinct approaches a specific problem persists—the lack of reliable data sources to validate the results. Furthermore, the results of different studies are not comparable because of the distinct clinical image sets used in each of them. In most cases it is a hard task to find where the images used in a particular research came from, due to an absence of information. The proposed methodology aims to design a dedicated platform (ADDI) to support the current lack of reliable and organized information sources. A ground-truth database like the one presented next is crucial to feed the researchers' algorithms and methods for several purposes (image segmentation, classification, lesion structures evaluation...). This platform adds a new stage (Reliable Data Sources) to the three phase's standard approach and gathers them all in one software. Moreover, a system like this one can provide a large amount of meaningful quantitative information to assist clinical evaluation. At a further level it may lead to a fully automatic CADS for early warning diagnosis of skin lesions. Collecting data and constructing a dedicated platform like this is a complex process, since it is not a straightforward collection of clinical cases from existent databases.

4 Database Development

Databases are powerful informatics tools, prepared to storage large collections of data and keep them organized. This way they allow fast and efficient access to the information saved. They also provide a user friendly interface and are easily implemented and adaptable to any professional area. So, implementing a tool based on a database system seemed the logical choice to develop a reliable data source component for the ADDI-Platform. This tool is composed by three database modules: Clinical Module (CM), Processing Module (PM) and Statistical Module (SM). The construction of each of these components is divided in four stages: system analysis, logical design, physical design and implementation. All stages enclose specific tasks and rules that must be followed strictly. So, in the end of the construction process, data organization, integrity and security will be accomplished.

4.1 System Analyses

In a first stage it was essential to fully understand the software used in the hospital as well as the daily clinical routine. Furthermore, it was necessary to aggregate all the possible information among clinical staff and specialist and gather opinions on possible improvements and development of additional features not existent in their current database system. Notice that, since this service is uncharged of all patients from Matosinhos County, there are two different sources of dermoscopic images. One face to face and another operated through a Telemedicine protocol. The work sessions in HPH provided and increased insight of the problem to be solved and allowed us to find some lacks to be corrected and improvements to implement in a new software platform, namely:

- Improve the database structure;
- Ensure data integrity;
- Decrease the subjectivity on the diagnosis;
- Compel the introduction of some important missing information;
- Restrict the permissions to update information;
- Implement a functionality to do the follow-up of lesions over time;
- Automatic introduction of diagnosis date by the system;
- Optimize the search tool;
- Keep clinical confidentiality of patients' identity.

This was a time consuming challenging task, dealing with sensitive issues, since it involved the transfer of confidential patient's information and the collaboration between multidisciplinary areas, with various sets of data with different storage places and different levels of accessibility. The biggest challenge was to understand the clinical mental model, almost completely qualitative, and translate it into a quantitative model [1].

The information collected was organized in different groups in a way it still reflects the real world concepts we are involved with. This drives us to the ER-model construction [4]. Figure 4 presents the three ER-model developed each one representing one module of the database system.

4.2 Logical Model

The next phase was to transform the ER-model into an R-model, which was done using normalization, the systematic process that takes the ER-model built and applies him several rules [4]. In this way a logical arrangement that guarantees the integrity of data and minimizes its redundancy is created. The R-model is the formal representation of each of our database modules. The R-model for this work is presented in Figs. 4, 5 and 6.

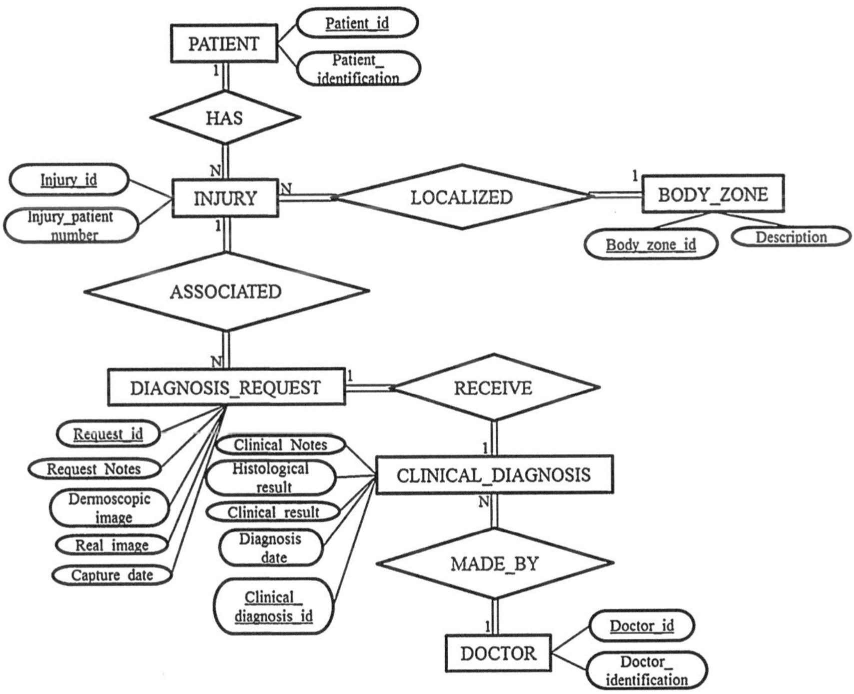

Fig. 4 ER-model representation of the Clinical Module from ADDI platform

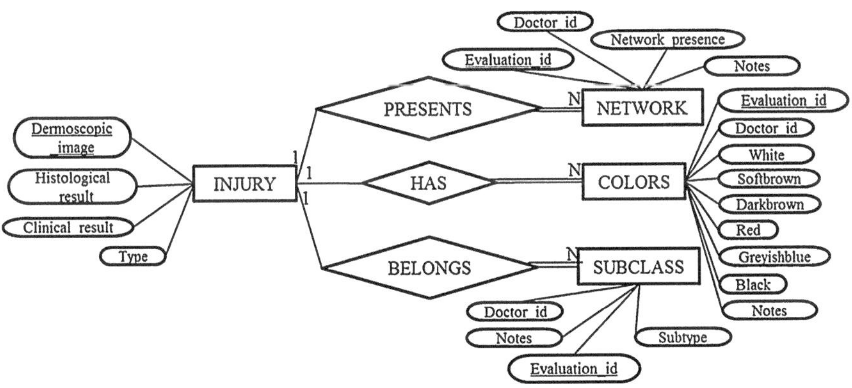

Fig. 5 ER-model representation of the Processing Module from ADDI platform

4.3 Physical Design and Implementation

The database modules presented were implemented with SQL language using the phpMyAdmin software. The access to clinical data is made using web applications. We chose to use web applications because they are independent from the

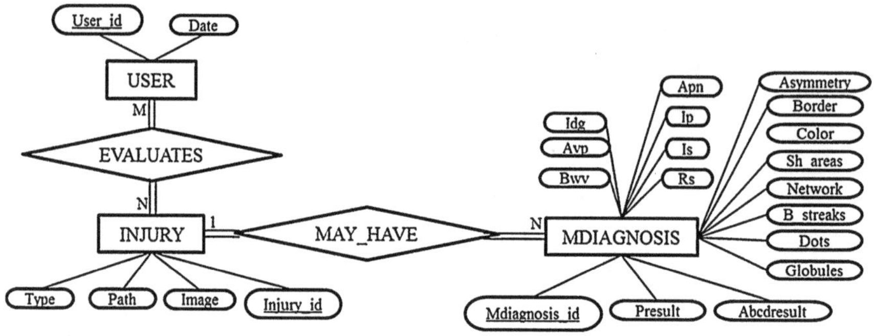

Fig. 6 ER-model representation of the Statistical Module from ADDI platform

operating system and can be accessed from any place around the world. The tools developed were implemented using HTML and CSS to design and organize its interfaces, JS to do the information processing in the client side and PHP to do information processing in the server side, including the implementation of SQL queries to the database (Figs. 7, 8, 9).

5 ADDI Platform

The database system prototype developed will be integrated in a software platform still in progress. The great advantage of having a reliable data source component structure in a platform like this relies on the independency of each module,

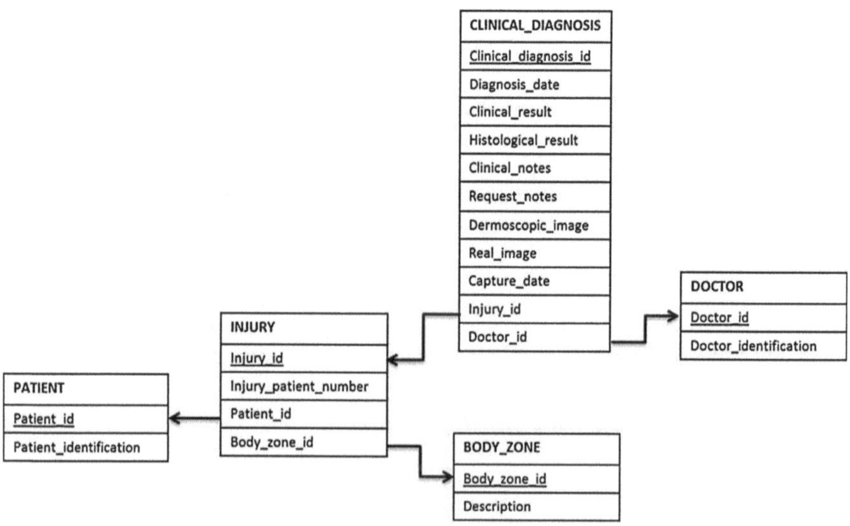

Fig. 7 R-model representation of the Clinical Module from ADDI platform

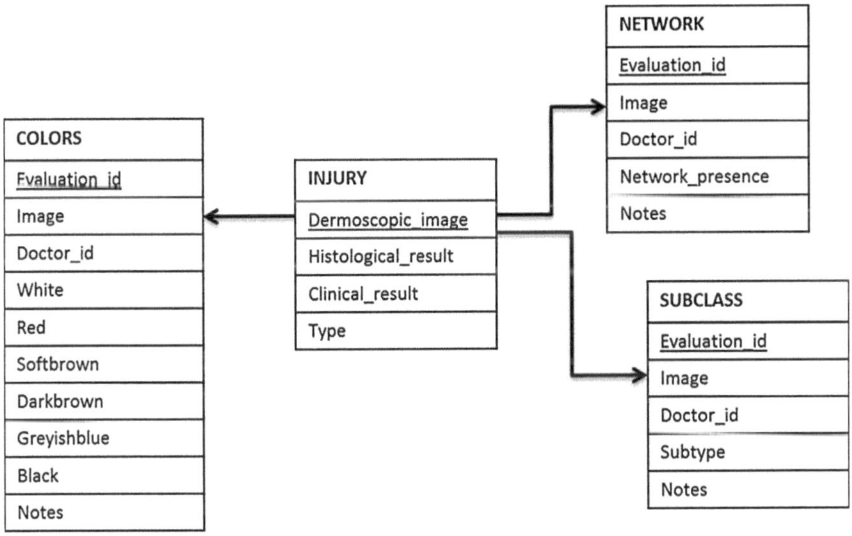

Fig. 8 R-model representation of the Processing Module from ADDI platform

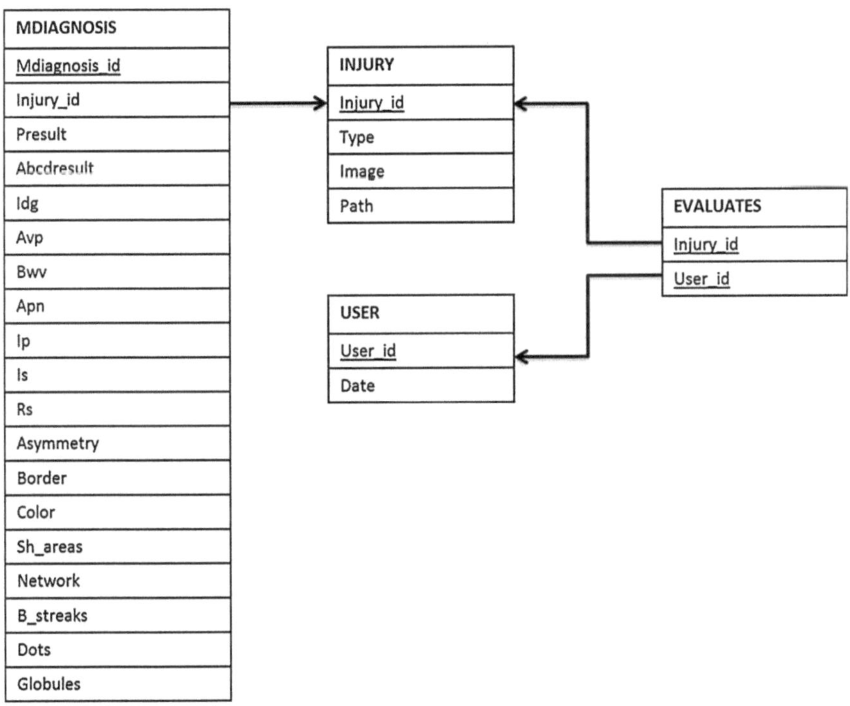

Fig. 9 R-model representation of the Statistical Module from ADDI platform

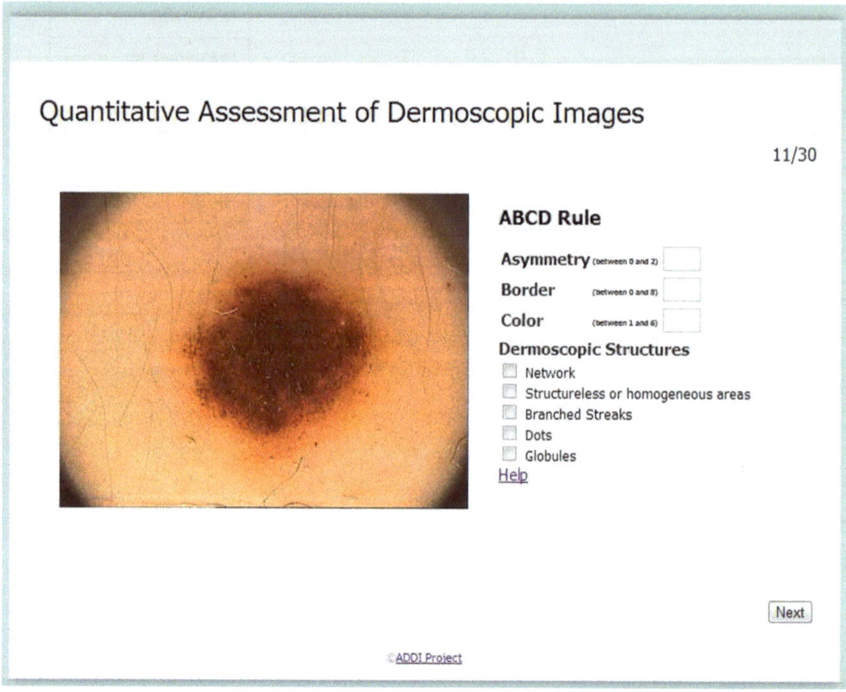

Fig. 10 Application to perform quantitative evaluation of lesions using ABCD Rule and 7 Point Checklist algorithms

meaning that, although the three of them are related, each of them works as a stand-alone tool too. The clinical staff will use the CM as a tool to collect, store and consult patient information's. At the same time researchers will access PM to obtain a bank of robust and reliable dermoscopic cases (both images and clinical diagnosis). PM receives a huge and permanent flow of information, since the hospital FotoFinder software collects daily the real cases and the correspondent dermoscopic and clinical diagnosis. The SM will be very useful for the image segmentation stage. This module uses a web application to collect, for each case, individual clinical classifications based upon available quantitative tests accepted by the International Dermoscopy Society (Fig. 10). In the image segmentation stage, researchers define a set of restrictions that dermoscopic images must respect in order to successfully integrate the image test group to be applied to the algorithms developed. Then they access PM to get those images. The research team may also access SM in this stage to help them to understand what images gather consensual opinion among specialists. This is a valuable issue, since the development of algorithms and their performance evaluation relies on the existence of well-defined subset of typical images.

A database tool like the one developed may also be useful to divide injuries into different sets, such as body zones and other clinical widely accepted standard

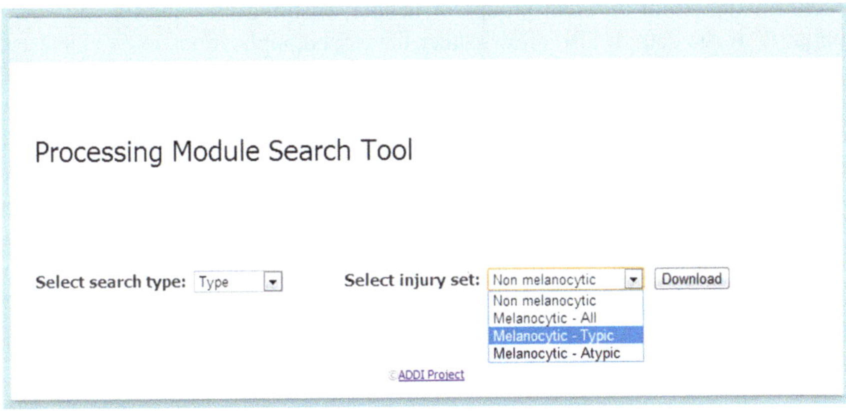

Fig. 11 Application to download images from database system

specifications. Afterward, feature selection and extraction has to be made. Researchers may apply statistical algorithms to the features information available in PM and SM, in order to choose which features are more likely to produce significant results in lesion classification. Notice that database structure may be easily modified and extended, since databases own a property called scalability. Furthermore, it may also complete itself, filing some lacks of information using machine learning and data mining algorithms based in all the knowledge acquired with the clinical specialists. The database is accessed through an application that allows all the research team members to have access to the clinical data collected from HPH database. It is a form where the user chooses the criteria he wants to evaluate and downloads automatically an image set respecting those criteria. An example of the use of this tool is presented in Fig. 6.

The download file is a text file including a list of image names present in PM database. This downloaded file is easily introduced into Matlab, which is the software used to develop the image processing algorithms. The txt extension can also be easily imported to algorithms developed in other lower level languages such as C or Java (Fig. 11).

6 Conclusion

Computer assisted diagnosis systems have great potential for dermoscopy. These systems provide meaningful quantitative information to assist clinical diagnosis and, at a further level, to perform an automatic early screening of skin lesions. A number of computer-assisted diagnosis systems are able to classify skin lesions with high sensitivity. The access to a reliable data source is a capital gain in terms of time and accessibility to clinical information. The development of a database divided in modules, like the one here presented, allows the access to different sets of information from different groups of people, ensuring the security and confidentiality of the data. It also allows other developed applications to be connected to the reliable data source with the purpose of increasing their computational power. A platform such as ADDI-Platform provides several benefits both to teledermoscopy and telemedicine, since computer assisted diagnosis systems are essential tools in these areas. However, further developments are still required in order to have a robust and reliable complete platform. In the near future other functionalities will be developed within the ADDI project. A synchronization tool will be implemented, which will allow PM and SM to be updated real-time every time a new case is introduced in CM at the hospital. PMST and PM will be extended to include information whether the lesions are acral, facial or other, since acral and facial lesions have an altogether different process of diagnosis.

References

1. Amorim B (2011) Database implementation for clinical and computer assisted diagnosis of dermoscopic images. VipImage 2011, Olhão, Portugal, 12–14 Oct 2011
2. Argenziano G (2001) Dermoscopy of pigmented skin lesions—a valuable tool for early diagnosis of melanoma. Lancet Oncol 2:443–449
3. Carli P (2003) Pattern analysis, not simplified algorithms, is the most reliable method for teaching dermoscopy for melanoma diagnosis to residents in dermatology. Br J Dermatol 148:981
4. Codd E (1990) The relational model for database management: version 2. Addison-Wesley Longman Publishing, Boston
5. Henning J (2007) The CASH (color, architecture, symmetry, and homogeneity) algorithm for dermoscopy. J Am Acad Dermatol 56:45–52
6. Johr R (2004) Dermoscopy: the essentials. Elsevier—Health Sciences Division, St. Louis
7. Marghoob A (2004) Atlas of dermoscopy. Taylor and Francis, London
8. Pehamberger H, Steiner A, Wolff K (1987) In vivo epiluminescence microscopy of pigmented skin lesions. I. Pattern analysis of pigmented skin lesions. J Am Acad Dermatol 17(4):571–583
9. Silveira M (2009) Comparison of segmentation methods for melanoma diagnosis in dermoscopy images. IEEE J Sel Top Sig Process 3(1):35–45

Segmentation Based Pattern Recognition for Peri-Urban Areas in X Band SAR Images

Bruno Cafaro, Silvia Canale, Alberto De Santis, Daniela Iacoviello, Fiora Pirri and Simone Sagratella

Abstract In this paper Synthetic Aperture Radar (SAR) images in X-band were analyzed in order to infer ground properties from data. The aim was to classify different zones in peri-urban forestries integrating information from different sources. In particular the X band is sensitive to the moisture content of the ground that can be therefore put into relation with the gray level of the image; moreover, the gray level is related to the smoothness and roughness of the ground. An integration of image segmentation and machine learning methods is studied to classify different zones of peri-urban forestries, such as trees canopies, lawns, water pounds, roads, etc., directly from the gray level signal properties. As case study the X-SAR data of a forest near Rome, the Castel Fusano area, are analyzed.

1 Introduction

The use of Synthetic Aperture Radar (SAR) images is well established for environment monitoring. As a matter of fact, in this last decade, more than 15 SAR satellites have been successfully launched for scientific, commercial, and security-related applications. Various methods [2, 18] have been devised to recognize areas of different soil and vegetation types, by mainly exploiting regression analysis of backscattering models relating the measured signal to some parameters characterizing the soil conditions. In this context the use of the X band is quite recent and its capability in environmental monitoring is yet to be fully evaluated.

A crucial scientific contribution to urban management in European metropolis, where large peri-urban forests and parks form a beautiful interface with the metropolitan settlement, is to provide a strategic tool for fire risk management based

B. Cafaro · S. Canale · A. De Santis · D. Iacoviello (✉) · F. Pirri · S. Sagratella
Department of Computer, Control and Management Engineering "A. Ruberti",
Sapienza University of Rome, Via Ariosto 25, 00185 Rome, Italy
e-mail: iacoviello@dis.uniroma1.it; iacoviel@dis.uniroma1.it

J. M. R. S. Tavares and R. M. Natal Jorge (eds.), *Topics in Medical Image Processing and Computational Vision*, Lecture Notes in Computational Vision and Biomechanics 8,
DOI: 10.1007/978-94-007-0726-9_15,

on X band image analysis. From several studies on European fires (e.g. [1, 14]) image analysis turns out to be very useful for detecting changes in land covers and define accurate fire risk indexes. The main difficulty in these studies is to conceal different data sources providing a suitable integration methodology that can face such a complex data structure. In fact, higher resolution datasets usually suffer a loss in favor of the lowest common resolution available.

In this paper an integration of image segmentation and machine learning methods is studied to classify different zones of peri-urban forestries, such as trees canopies, lawns, water pounds, roads, etc., directly from the gray level signal properties. The images were segmented by a discrete level set method [8], applied to a suitable transformation of the data. In fact the different regions in the X-SAR image differ mainly for the texture, that is the spatial relation between pixels [13]. Therefore the difficulty was to determine the best transformation that enhanced the differences between the regions.

The X band is known to be sensitive to the ground roughness and the moisture content [9, 12, 19, 20]. For identifying accurate classification rules starting from segmented X band SAR images a Support Vector Machine (SVM) based approach was adopted. SVMs [7, 17, 21] have been successfully adopted in a number of image processing applications, including target recognition in SAR images [11, 22]. In this paper the aim was to automatically recognize the structure of particular kinds of areas and land covers in peri-urban forestry, e.g. burned areas, lakes, roads, and so on.

One of the goal of land and urban data analysis is to define accurate classification layers for the data of the Region of Interest (ROI) to aggregate different resolution levels. Different levels of knowledge may be considered according to the particular application: the soil characteristics, vegetation, land use, fire hazard, water river basins, administrative boundaries, etc.

As area test the Castel Fusano region was considered, a large urban forest near Rome (Italy). It contains a quite complete set of forestry items, such as canopies, brushwood, Mediterranean maquis, roads, buildings, rivers, burned areas, sea shore and so on.

The paper is organized as follows. In Sect. 2 the characteristics of X band SAR images are described along with the adopted method for their processing. In Sect. 3 as an example of a classification layer the moisture feature extraction procedure is presented, whereas in Sect. 4 data representation and classification procedures are outlined. In Sect. 5 a case study is presented; the results are shown on the urban forestry of Castel Fusano. Some conclusions and future development are illustrated.

2 Data Characteristics and Image Analysis

Synthetic Aperture Radar (SAR) data have a great potential as a source of relevant and near real time information for change detection, early warning, mitigation, and forecast and management of natural disasters. That is because of its observation capability regardless climate conditions and solar illumination. Indeed, SAR is an active form of remote sensing. The surface is illuminated by a beam of energy with a fixed wavelength within the range from 1 cm (K band) to approximately 70 cm (P band).

These long wavelengths penetrate clouds and atmospheric interferences common to optical imagery and therefore are not limited spatially or temporally because of solar illumination or atmospheric interferences. The images considered for the present paper are Cosmo-SkyMed products delivered by the Italian Space Agency [3]. They are high quality and high spatial definition, with resolution ranging from 0.6 to 1 m in the SpotLight mode, level 1C-GEC, speckle filtered, only obtained in the X band (wavelength ranging from 2.4 to 3.8 cm). As well known, smooth surfaces have a darker response to X band than ragged ones. Indeed, the X band is known to be sensitive to changes in the target moisture content, namely the response is lighter on increasing humidity. On the other hand different patterns on X-SAR images, corresponding to regions with different characteristics, are only distinguishable by the gray level spatial distribution (texture). See Fig. 1 as an example of a median filtered X-SAR data; in the image regions of different nature are present and the resulting gray level is due to the moisture content and the smoothness of the ground.

A first step in the interpretation of SAR images is achieved by a segmentation procedure based on a discrete level set method, see [8], applied to a suitable transformation of the data. The regions with different characteristics have different textures and therefore are distinguishable by some properties of the gray level spatial distribution. Following a statistical approach [13], the most effective transformation to deal with this kind of data was the local contrast. It is based on the local signal variance evaluated on a square neighborhood with chosen size;

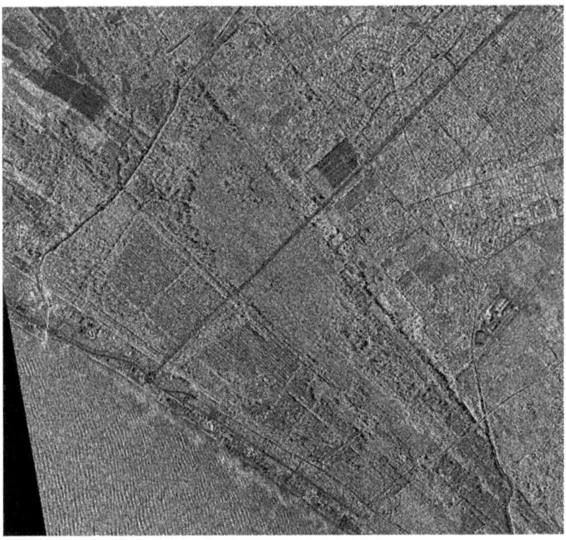

Fig. 1 An example of a median filtered X-SAR data

furthermore the contrast image is processed by a bank of rank filters obtained by varying kernel size and rank order, aiming at the enhancement of the texture properties that better describe the characteristics of the zones to be identified.

A four levels discrete level set segmentation of the region of interest applied to the transformed data provides a simplified representation of the original image preserving the information to be retrieved. It is obtained by successive image binarizations. Let I be the image transformed data; first the image I is partitioned into two distinct subregions (not necessarily simply connected), A_1, A_2 and represented, for any pixel (i, j) of the image domain D, as follows:

$$I_b(i, j) = c_1 \chi_{A_1}(i, j) + c_2 \chi_{A_2}(i, j)$$

where I_b is the piecewise constant image binarization and the constants c_1, c_2 are the signal mean values within the sets A_1, A_2 respectively. Function χ_A is the characteristic function of a set A. The sets A_1,A_2 are described by the level set function $\phi : D \to R$ as follows:

$$A_1 = \{(i, j) \in D : \phi(i, j) \geq 0\}$$
$$A_2 = \{(i, j) \in D : \phi(i, j) < 0\}$$

.

To obtain the binarization elements $(c_1, c_2, \{\phi(i,j)\})$, a suitable cost function is minimized: it contains the fit error between the image and its binary representation and a regularization term for the level set function:

$$\begin{aligned} F(c_1, c_2, \phi) = \lambda \sum_{(i,j)} (I(i, j) - c_1)^2 \chi_{A_i}(i, j) \\ + \lambda \sum_{(i,j)} (I(i, j) - c_2)^2 \chi_{A_2}(i, j) + \sum_{(i,j)} \phi(i, j)^2 \end{aligned} \quad (1)$$

Parameter λ is chosen to enhance the fit error influence over the optimal solution. In [8] it has been shown that the problem of minimizing the cost function (1) has a unique optimal solution; this is due to the presence of the latter term in (1), that makes the cost functional convex.

Once the first level optimal binarization is obtained, the regions A_1, A_2 are further binarized with the same procedure. Thus a four levels optimal segmentation is finally obtained.

The discrete level set algorithm was tested versus the analogous continuous one in [8], showing a more efficient converging rate and a generally more accurate segmentation result.

In the next section, by exploiting the zones identified by the segmentation, an example of moisture feature extraction procedure is presented. In this way the local humidity level can be sensed on the base of global meteorological data acquired over a larger area containing the test zone.

3 Layer Analysis: Moisture Content

The goal of land and urban data analysis is to define accurate classification layers for the data of the ROI to aggregate different resolution levels. These steps are needed, for example, for training a classifier that can provide specific thematic maps. Once the different areas of the ROI are specified on the basic tessellation, they can be assigned various tags, according to ancillary data. Different levels of knowledge may be considered, according to the particular application: the soil characteristics, vegetation, land use, fire hazard, water river basins, administrative boundaries, etc.

One possible layer is the moisture content, that is, as already noted, strictly related to the gray level of the image.

Usually, empirical models are used for soil moisture evaluation by estimating dielectric constant [15]. The soil moisture of vegetated area may be estimated by considering the vegetation and soil backscattering coefficients [16].

In this paper a different approach is considered. The homogeneous zones identified by the segmentation step can be monitored by a periodical acquisition of X-SAR images: their average gray level value can be correlated with ground truth data obtained by the meteorological stations. They provide the daily temperature and the dew point. The latter value represents the temperature to which a given parcel of air or, more precisely, water vapor, must be cooled down to condense into water at constant barometric pressure. It is strictly related to the humidity value *RH*. To retrieve this value we can consider a psychrometric chart or a look-up table, or by means of empirical relations such as the following:

$$RH = \frac{E}{E_s} 100 \tag{2}$$

where E is the actual water vapor pressure and E_s is the saturated water vapor pressure, in units of millibar. These quantities can be evaluated using the dew point values T_d and the temperature values T, both in Celsius scale:

$$\begin{aligned} E_s &= 6.11 \cdot 10^{(7.5 \cdot T/(237.7+T))} \\ E &= 6.11 \cdot 10^{(7.5 \cdot T_d/(237.7+T_d))} \end{aligned} \tag{3}$$

From the above relations the average relative humidity of the considered target area is obtained, and the values correlated with the identified subregions can be found by a simple proportion, using their average gray level value, evaluated over the zones identified according to the procedure of Sect. 2.

Periodical image acquisition provides a time series *RH* moisture values for every subregions. The moisture content of each zone is strictly related with the weather conditions but also on the soil and vegetation characteristics.

4 Area Classification and Pattern Recognition

In this section we present the data model and the machine learning based approach for data analysis and pattern recognition in X-SAR images. The goal is that of defining an accurate area classification on the base of information extracted directly from X-SAR images provided by Cosmo-SkyMed. Once different areas have been identified by the segmentation algorithm described in Sect. 2, the aim is that of identifying accurate classification rules in order to recognize the structure of particular kinds of subregions and land covers in peri-urban forestry, e.g. burned areas, lakes, roads, and so on. These classification rules will be then used to recognize automatically the areas of interest in different images.

As customary in supervised machine learning, the first step is that of defining a set of features describing the X-SAR images and the correlation between each pixel and the others in the same image. This matter is still an open topic in research concerning X-SAR images, while several approaches have been presented for generic SAR images (e.g. [10]). The data integration model we consider allows to describe each pixel by a set of quantitative features based on the gray level in the X-SAR image. These features define the spatial cross correlations among the closest pixels in terms of gray level. In particular, the features of interest in this work are characteristics of the image texture and we have taken into account:

- differential features: first and second order derivatives at different scales. The derivatives are computed by the image convolution with the derivatives of a Gaussian kernel. The different scale are obtained by changing the kernel variance.
- textural features: contrast, uniformity, entropy. They are obtained by computing the gray level histogram over the pixel within a neighborhood of a given size. So far, in our experiments the contrast has given the best results.

Hence the pixel features are: gray level value, local mean, five derivatives at three scales, contrast rank filtering at different ranks. Accordingly we define an input space where each record of quantitative attributes describes one pixel area of the image. For each segmentation level we define a pattern recognition problem and assign to each record x a binary label y according to the segmentation level. The set of these records and their labels represents the training set $\{(x^1, y_1), \ldots, (x^m, y_m)\}$ where x^i is the vector of features describing the pixel i and y_i is the binary label indicating if the pixel i represents a given kind of area according to image segmentation. Of course, we have as many training sets as the possible kinds of subregions we are interested in identifying automatically. For each of them, our aim is that of identifying the classification rule defined over the training set and using this rule to assign the correct class to areas that have not been classified yet (test set).

After selecting the features of interest we have selected one of the most popular pattern recognition models currently adopted in real world application: the Support Vector Machine (SVM). For a complete survey on SVMs we refer to [4] and to the seminal papers by Vapnik [4] and to the seminal papers by Vapnik [6, 21] and the recent literature concerning the so called "kernel methods" [7, 17]. This learning model has been successfully adopted in literature in several domains including SAR image analysis [11, 22]. As far as we know, this paper represents the first attempt to adopt SVM based pattern recognition to X band SAR images, that are high resolution images and provide very large dataset.

As well known, training a 2-norm SVM yields the optimal separating hyperplane between two sets of instances with different labels. From the operative point of view, it implies solving the following quadratic optimization problems where m is the cardinality of the training set, Φ_k is the kernel mapping induced by a Radial Basis Function, e is the vector of ones and (w,b,ξ) are the variables of the problems.

$$\begin{aligned} &\min_{w,b,\xi} \|w\|_2^2 + Ce^T\xi \\ &\Phi_k(x^i)^T w + \xi_i \geq b+1 \qquad x^i : y_i = 1 \qquad i = 1,\ldots,m \\ &\Phi_k(x^i)^T w - \xi_i \leq b-1 \qquad x^i : y_i = -1, \qquad i = 1,\ldots,m \\ &\xi_i \geq 0 \qquad i = 1,\ldots,m \end{aligned} \tag{4}$$

The set of all possible vectors $(w, b) \in \Re^{n+1}$ represents the family of hyperplanes in $\Re^{n+1}$, while the slack variables $\xi \in \Re^m$ measure the violation of each linear constraints. C is the trade-off parameter between the classification error and the regularization term. In 2-norm SVM, the hinge loss function is used to measure the classification error. The regularization term controlling the size of the coefficients in the model is given by the 2-norm of the vector w appearing in the objective function. We made several experiments in order to choose the best kernel mapping Φ_k and in the end we selected the kernel mapping induced by a Radial Basis Function. We have used the well known software LIBSVM [5] to solve the optimization problem and to select the best parameter C and have obtained the results shown in the next section.

5 Case Study: The Castel Fusano Area

As case study the Castel Fusano urban forest near Rome (Italy) was chosen, see Fig. 2.

This area suits well for the purposes of this work; in fact it contains a quite complete set of typical urban and peri-urban forestry items, such as canopies, brushwood, Mediterranean marquis, roads, buildings, rivers, burned areas, sea shore and so on. In 2000 year it suffered a great fire event that destroyed a significant percentage of the area. The choice of the Castel Fusano area as ROI was motivated also on the large amount of ground truth data made available by the Civil Protection.

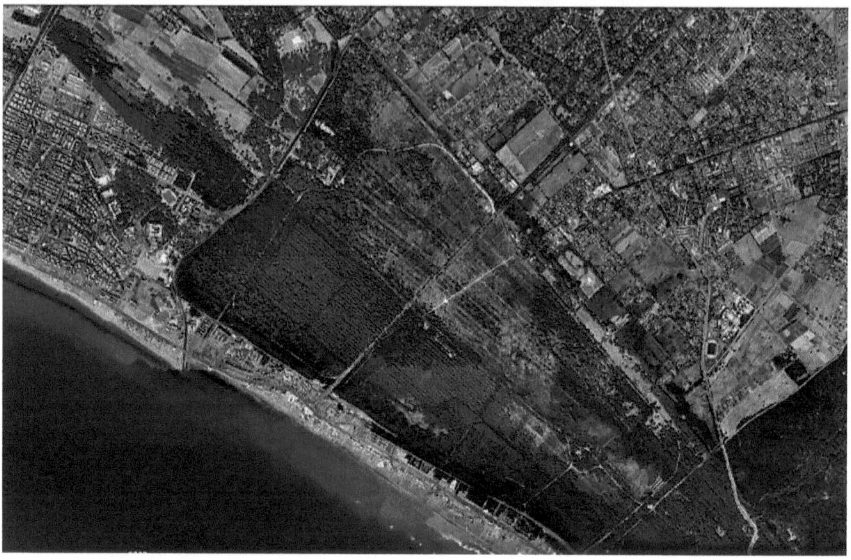

Fig. 2 The ROI (Google Earth, 41.762054 -12.287140/41.701957 -12.362341)

The original data showed a very noisy-like behavior, that was reduced by rank filtering (5,12), that is a filter with kernel size 5 $\times$ 5 and taking the 12-th rank (i.e. a median filter).

As already noted, the different ROI subregions did not differ just for the gray level value, but rather for their texture. Contrast was found to be a convenient data transformation to enhance the dissimilarities between the area subregions. For any image pixel, the contrast is a measure of the signal variance computed in a neighborhood of a given size, in our case 5. On the contrast image a bank of rank filter was used: (10, 50), (10, 80), (5, 5), (5, 20), (20, 200). The application of the level set segmentation to these rank filtered contrast images yielded the complete ROI partition. For instance the burned area was obtained by segmenting the contrast image, Fig. 3, processed by a rank filter (5, 20), as shown in Fig. 4.

In Fig. 4 the burned area obtained by segmenting the rank filtered contrast image is represented. The measure of the local contrast allowed in the chosen zone of Castel Fusano the identification of subregions like the typical canopy of the old oak forest, planted in rows, see Fig. 5.

About ten different subregions can be identified in the ROI, using different rank filters of the contrast image as data to be segmented, see Fig. 6. For each of the identified zone an accurate determination of the contour coordinates and extension is provided.

The gray level mean value is correlated with the local moisture content, one of the relevant physical parameter in the fire susceptibility model. The Aviation Digital Data Service (http://www.aviationweather.gov) provides the daily temperature and dew point values of the ROI; by a simple proportional operation it is

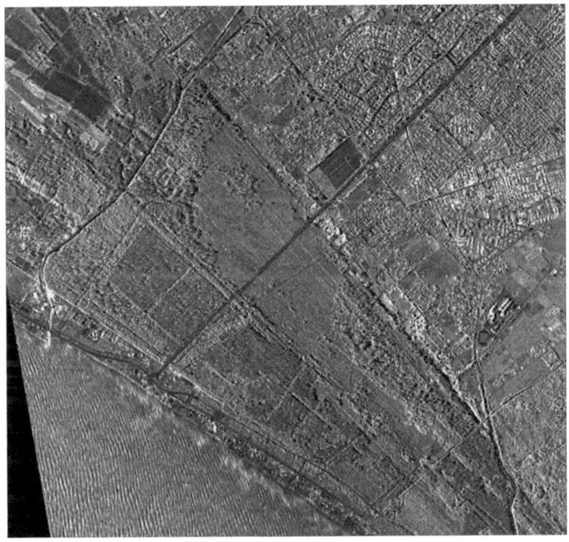

Fig. 3 The image transformation used to detect the burned area: the original data is first processed by a rank filter (5, 12); then the contrast image of these data is computed over a neighborhood of size 5 × 5

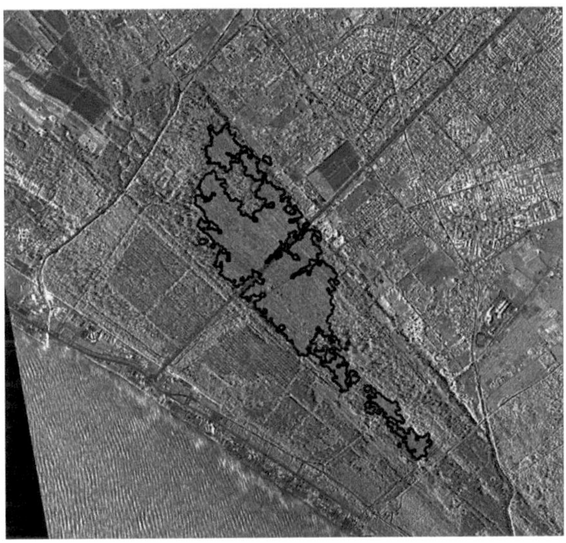

Fig. 4 The burned area obtained by segmenting the contrast image on Fig. 3, processed by a rank filter (5, 20)

possible to retrieve an estimation of the humidity value in all the identified subregions. More precisely, with reference to the image of May 14th 2010 (Fig. 1), from the unique data of the dew point and of the temperature of the ROI, it was possible to estimate the humidity by (2) and (3), obtaining 77.63 %, and therefore by the global mean value of the gray level, 122.98. Knowing the mean value of the gray level in the regions identified by the segmentation procedure, it was possible to estimate the relative humidity value in all the subregions; for example the relative humidity in the area burned in the fire event of 2000 year was of 78 %, whereas it was of 76 % in the oak tree forest.

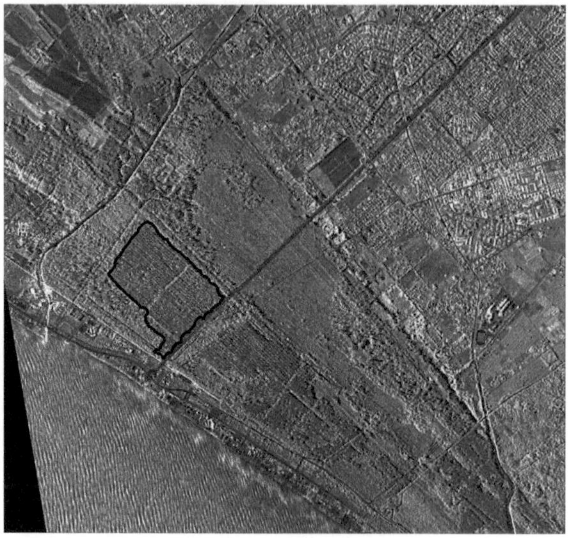

Fig. 5 The oak forest obtained by segmenting the contrast image of Fig. 3, processed by a rank filter (10, 80)

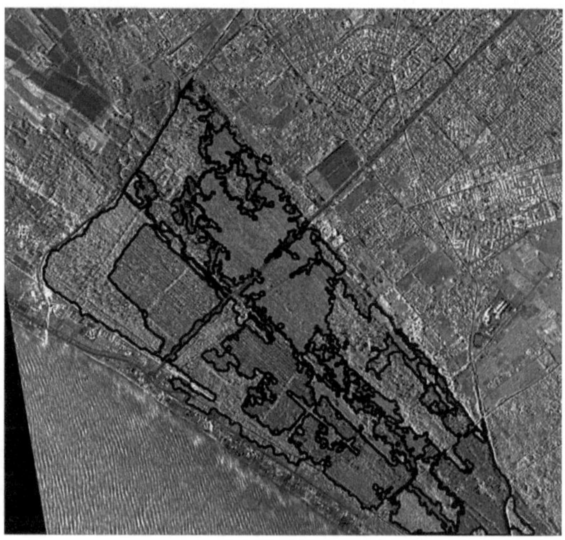

Fig. 6 The identified zones

As regards the area classification and pattern recognition task, the set of pixels indicated in Fig. 7 were selected: the pixels within the square and circle markers are extracted from one segment identified by the segmentation algorithm as the segment of "oak trees", whereas the pixels within the triangle and the diamond markers are extracted from a second segment, corresponding to the "burned area" in Castel Fusano. Each pixel has been mapped in a vector of 20 significant features as described above. The size of the neighbor for the textural features extraction is 100.

Then the five derivatives have been calculated at three scales and the contrast rank filtering at three different ranks (size 30 × 30, ranks 200, 450, 700).

For the oak trees area the training set consists of 20000 pixels within the square markers and the test set of 30000 pixels within the circle markers, shown in Fig. 7. For the burned area the training set consist of 10000 pixels within the triangle marker and the test set of 10000 pixels within the diamond marker.

We have performed three different experiments in order to investigate both the effectiveness of the pattern recognition approach and the quality of the set of features of interest selected for the preliminary analysis.

In the first one, the pixels in the test set (the ones in the circle and diamond markers in Fig. 7) have been extracted from the same image with respect to the training set (pixels in square and triangle markers in Fig. 7). The corresponding experimental results on the test set are shown in Fig. 8a. The pixels within the circle markers have been labeled as "oak tree" by the SVM trained on the training set, while the pixels within the diamond marker have been labeled as "burned area". The four test areas show that the classification of the "burned area" pixels is good with an accuracy of 79.08 %. The remaining 20.92 % error is due to sparse local green areas of tree grew up after the last fire that interested this area in 2006. The three sets of "oak tree" pixels have been identified with an accuracy greater than 80 % in two cases and less than 60 % in one case. The classification accuracy has been rendered by filling the markers with gray tones (0 % black, 100 % white).

In the second experiment, the pixels in the test set (the ones in the circle and diamond markers in Fig. 7) have been extracted from a different image with respect to the training set (pixels in square and triangle markers in Fig. 7). In particular, they have been drawn from a X-SAR image taken the following day with a different polarization. The corresponding experimental results on the test set are shown in Fig. 8b. The pixels within the circle markers have been labeled as

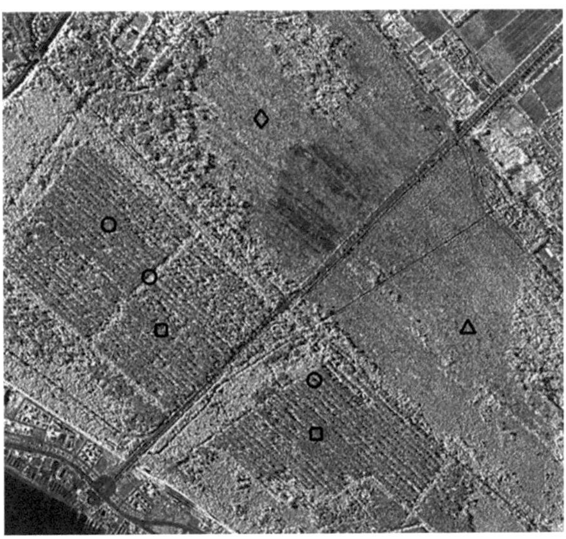

Fig. 7 Sample set selection: the pixels in the square and triangle markers have been selected as training set (the former group is labeled as "oak tree", the latter as "burned") and the pixels in the circle and diamond markers as test set (the former group is labeled as the ones in the square markers and the latter as the ones in the triangle markers)

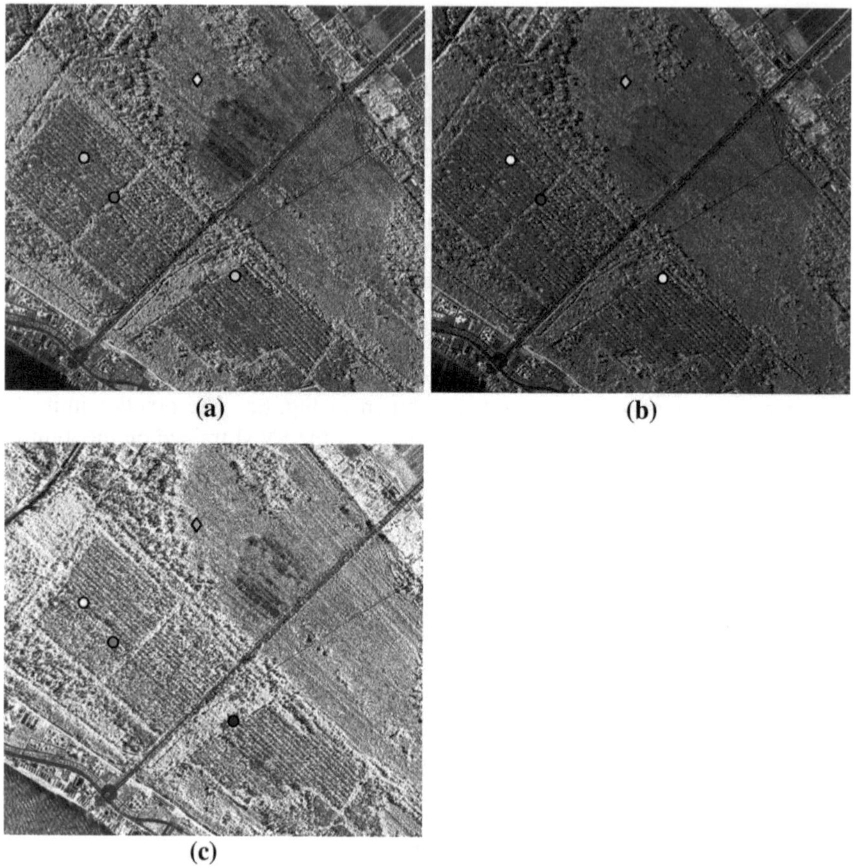

Fig. 8 Experimental results obtained by three different experiments concerning four test areas

"oak tree" by the SVM trained on the training set, while the pixels within the diamond marker have been labeled as "burned area". The four test areas show that the classification of the "burned area" pixels is good with an accuracy of 82.39 %. The remaining error, due to sparse local green areas of tree grew up after the last fire that interested this area in 2006 as in the first experiment, is a more precise measure of the fresh growth of oak trees after the fire. The three sets of "oak tree" pixels have been identified with an accuracy greater than 79 % in two cases and less than 40 % in one case. It is interesting to note that this case includes an area with a track that goes across the oak tree forest and that this aspect has not been recognized in the first experiment, probably because of the effect of the different polarization and soil moisture.

In the third experiment, the test set has been extracted from a different image with respect to the training set (pixels within square and triangle markers in Fig. 7) and from a different location with respect to the test set of Fig. 7 (circle and diamond markers). In particular, the four test areas have been moved to south-west and hence may now cover different segments. In two cases, these areas are now near the boundary of the two segments of oak tree forest and burned area. The corresponding experimental results on the test set are shown in Fig. 8c. The pixels within the circle markers have been labeled as "oak tree" by the SVM trained on the training set, while the pixels within the diamond marker have been labeled as "burned area". The four test areas show that the classification of the "burned area" pixels is good with an accuracy of 77.08 %. The remaining error, due to sparse local green areas as in the previous experiments, indicates that the fresh growth of oak trees after the fire has been faster on the boundary of the segment identifying the burned area, as we can expect. The three sets of "oak tree" pixels have been identified with an accuracy greater than 80 % in the one case where the pixels are still in the segment after moving and less than 70 % in the cases where moved pixels are now on the boundary of the segment that identifies the oak tree forest, as it is reasonable.

These experimental results show that the information does not rely only on the X-SAR signal but on appropriate signal transformations that characterize its texture. The features describing the spatial characteristics of each single pixels are important and must be investigated in the case of X band SAR images, providing further research on the adoption of more sophisticated features, e.g. SURF. Nonetheless, these encouraging classification results prove that the adopted data model yields useful information about the different kinds of areas of interest and that an accurate pattern recognition method can play a fundamental role for extracting useful information from X-SAR images. Classification results obtained so far by training a standard 2-norm SVM can be improved by adopting both more promising kernel functions and more accurate learning models as well as efficient training algorithms.

6 Conclusions

In this paper Synthetic Aperture Radar images in X band were analyzed in order to infer ground properties from data. The aim is to segment and classify different zones of urban forestry integrating information from different sources. In particular the X band is sensitive to the moisture content of the ground that can be therefore put into relation with the gray level of the image. A segmentation with respect to the texture content of the image is provided and integrated with a pattern recognition method in order to identify interesting zones in peri-urban areas, such as lawns, water pounds, trees canopies, roads and so on.

The integration of image segmentation and machine learning methods provides a finite partition of the target zone in areas of different characteristics. This is obtained by a suitable characterization of the signal properties that constitute a SAR label for each area. It is of great interest to evaluate if such a set of features easily generalizes to different urban forestries in the world. In this case the X-SAR databases could be endowed with semantic queries utilities, searching directly for "canopies", "roads", "ponds", etc. As a further application the problem of forests fires can be addressed by studying the fire susceptibility of a zone of interest by classifying the fuel characteristics within each subarea. In this case the segmentation/classification is just one of the layer of a database that includes land use data, meteorological data, human intervention and anthropic factors, including past fires histories. This could help land management authorities in defining thematic maps taking into account particular behaviors in the signal statistics. From the theoretical point of view, our approach can be considered a promising starting point for a deeper analysis on the statistical nature of X-SAR signal distribution for which a suitable implicit representation is still missing. The first encouraging results are shown on the test area of Castel Fusano, a large urban forest near Rome.

Acknowledgments The work reported in this paper has been supported by the Italian Space Agency (ASI) within the Cosmo-SkyMed Announcement of Opportunity (DCOST-2009-116). Data have been provided by ASI Cosmo-SkyMed constellation.

References

1. Alonso-Betanzos A et al (2003) An intelligent system for forest risk prediction and fire fighting management in Galicia. Expert Syst Appl 4(545):554
2. Anguela TP, Zribi M, Baghdadi N, Loumagne C (2010) Analysis of local variation of soil surface parameters with TerraSAR-X Radar data over bare agricultural fields. IEEE Trans Geosci Remote Sens 48:874–881
3. ASI (2010) Italian space agency COSMO-skymed system description & user guide doc. no: ASI-CSM-ENG-RS-093-A. http://www.cosmo-skymed.it/docs/ASI-CSM-ENG-RS-093-A-CSKSysDescriptionAndUserGuide.pdf
4. Burges CJC (1998) A tutorial on support vector machines for pattern recognition. Data Min Knowl Discov 2:121–167
5. Chang CC, Lin CJ (2001). LIBSVM: a library for support vector machines (www.csie.ntu.edu.tw/ ~ cjlin/libsvm/)
6. Cortes C, Vapnik V (1995) Support-vector networks. Mach Learn. 20:273–297
7. Cristianini N, Shawe-Taylor J (2000) An introduction to support vector machines. Cambridge University Press, Cambridge
8. De Santis A, Iacoviello D (2007) Discrete level set approach to image segmentation. Signal Image Video Process 1:303–320
9. Dobson MC, Ulaby FT (1986) Active microwave soil moisture research. IEEE Trans Geosci Remote Sens 24:23–36
10. Frost VS, Yurovsky LS (1985) Maximum likelihood classification of synthetic aperture radar imagery. Comp Vis Graph Image Proc 32:291–313
11. Fukuda S, Hirosawa H (2001) Support vector machine classification of land cover: application to polarimetric SAR data. In: IEEE geoscience and remote sensing society (IGARSS), vol 1, pp 187–189
12. Fung AK (1994) Microwave scattering and emission models and their applications. Artech House, Boston
13. Gonzales RC, Woods RE (2001) Digital image processing, Prentice Hall, Upper Saddle River
14. Iliadis LS, Papastavrou AK, Lefakis PD (2002) A computer system that classifies the prefectures of Greece in forest fire risk zones using fuzzy sets. Forest Policy Econ 4

15. Kseneman M, Gleich D (2009) Soil moisture estimation with TerraSAR-X: with Dubois empirical model. 16th international conference on systems, signals and image processing, Chalkida, pp 1–4
16. Kseneman M, Gleich D, Cucej Z (2011) Soil moisture estimation using high-resolution spotlight TerraSAR- X data. IEEE Geosci Remote Sens Lett 8:686–690
17. Schölkopf B, Smola A (2001) Learning with kernels. Support vector machines, regularization, optimization, and beyond. MIT Press, Cambridge
18. Tanase MA, Pérez-Cabello F, de la Juan Riva, Santoro M (2010) TerraSAR-X Data for burn severity evaluation in mediterranean forests on sloped terrain. IEEE Trans Geosci Remote Sens 48:917–928
19. Ulaby FT, Moore RK, Fung AK (1982) Microwave remote sensing: active and passive. Radar remote sensing and surface scattering and emission theory, vol 2. Wesley, Reading
20. Ulaby FT, Moore RK, Fung AK (1986) Microwave remote tensing: active and passive. from theory to applications, vol 4. Artech House, Boston
21. Vapnik V (1995) The nature of statistical learning theory. Springer-Verlag, New York
22. Zhao Q, Principe J (2001) Support vector machines for SAR automatic target recognition. IEEE Trans Aer El Syst 37:643–654

Improving Flood Risk Management in the City of Lisbon: Developing a Detailed and Updated Map of Imperviousness Using Satellite Imagery

T. Santos and S. Freire

Abstract The spatial distribution and extent of pervious and impervious areas in the city are important variables for planning, mitigating, preparing and responding to potential urban flooding events. Remote sensing constitutes a valuable data source to derive land cover information required for flood risk assessment. The present paper describes the generation of a Land Cover Map for the city of Lisbon, Portugal. The data source is an IKONOS-2 pansharp image, from 2008, with a spatial resolution of 1 m, and a normalized Digital Surface Model (nDSM) from 2006. The methodology was based on the extraction of features of interest, namely: vegetation, soil and impervious surfaces. It is demonstrated that using a methodology based on Very-High Resolution (VHR) images, quick updating of detailed land cover information is possible and can be used to support decisions in a crisis situation where official maps are generally outdated.

1 Introduction

Natural disasters such as urban floods are a major problem, often resulting in extensive damage to private and public property and sometimes claiming human lives. Urban floods are a good example of a 'natural hazard' compounded by human action, thus more appropriately classified as a 'semi-natural' disaster [28]. In fact, the urbanization process results in the impermeabilization of land surfaces, thus increasing soil sealing, which contributes to elevate the risk of flooding. Impervious surfaces generate intense rainwater run-off which the drainage network

T. Santos (✉) · S. Freire
Faculdade de Ciências Sociais e Humanas, FCSH, e-GEO—Research Centre for Geography and Regional Planning, Universidade Nova de Lisboa, Lisbon, Portugal
e-mail: teresasantos@fcsh.unl.pt

S. Freire
e-mail: sfreire@fcsh.unl.pt

J. M. R. S. Tavares and R. M. Natal Jorge (eds.), *Topics in Medical Image Processing and Computational Vision*, Lecture Notes in Computational Vision and Biomechanics 8,
DOI: 10.1007/978-94-007-0726-9_16, © Springer Science+Business Media Dordrecht 2013

cannot accommodate, thus contributing to flooding events. The availability of appropriate flood risk maps is important to support decisions in most phases of the emergency management cycle:

- Planning: flood risk maps are essential to locate, assess and rank areas at risk of flooding;
- Mitigation: flood risk maps should be used to implement mitigation measures in areas of higher risk in order to decrease severity of potential outcomes;
- Preparation: flood risk maps can be used to locate response means and resources close to areas at higher risk and to monitor those areas before and during events;
- Response: flood risk maps can assist response after events of heavy rainfall by giving indication on the areas that were worst hit and possible water depth and thus help to tailor means and resources.

Some areas in the city of Lisbon, Portugal, are subject to cyclical flooding due to a combination of factors: intense rainfall, inappropriate draining infrastructure, and other geographic conditions (e.g., effect of ocean tide) [9]. This urban flooding causes damages in infrastructures, disruption in normal city activities and economic losses [20]. Also the human intervention (including artificial fills and river channel diversion) as a consequence of urban development has contributed to the flooding phenomenon [21].

Studies on impacts of urbanization, responses to natural and man-made disasters, vulnerability analysis or housing conditions, all require updated land cover information. Efficient management of urban flooding is based on mapping its risk, for which maps of ground imperviousness are essential [16]. Highly permeable landscapes reduce erosion and flood risk, recharge groundwater and stabilize stream flows over time. However, when soil permeability is reduced, surface runoff, erosion and flood risk increase, groundwater recharge is reduced, and stream flows fluctuate more over time. Frequently, cadastral information on land cover is not available with sufficient spatial resolution. This information is difficult to obtain and rapidly becomes outdated in cities having a dynamic development. Instead, satellite data can be used for mapping and quantifying sealed surfaces in a quick way and at low costs. Furthermore, continuous acquisition of satellite data allows updating already existing land cover maps, contributing to a more accurate estimate of the actual proportion of impervious ground within city areas.

Remote sensing imagery due to its spectral and temporal characteristics, can be used in flood risk analysis, as a source of related information like land use and land cover, surface roughness, terrain relief or soil moisture. Ebert et al. [10] modeled the influence of land use types and their spatial patterns on the flood risk, using satellite data (Landsat, SPOT and ASTER). Chormanski et al. [6] and Canters et al. [3] examined the impact of different methods for estimating impervious surface cover from satellite data (IKONOS and Landsat), on the outcome of a distributed rainfall-runoff model. Aponte [1] used a QuickBird image in order to detect different types of impervious surfaces, and studied the relationship between the rainfall-infiltration-runoff rates, the land cover and the geomorphologic susceptibility. Nirupama et al. [19] studied the increase of flood risk due to urbanization, based on land use classification derived from Landsat imagery. Forte et al. [13] conducted loss estimation and flood vulnerability analysis based on aerial photos, Landsat imagery and historic records of major floods. Shamaoma et al. [25] extracted building footprints and boundaries of informal settlements from QuickBird imagery and laser scanning data, and tested its potential in providing the information required to run flood risk models. Van der Sande et al. [26] used a land cover map derived from an IKONOS-2 image, as input for a flood simulation model.

Land cover mapping is generally made by processing imagery obtained from remote sensing instruments, like aerial photographs or satellite images. The current and future VHR satellite imagery provides an advantageous alternative to detect and map urban features. However, their effective use requires the development of novel approaches that enable a timely and consistent discrimination, classification and delineation of these specific land uses with quality [14]. In this context, Geographic Object-Based Image Analysis (GEOBIA) approaches are the recent response to these expectations on geographic information products [15], and constitute an alternative to the pixel-based classifiers. The concept behind GEOBIA is that information relevant to the interpretation of an image is not represented in single pixels but in meaningful image objects, which reflect real patterns and their mutual relations [5]. Although sometimes there may be objects with the size of one pixel, the applications typically seek to identify elements that are composed of multiple pixels such as roads, buildings, crops, etc. The construction of these image-objects is based on the concept of spatial patchiness. A landscape object is a patch, defined as a discrete spatial unit having a certain minimum extension and differing from its surroundings in nature or appearance, like size, shape and internal consistency [17, 27]. Therefore, the partitioning of the image into sets of useful objects is key to the success of the automatic image analysis [2].

GEOBIA classifiers have performed better than the traditional ones at the pixel level, particularly with higher spatial resolution data [2, 4, 18].

The present work details the development of an updated and detailed map of imperviousness for the city of Lisbon using IKONOS-2 satellite imagery, and an nDSM from 2006. The imagery classification for extracting land cover information at the city-scale was based on a GEOBIA approach.

The information on land cover collected from remote sensing data can be useful for many applications. Indicators of land-sealing areas and the quantification of green areas and available vacant land in the city are ecological measures that can be used as tools for monitoring and analyzing trends over the territory [24].

2 Data and Study Area

The dataset explored in this paper includes spectral and altimetric data. The spectral data includes an image, acquired by the IKONOS-2 satellite, in June, 30, 2008. This image has a spatial resolution of 4 m in the multispectral mode (visible and near-infrared bands) and 1 m in the panchromatic mode, and a radiometric resolution of 11 bits.

The altimetric data is composed of two sets. One set is derived from a Light Detection And Ranging (LiDAR) point cloud, and the other is derived from cartography. From a flight with a LiDAR camera performed in 2006, a surface image was produced based on the 2nd return, with 1 m resolution. This image represents the Digital Surface Model (DSM) of the area. Another source of altimetric information was a set of elevation mass points and contours, retrieved from 1:1000 scale altimetric cartography of 1998.

The study area is the city of Lisbon (Fig. 1). The municipality occupies an area of 84 Km^2, and is a typical European capital city, with a very diverse land use dynamics, varying from historical neighborhoods where the street-network is dense and most of the area is built-up, to modern residential ones, with on-going construction of roads and multi-family buildings. Between these two situations, there are more heterogeneous places with land uses such as residential, parks, agriculture, vacant land, industrial, utilities, and schools. The fact that Lisbon has such a diverse land use, gathered with the fact that it is a riverside city, makes it a good study area.

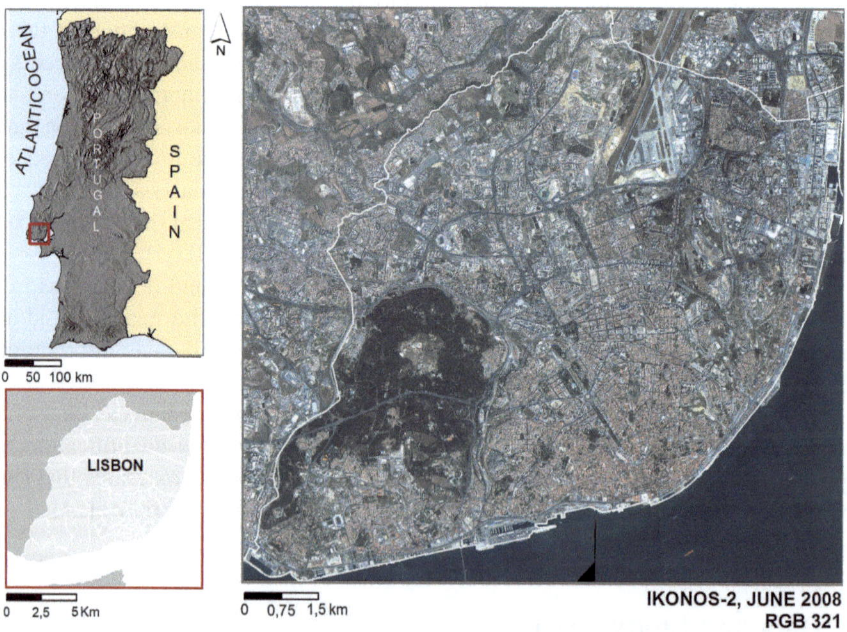

Fig. 1 Study area and IKONOS-2 imagery used to produce Lisbon's impervious surface map

3 Methodology

The cartographic workflow based on remote sensing data, begins with the pre-processing stage where several tasks are applied to geometrically correct the data sets and to attribute a common coordinate system. The altimetric information is also processed in this stage, in order to produce a normalized Digital Surface Model (nDSM). Afterwards, the feature extraction takes place to produce a map with the distribution of the land cover features. The final step includes accuracy assessment of the produced land cover map.

3.1 Pre-processing

The altimetric data suffered several operations in order to generate the final maps describing the terrain and the surface.

A Digital Terrain Model (DTM) for the city of Lisbon was produced from the elevation mass points and contours of the 1:1000 scale altimetry. Firstly, a Triangulated Irregular Network (TIN) was generated and then converted to a grid with 1 m of resolution. This final data set corresponds to the DTM for the area. The DTM was then used to orthorectify the IKONOS-2 image, and to derive the normalized Digital Surface Model (nDSM). The nDSM was obtained by subtracting the DTM from the DSM image. This raster file stores the height of all elements above and, due to the temporal different between both altimetric data sets, also some elements below the terrain. All files were geometrically corrected to attribute a common coordinate system (PT-TM06/ETRS89).

The Lisbon city area was captured in four IKONOS-2 images, which were mosaicked into a single large image. The mosaic was then orthorectified in order to reduce the geometric distortions caused by the terrain and to attribute a national coordinate system (PT-TM06/ETRS89). Previously, a pansharp image of the visible and panchromatic bands was produced, using the method available at PCI Geomatica [29].

The imagery orthorectification was performed based on the Rational Function Coefficients (RFCs), available with the image, and a set of 48 ground control points retrieved from the 1:1 000 planimetric and altimetric cartography of 1998, obtained from the Lisbon City Hall. The DTM was used as reference for the elevation. A 2nd order polynomial was selected for the transformation. To validate the process, 55 check points, well distributed across the image, were used. The obtained Root Mean Square Error RMSE was less than one pixel.

Afterwards, a Normalized Difference Vegetation Index (NDVI) [22] layer was produced to integrate the dataset for feature extraction.

3.2 Feature Extraction

Feature extraction algorithms extract geo-information using object-based methodologies. In this work, all feature extraction was performed using Feature Analyst (FA) v4.2 (by Visual Learning Systems, now Overwatch Systems) for ArcGIS (ESRI). FA uses a combination of object segmentation and neural network technology. The selected FA classification setup is similar to a standard supervised classification, where the user needs to supply training sites of each feature class of interest. The FA classification scheme incorporates a contextual classifier, defined by the user, according to the configuration of the image features to be extracted. To take the spatial context into account, FA uses predefined patterns that can be parameterized (e.g., Manhattan, Bull's Eye). These patterns are knowledge-based criteria, allowing to specify whether the feature of interest is long and narrow (e.g., roads) or small and boxy (e.g., buildings). It is during the training stage that the user indicates the pattern that best fits the feature target. The user controls the shape and size of the moving window through which FA looks to gather information in a pixel basis, and to determine if it is part of the target feature. Besides the classification pattern, it is also possible to indicate a minimum area to be extracted. In the supervised mode, the program analyzes the training set and creates distinct segments based on the training data and the input knowledge. The results of this first pass can be corrected and added back into the system as knowledge, in an interactive learning process.

The land cover nomenclature is organized in two levels of detail. The 1st level includes the classes "Vegetation", "Impervious Surfaces", "Soil" and "Shadow and Water". On the 2nd level, seven classes were defined: "Trees", "Low Vegetation", "Buildings", "Roads", "Other impervious surfaces", "Soil", and "Shadows and Water" (Table 1):

- Vegetation cover corresponds to maintained and 'natural' green areas. These are an important land use type in urban areas which perform relevant environmental functions, such as improving urban climate, reducing atmospheric pollution, providing amenities, aesthetical benefits and a good environment for urban population. Green land cover includes trees, shrubland, herbaceous vegetation, parks, private gardens, and agricultural plots;

Table 1 Land cover nomenclature

Level 1	Level 2
Vegetation	Trees
	Low vegetation
Impervious surface	Buildings
	Roads
	Other impervious surfaces
Soil	Soil
Shadow and water	Shadow and water

- Impervious surfaces can generally be defined as anthropogenic features, such as roads, buildings, sidewalks and parking lots, through which water cannot infiltrate into the soil. The artificial surface cover can be used to evaluate the quality of urban streams, and to study effects of runoff. Impervious surface is increasingly recognized as a key indicator for assessing the sustainability of land use changes due to urban growth [11];
- Soil is vacant land and is usually comprised of bare ground or with little vegetation, thin soil, sand or rocks;
- Shadows occur in remotely sensed imagery when objects totally or partially occlude the direct light coming from a source of illumination, which include cast shadows (shadows cast on the ground, or on other objects, by high-rise objects), and self-shadows (the part of the object that is not illuminated) [23]. Great difficulty arises in the classification and interpretation of shaded objects in an image due to the reduction or total loss of spectral information of those shaded objects [8]. This issue is particularly significant in urban environments where tall buildings are often present. Water is included in the same class as shadow, since both are dark objects in the image that will not be used for producing land-based indicators.

The classification is based on a supervised approach and aims at extracting the three main components of land cover: "Vegetation", "Impervious Surfaces" and "Soil" (Fig. 2).

3.2.1 Extracting Vegetation

After extracting shadows and water elements, the next steps explored the possibility of classifying the study area in two major classes—"Vegetation", "No-vegetation"—and in the subsequent stages, each individual 2nd level class of the nomenclature was extracted independently.

The vegetation extraction was conducted for the unclassified areas (i.e., no "Shadow and Water" elements). In order to separate vegetated from non-vegetated surfaces in the urban environment, the NDVI was computed for the pansharp image. A threshold of 0.22 was determined to mask the vegetated regions. This layer stands for the level 1 class "Vegetation" and includes the city's green surface. In the 2nd level of the nomenclature, two classes were distinguished: "Trees" and "Low Vegetation". The first class identifies trees and tall shrubs whereas the other class identifies lawns and other herbaceous vegetation. The "Trees" were extracted with FA using the pansharp and the NDVI image, Bull's Eye 3 pattern, width 5, for the input representation, using as inside mask the level 1 class "Vegetation", and 5 pixels of aggregation. After training the classifier, the final map was obtained after one 'add missing areas' process. The low vegetation class was the remaining vegetation.

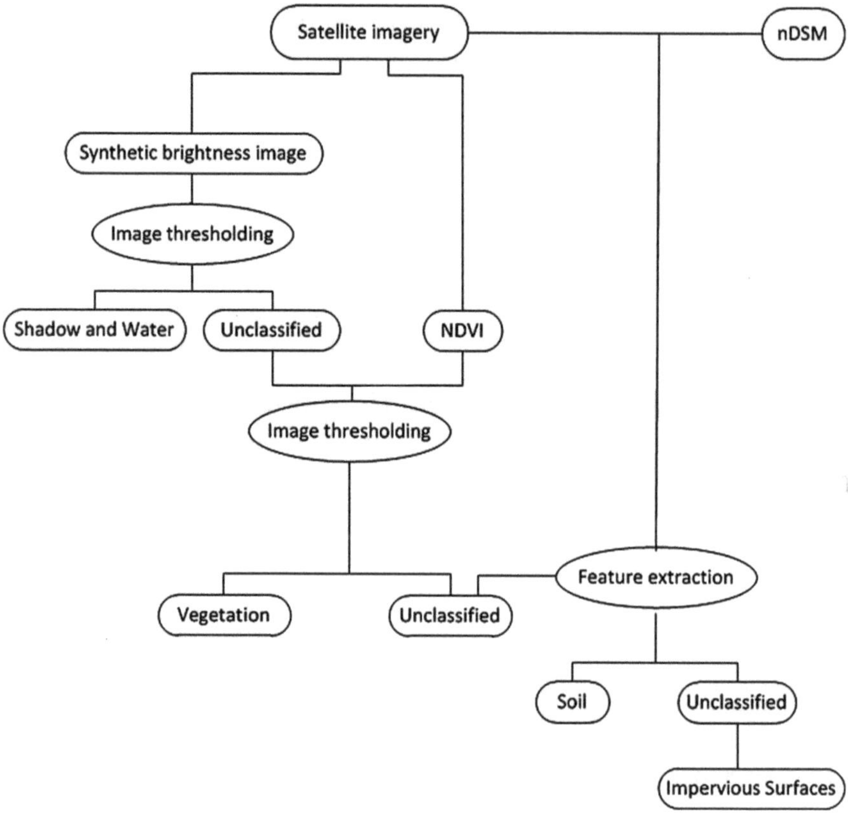

Fig. 2 Flowchart of the land cover information obtained from remote sensing data

3.2.2 Extracting Soil

The next major class to be extracted was "Soil", and was extracted in the remaining unclassified areas (i.e., no "Shadow and Water", and no "Vegetation"). The input dataset included the pansharp image and the nDSM. The classifiers' learning was performed in two independent extractions, considering two types of soil classes. The extraction was made with the Manhattan pattern, width 3, and considering 50 and 100 pixels of aggregation. The bare soil was subject to an iteration process for clutter removal. The final step was the generalization of the soil polygons using the "aggregate polygons" tool from ArcGIS, aiming at merging polygons that were closer than 2 m, and considering areas grater or equal to 100 m^2.

3.2.3 Extracting Impervious Surface

The map of impervious areas includes a wide range of materials, some of which have very different spectral properties (e.g., asphalt, concrete, roof tiles, etc.). The level 1 class "Impervious Surface" corresponds to the land surface after masking out the "Vegetation", "Soil", and "Shadow and Water" classes. In the 2nd level of the nomenclature, three classes were distinguished: "Buildings", "Roads" and "Other impervious surfaces", based on the pansharp image and the nDSM.

"Buildings" were extracted in three stages, considering different roof materials. For red tiles, the parameters used were Manhattan pattern, width 7, and 75 pixels of aggregation. For darker roof materials and for the brighter ones, Manhattan pattern, width 7, and 100 pixels of aggregation were the selected parameters. For all these feature types the learning stages were followed by "remove clutter" and "add missing data" iterations to extract three types of roofs which were merged to obtain the "Buildings" class. The last step included generalizing the building polygons using the same parameters as for the "Soil" class: merging with distance between lines inferior to 2 m, and considering areas grater or equal to 100 m^2.

The class "Roads" was extracted in three independent processes, using different parameters. For wide roads, Bull's Eye 2, width 25, and 1100 pixels of aggregation were considered. For narrow roads, Bull's Eye 2, width 19, and 500 pixels of aggregation were considered. The remaining asphalt pavement was extracted with Bull's Eye 2 pattern, width 25, and 500 pixels of aggregation. These three layers were then merged to produce the "Roads" class. The final layer was obtained by generalization, using 2 m as merging distance and 100 m^2 as minimum area.

The "Other impervious surfaces" (like sidewalks or railroads), were the remaining areas within the "Impervious surface" class, after masking out the "Buildings" and "Roads" classes.

The selected parameters that produced the best extraction results for each land cover class are presented in Table 2.

Table 2 Parameters used for extraction of land cover classes

Level 2 class	Land cover	Mask	Pattern and width	Aggregation (pixels)
Shadow and water	Shadows and deep water bodies	Threshold value	n.a	n.a
Trees	Trees and tall shrubs	NDVI threshold	Bull's Eye 3, 5	5
Low vegetation	Herbaceous vegetation	NDVI threshold	n.a	n.a
Soil	Bare land_1	Unclassified areas	Manhattan, 3	100
	Bare land_2	Unclassified areas	Manhattan, 3	50
Buildings	Red tiles	Unclassified areas	Manhattan, 7	75
	Other roof materials	Unclassified areas	Manhattan, 7	100
Roads	Wide roads	Unclassified areas	Bull's Eye 2, 25	1100
	Narrow roads	Unclassified areas	Bull's Eye 2, 19	500
	Asphalt pavement	Unclassified areas	Bull's Eye 2, 25	500
Other impervious surfaces	Sidewalks and railroads	Unclassified areas	n.a	n.a

Figure 3 shows the Land Cover Map produced for 2008, with seven classes, for the city of Lisbon, using satellite and LiDAR data.

3.3 Accuracy Assessment of Land Cover Map 2008

After extracting the land cover classes, the thematic accuracy of the Land Cover Map of 2008 must be evaluated. The evaluation of the thematic accuracy is usually carried out by filling an error matrix. In order to properly generate an error matrix, one must consider sampling since it is not reasonable to investigate every place on the ground [7]. The sampling scheme defined for selecting reference information

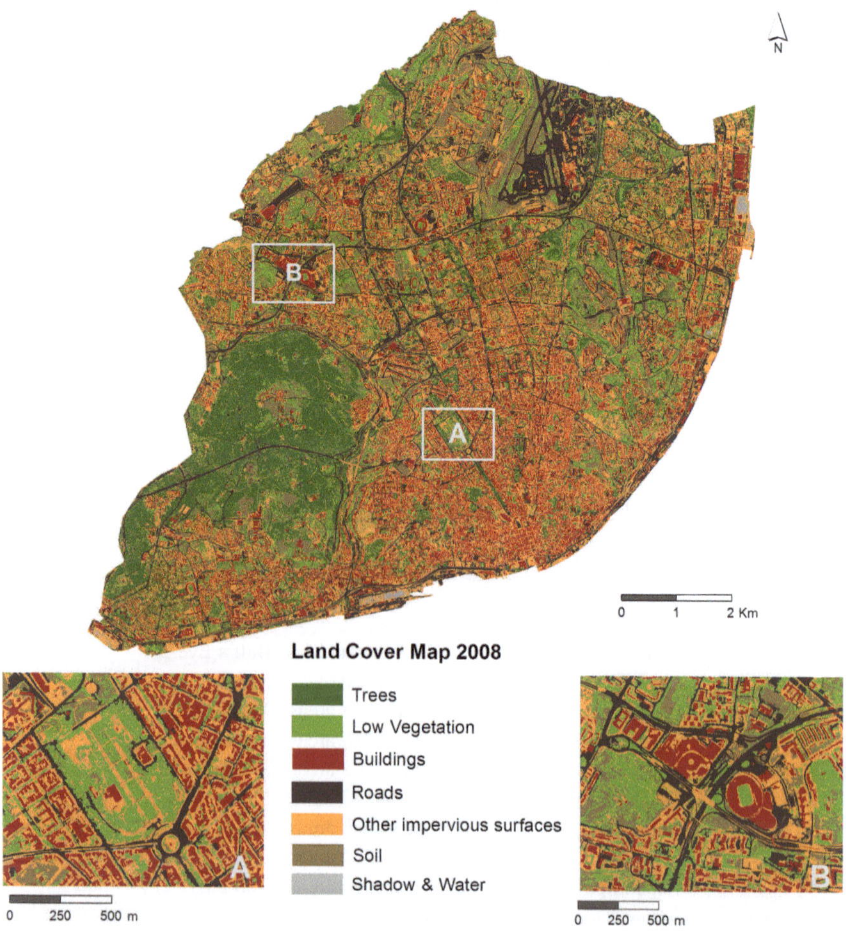

Fig. 3 Land cover map of the city of Lisbon for 2008

for accuracy assessment is simple random sampling, which is commonly applied for evaluating land cover maps [12]. The number of samples to be collected is calculated based on the multinomial distribution as proposed by Congalton and Green [7] and the adopted sample unit is a point. The ground truth is obtained from visual analysis of the IKONOS-2 image supported by auxiliary information like the oblique images available at www.bing.com/maps, and field work done in 2008.

Based on the previous considerations, for each strata (i.e., each level 2 land cover class), 100 random points were analyzed through visual analysis of the imagery and ancillary data (oblique images). From the 700 samples, 2 were excluded from the evaluation because it was not possible to correctly identify the class.

The samples are then used to fill the error matrix. The matrix's columns usually represent the reference data, while the rows indicate the classification generated from the remotely sensed data (i.e., the map). From this matrix it is possible to calculate a series of quality indices: global indices like the KHAT statistic (obtain in a Kappa analysis) and the Overall Accuracy, and individual class's indices like the Producer's and User's Accuracy.

4 Results and Discussion

For assessing the quality of the Land Cover Map of 2008, the sampling schema presented in Sect. 3.3 was applied, and the results were used to fill the error matrix and to calculate quality indices (Tables 3 and 4).

The main problems detected in the map are commission errors in "Low vegetation" and "Trees", and with "Other impervious surfaces" and "Shadow and Water" and "Buildings". Omission errors were also detected with "Trees" and "Low vegetation", and with "Buildings" with "Other impervious surfaces". These confusions were due to spectral heterogeneity of the classes.

Table 3 Error matrix for the land cover map of 2008

Reference map	Trees	Low veg.	Buildings	Roads	Other imp. surfaces	Soil	Shadow water	Total row
Trees	96	4	0	0	0	0	0	100
Low vegetation	23	72	0	1	2	2	1	101
Buildings	0	0	98	0	0	2	0	100
Roads	0	0	4	91	5		0	100
Other imp. surfaces	0	1	8	2	72	3	13	99
Soil	0	2	4	0	1	91	0	98
Shadow and water	0	0	0	0	0	0	100	0
Total column	119	79	114	94	80	98	114	698

Table 4 Results of thematic accuracies of the land cover map of 2008

Overall Accuracy = 89 %, KHAT = 87 %

Level 2 class	Commission error (%)	Omission error (%)
Trees	4	19
Low vegetation	29	9
Buildings	2	14
Roads	9	3
Other impervious surfaces	27	10
Soil	7	7
Shadow and water	0	12

Table 5 Areas of the level 1 and 2 land cover classes in the city of Lisbon

Level 1	Area (ha)	Area (%)	Level 2	Area (ha)	Area (%)
Vegetation	2428	29	Trees	1101	13
			Low vegetation	1327	16
Impervious surface	4907	58	Buildings	1213	14
			Roads	1352	16
			Other impervious surfaces	2342	28
Soil	839	10	Soil	839	10
Shadow and water	299	4	Shadow and water	299	4

From this analysis, we conclude that the Land Cover Map of 2008 has an Overall Accuracy of 89 % and a KHAT statistic of 87 %, in the most detailed level. These values indicate a high degree of agreement between the reference data and the classified map.

From the Land Cover Map of 2008, two variables are extracted: the area (Table 5) and the spatial distribution of each land cover class in the city (Fig. 3). According to this map, the impervious surface occupies 4907 ha, corresponding to 58 % of the city's area (Fig. 4).

5 Conclusions

A methodology for mapping impervious surfaces in the riverside city of Lisbon was presented, combining high-resolution optical satellite imagery and a GEOBIA approach. The land cover map is currently the most detailed and updated such dataset for the city. The case study demonstrates that semi-automatic classification of remote sensing data can produce fast updating of detailed land cover information and can be used to support land planning decisions or to aid in the response to a crisis situation where official maps are generally outdated. Results show that in Lisbon most of the surface is impervious, fact that contributes to the occurrence of

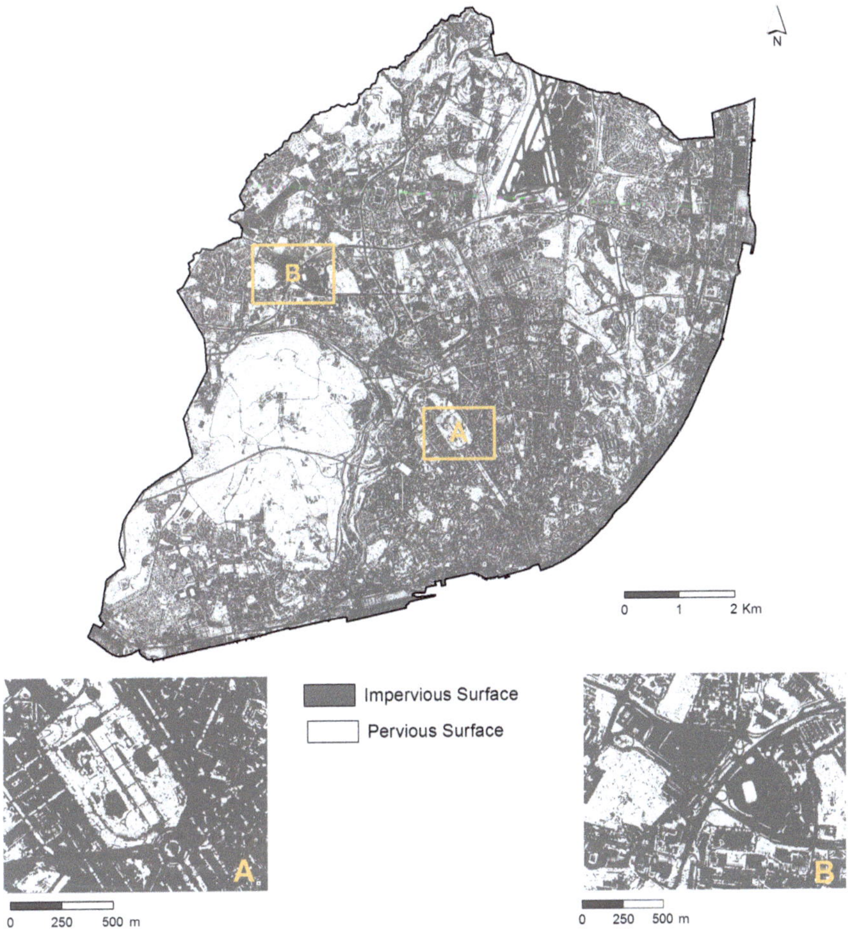

Fig. 4 Impervious map for the city of Lisbon in 2008 derived from IKONOS-2 imagery

urban flooding. It is expected that such a dataset will aid in improving all phases of flood risk management at the municipal level, from planning to response and rehabilitation.

Furthermore, all land cover layers produced in this work are eminently suitable for diverse urban applications and planning functions due to its very high geometric resolution. They can be used, for example, to support decision-making and identifying major areas for policy intervention, to update the land use inventory as well as biotope mapping.

Future work includes comparing the evolution of land cover and the degree of imperviousness at the city scale, using change detection methods with multi-temporal images.

Acknowledgments This work was conducted in the framework of project GeoSat—Methodologies to extract large scale GEOgraphical information from very high resolution SATellite images, funded by the Portuguese Foundation for Science and Technology (PTDC/GEO/64826/2006).

The authors would like to thank Logica for the opportunity of using the LiDAR data set.

References

1. Aponte AGP (2007) Runoff coefficients using a quickbird image for mapping flood hazard in a Tropical Coastal City, Campeche, Mexico. In: Geoscience and remote sensing symposium 2007 IGARSS 2007 IEEE international, Barcelona, Spain, 23–28 July 2007
2. Blaschke T, Lang S, Möller M (2005) Object-based analysis of remote sensing data for landscape monitoring: Recent developments. Anais XII Simpósio Brasileiro de Sensoriamento Remoto, Goiania
3. Canters F, Chormanski J, van de Voorde T, and Batelaan O (2006) Effects of different methods for estimating impervious surface cover on runoff estimation at catchment level. In: 7th international symposium on spatial accuracy assessment in natural resources and environmental sciences, Lisbon, Portugal, 5–7 July 2006
4. Caprioli M, Tarantino E (2003) Urban features recognition from VHR satellite data with an object-oriented approach. Commission IV joint workshop, challenges in geospatial analysis, integration and visualization II, Stuttgart, Germany, 8–9 September 2003
5. Chen Q, Luo J, Zhou GH, Pei T (2003) A hybrid multi-scale segmentation approach for remotely sensed imagery. In: Geoscience and remote sensing symposium 2003 IGARSS 2003 IEEE 2003 international, Toulouse, France, 21–25 July 2003
6. Chormanski J, van de Voorde T, Batelaan O, Canters F (2008) Improving distributed runoff prediction in urbanized catchments with remote sensing based estimates of impervious surface cover. Sensors 8:910–932
7. Congalton R, Green K (2009) Assessing the accuracy of remotely sensed data: principles and practices, 2nd edn. CRC/Lewis Press, Boca Raton
8. Dare P (2005) Shadow Analysis in high-resolution satellite imagery of urban areas. Photogramm Eng Remote Sens 71(2):169–177
9. Duarte A, Borges B, Ramos C, Pedro P, Pancad R (2005) Cheias rápidas em áreas urbanas e sua percepção: o caso da bacia de r[a] de Odivelas. X Colóquio Ibérico de Geografia, Évora
10. Ebert A, Banzhaf E, McPhee J (2009) The influence of urban expansion on the flood hazard in Santiago de Chile, 2009 Urban Remote Sensing Joint Event, Shanghai, China, 20–22 May 2009
11. Esch T, Conrad C, Schorcht G, Thiel M, Wehrmann T, Dech S (2008) Model-based estimation of impervious surface by application of support vector machines. In: Proceedings of the international archives of the photogrammetry, remote sensing and spatial information sciences ISPRS, Part B8, Beijing, China
12. Foody G (2002) Status of land cover classification accuracy assessment. Remote Sens Environ 80:185–201
13. Forte F, Strobl R, Pennetta L (2006) A methodology using GIS, aerial photos and remote sensing for loss estimation and flood vulnerability analysis in the Supersano-Ruffano-Nociglia Graben, southern Italy. Environ Geol 50(4):581–594
14. Freire S, Santos T, Navarro A, Silva J, Soares F, Fonseca A (2010) Extraction of buildings from QuickBird imagery for municipal planning purposes: quality assessment considering existing mapping standards. In: Proceedings of GEOBIA—GEOgraphic object-based image analysis, Ghent, Belgium, 29 June–2 July

15. Hay GJ, Castilla G (2008) Geographic object-based image analysis (GEOBIA): a new name for a new discipline? In: Blaschke T, Lang S, Hay GJ (eds) Object-based image analysis—spatial concepts for knowledge-driven remote sensing applications. Springer, Berlin, pp 75–89
16. Jha A K, Bloch R, Lamond J (2012) Cities and flooding: a guide to integrated urban flood risk management for the 21st century. World Bank Publications, Washington
17. Kotliar NB, Wiens JA (1990) Multiple scales of patchiness and patch structure: a hierarchical framework for the study of heterogeneity. Oikos 59:253–260
18. Lu D, Weng Q (2007) A survey of image classification methods and techniques for improving classification performance. Int J Remote Sens 28(5):823–870
19. Nirupama N, Simonovic S (2007) Increase of flood risk due to urbanisation: a canadian example. Nat Hazards 40(1):25–41
20. Ramos C, Reis E (2001) The floods in the south of Portugal in different kinds of drainage basins. Finisterra 71:61–82
21. Rebelo F (2008) Um novo olhar sobre os riscos? O exemplo das cheias rápidas (flash floods) em domínio mediterrâneo. Territorium—Revista da Associação Portuguesa de Riscos, Prevenção e Segurança 15:7–14
22. Rouse JW, Hass RH, Schell JA, Deering DW (1973) Monitoring vegetation systems in the great plains with ERTS. Third NASA ERTS Symposium, vol 1, pp 309–317
23. Salvador E, Cavallaro A, Ebrahimi T (2001) Shadow identification and classification using invariant color models. IEEE Int Conf Acoust Speech Signal Process 3:1545–1548
24. Santos T, Freire S, Tenedório J A, Fonseca A, Afonso N, Navarro A, Soares F (2011) The GeoSat project: using remote sensing to keep pace with urban dynamics. Earthzine (www.Earthzine.org), IEEE committee on earth observation. Posted on 9 November 2011
25. Shamaoma H, Kerle N, Alkema D (2006) Extraction of flood-modelling related base-data from multi-source remote sensing imagery. In: ISPRS mid-term symposium 2006, remote sensing: from pixels to processes, Enschede, the Netherlands, 8-11 May 2006
26. Van der Sande CJ, de Jong SM, de Roo APJ (2003) A segmentation and classification approach of IKONOS-2 imagery for land cover mapping to assist flood risk and flood damage assessment. Int J Appl Earth Obs Geoinf 4:217–229
27. Wiens JA (1976) Population responses to patchy environments. Annu Rev Ecol Syst 7:81–120
28. WMO (World Meteorological Organization) (2008) Urban flood risk management. A tool for integrated flood management. APFM technical document No.11, Flood management tools series
29. Zhang Y (2002) A new automatic approach for effectively fusing landsat 7 images and IKONOS images. In: Geoscience and remote sensing symposium 2002 IGARSS '02 2002 IEEE international, Toronto, Canada, 24–28 June 2002

Author Biography

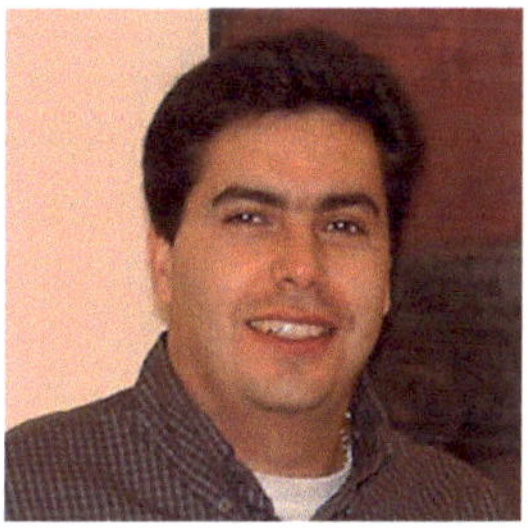

João Manuel R. S. Tavares
Faculdade de Engenharia da
Universidade do Porto (FEUP),
Rua Dr. Roberto Frias, s/n,
4200-465 Porto,
PORTUGAL,
Email: tavares@fe.up.pt,
url: www.fe.up.pt/~tavares

João Manuel R. S. Tavares graduated in Mechanical Engineering from the University of Porto-Portugal (1992); MSc in Electrical and Computer Engineering, in the field of Industrial Informatics, University of Porto (1995); PhD in Electrical and Computer Engineering, University of Porto (2001). From 1995 to 2000 he was a researcher at the Institute of Biomedical Engineering (INEB).

He has been senior researcher and project coordinator at the Laboratory of Optical and Experimental Mechanics (LOME) at the Institute of Mechanical Engineering and Industrial Management (INEGI) since 2001. Between 2001 and 2011, he was Assistant Professor at the Department of Mechanical Engineering (DEMec) of the Engineering Faculty of the University of Porto (FEUP), and he has been Associate Professor at DEMec since 2011.

He is co-author of more than 350 scientific papers in national and international journals and conferences, co-editor of 18 international books and guest-editor of several special issues of international journals. In addition, he is Editor-in-Chief of the Computer Methods in Biomechanics and Biomedical Engineering: Imaging & Visualization (CMBBE: Imaging & Visualization); Editor-in-Chief of the International Journal of Biometrics and Bioinformatics (IJBB); Co-Editor-in-Chief of the International Journal for Computational Vision and Biomechanics (IJCV&B); Co-Editor of the Lecture Notes in Computational Vision and Biomechanics (LNCV&B); Associate Editor of the EURASIP Journal on Advances in Signal Processing (JASP), Journal of Engineering, ISRN Machine

J. M. R. S. Tavares and R. M. Natal Jorge (eds.), *Topics in Medical Image Processing and Computational Vision*, Lecture Notes in Computational Vision and Biomechanics 8,
DOI: 10.1007/978-94-007-0726-9, © Springer Science+Business Media Dordrecht 2013

Vision, Advances in Biomechanics & Applications, and of the Journal of Computer Science (INFOCOMP), and reviewer of several international scientific journals.

Since 2001, he has been Supervisor and Co-Supervisor of several MSc and PhD thesis and involved in several research projects, both as researcher and as scientific coordinator. Additionally, he is co-author of three international patents and two national patents.

He has been Co-Chairman of various international conferences, such as: CompIMAGE 2006/2010/2012, VipIMAGE 2007/2009/2011/2013, CIBEM 2011, BioDENTAL 2009/2012, TMSi 2010, IMAGAPP 2009 and EUROMEDIA 2008; and of numerous mini-symposia, workshops and thematic sessions. In addition, he has been a member of scientific and organizing committees of several national and international conferences.

His main research areas include Computational Vision, Medical Imaging, Computational Mechanics, Scientific Visualization, Human-Computer Interaction and New Product Development.

Renato Natal Jorge (rnatal@fe.up.pt)
IDMEC—Pole FEUP,
Faculty of Engineering,
University of Porto,
Rua Dr. Roberto Frias,
4200-465 Porto, Portugal

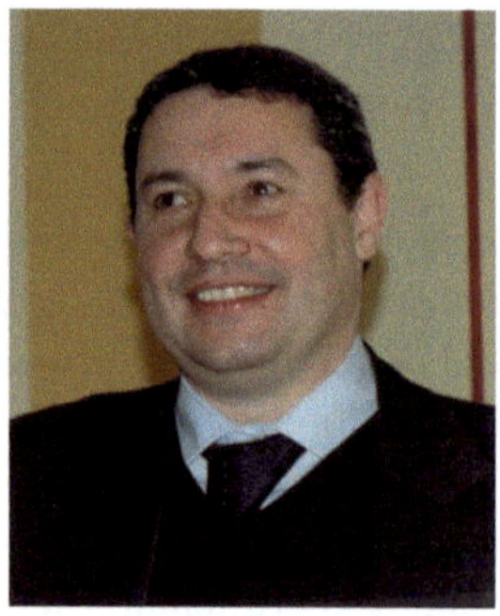

Associate Professor at the Faculty of Engineering, University of Porto (FEUP); Mechanical Engineer from the University of Porto, 1987; MSc from the University of Porto, 1991; PhD from the University of Porto, 1999.

Present teaching and research interests: Computational methods in applied mechanics and engineering; New product development; Biomechanics and mechanobiology; Computational vision and medical image processing.

Between 2007 and 2011 was the Director of the "Structural Integrity Unit" research group of the Institute of Mechanical Engineering at FEUP (IDMEC—a R & D non-profit, private Research Institute). Member of the executive board of IDMEC-FEUP.

Responsible for the Supervision or Co-supervision of twelve PhD students.

Co-chair of the following conferences: CompIMAGE; 14th International Product Development Management; VIPIMAGE; Fourteenth Annual Scientific Conference on WEB Technology, New Media, Communications and Telematics

Theory, Methods, Tools and Applications; VIPIMAGE 2009; CompIMAGE 2010; Biodental; iDEMi'09; 6th International Conference on Technology and Medical Sciences, CIBEM 2011, VIPIMAGE 2011; among other mini-symposia within conferences.

Founder and Editor of the International Journal for Computational Vision and Biomechanics. Guest editor of several scientific journals.

Principal Investigator for several national and European scientific projects.

Co-author of more than 90 papers in international journals and more than 300 publications in international conferences.

MIX
Papier aus verantwortungsvollen Quellen
Paper from responsible sources
FSC® C105338

If you have any concerns about our products,
you can contact us on
ProductSafety@springernature.com

In case Publisher is established outside the EU,
the EU authorized representative is:
Springer Nature Customer Service Center GmbH
Europaplatz 3, 69115 Heidelberg, Germany

Printed by Libri Plureos GmbH
in Hamburg, Germany